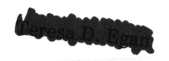

Getting Health Reform Right

Getting Health Reform Right

A GUIDE TO IMPROVING PERFORMANCE AND EQUITY

Marc J. Roberts

William Hsiao

Peter Berman

Michael R. Reich

OXFORD
UNIVERSITY PRESS
2004

OXFORD
UNIVERSITY PRESS

Oxford   New York
Auckland   Bangkok   Buenos Aires   Cape Town   Chennai
Dar es Salaam   Delhi   Hong Kong   Istanbul   Karachi   Kolkata
Kuala Lumpur   Madrid   Melbourne   Mexico City   Mumbai
Nairobi   São Paulo   Shanghai   Taipei   Tokyo   Toronto

Published by Oxford University Press, Inc.
198 Madison Avenue, New York, New York 10016
http:www.oup.org

Library of Congress Cataloging-in-Publication Data
Getting health reform right : a guide to improving performance and equity /
Marc J. Roberts . . . [et al.].
p. cm.   Includes bibliographical references and index.
ISBN 0-19-516232-3
1. Health care reform—Developing countries. 2. Health policy—Developing countries.
3. Medical care—Developing countries. 4. Public health—Developing countries.
I. Roberts, Marc J.
RA395.D44G48 2003   362.1'09172'4—dc21   2003050437

9 8 7 6 5 4 3 2 1

Printed in the United States of America
on acid-free paper

Preface

In recent decades many governments have undertaken efforts to reform and reorganize their health-care systems. They have created new insurance systems, changed how primary care is delivered, restructured hospital governance, decentralized the government's health-delivery system—all in pursuit of better performance and equity. Yet many of these reform efforts have yielded disappointing results. Patients still complain about poor service, doctors about low salaries, and budget-makers about the costs of the health sector. Some countries have enacted successive rounds of reform, while others have struggled to implement the plans they adopted. Still others wonder what to do next.

This book is intended to help those who find themselves caught up in health-sector reform. As our title suggests, it is a guide book designed to provide practical advice that will help reformers improve the performance of their health systems, with special attention to the equity of those results. While we make extensive use of the academic literature, we have not pursued this project as an academic exercise. Instead, the book emerges from many years of courses and seminars for health-sector decision-makers around the world and from our extensive involvement in consulting and advisory relationships with various governments.

There are four critical features in our approach to health-sector reform. The first is that we see the health sector as a means to an end. We urge reformers to judge their systems by the consequences, to define problems in terms of performance deficiencies, and to assess proposed solutions by whether they promise to remedy those deficiencies. This approach leads to an analytically rigorous method for problem definition, causal diagnosis, and policy development. This kind of method has often been lacking in health reform efforts, and its lack is partially responsible for the disappointing results.

A second major feature of our approach is a commitment to combining international experience with deep sensitivity to local circumstances. In this book we do *not* tell reformers what we think is the one "right answer." Instead, we offer methods and tools they can use to develop answers that will fit the economic resources, political circumstances, and administrative capacities of their own national situations. We do offer guidance for those choices, based on reform experience around the world, but it should always be conditioned by the local context. Again, we believe many recent disappointments can be traced to the uncritical advocacy of some favored policy solution by international experts or agencies—without an adequate understanding of local conditions.

Our third major commitment is to a multidisciplinary approach to the problems of health-sector reform. Admittedly, the range of relevant concepts and methods is dauntingly wide. But narrow analyses, which ignore important features of the situation, only invite failure from unanticipated consequences or unforeseen difficulties. Because money flows and incentives are so important in understanding any health system, we make extensive use of economic analysis. But we also believe that incentives alone do not explain everything, therefore we rely heavily on organizational theory and social psychology to explain the behavior of doctors, hospitals, patients, and other actors. In addition, we argue that attention to technical issues alone will never allow a reformer to fully understand and be effective in real situations. Hence, we devote much attention to understanding the political context for health-sector reform and to developing political strategies that can move reform forward. Finally, we argue that health-sector policy inevitably involves ethical choices. Thus, a grounding in basic political and moral philosophy is essential for reformers to understand and make those choices in a reasoned way.

This point about ethics leads to the final critical feature of our approach. The equity aspects of health-sector reform efforts are a continuing theme in this book, reflecting both our own personal values and the concerns expressed in the Millennium Development Goals adopted by the international community. We explicitly acknowledge and discuss how views about equity vary around the world. At the same time, we offer our own ethical views and indicate how equity in health system performance is influenced by various kinds of reform efforts.

While we believe that more systematic analysis can make a difference in health-sector reform efforts, we are not naïve about the difficulties. Health systems are extremely complex, and they often react in unanticipated ways to policy initiatives. Those who benefit from the status quo will continue to resist change. Advocates for reform often ignore local realities, and international agencies respond to their own internal dynamics and incentives. Still, we believe that an increase in both the breadth and the depth of thinking about reform can lead to better performance outcomes, and that is what we seek to facilitate in this book.

Producing a work aimed at these objectives has required six years of intense collaboration—the product of innumerable meetings, memos, conversations, and confrontations. Chapters have been drafted and critiqued, edited and revised, often many times. Some did more writing, others more critiquing. Some focused on crafting our concepts, while others contributed wisdom from years of hard-won experience. No two or three of us could have produced what the four of us have produced together.

The credit for initiating the project goes to Paul Shaw at the World Bank Institute, who, in 1996, began organizing a major teaching program that became known as the "Flagship Course on Health Sector Reform and Sustainable Financing." Shaw asked Hsiao to take responsibility for an introductory module on health systems assessment and diagnosis. Hsiao then recruited Berman, Reich, and Roberts, and our collaboration began.

In the summer of 1997, we produced a six-chapter set of background notes and teaching materials for the first offering of the course, which took place that fall in Washington, D.C., with 90 participants from many countries. Those background papers became the first draft of this book. In the summer of 1998, the World Bank retained Roberts to rewrite and expand those materials for the following year's course. After that offering, the four of us agreed to collaborate in turning the background papers into a book. We used subsequent versions of the manuscript each year in various Flagship courses—both in Washington and abroad. During the latter half of 2002 and the winter of 2003, Roberts and Reich, with critical input from Hsiao and Berman, revised the manuscript to highlight key themes, integrate various parts, ensure consistency, and give the text a common style.

The book relies on six key conceptual contributions, as identified in Chapter 1. Here we note the initial source for each of these.

The *policy cycle* formulation comes from work that Roberts did with a colleague, Christian Koeck, for a course they taught on health policy.

The *ethical framework* was developed by Roberts and Reich, together with a colleague, Karl Lauterbach, for a course they have taught on public-health ethics for more than a decade.

The *political analysis* we use was developed by Reich, along with software he has produced, called *Policymaker* (with David Cooper).

The concept that *health systems are means to ends* and the *performance goal formulation* were developed by Hsiao from his research and advisory role to many countries. Roberts and Berman elaborated these and their relationship to the ethical framework.

The *control knob* conceptualization was developed by Hsiao—with three of the specific "knobs" (organization, regulation, and behavior) extensively deepened and expanded from our conversations.

The *diagnostic tree* approach came from Roberts.

Now for some words about primary authorship for specific chapters. Chapters 1 (introduction) and 2 (policy cycle) were written by Roberts with input from Reich. Chapter 3 (ethics) is by Roberts and Reich. Chapter 4 (politics) is by Reich. Chapters 5 (goals) and 6 (performance) are by Roberts. Chapter 7 (diagnosis and policy development) is by Berman and Roberts. Chapter 8 (financing) is by Hsiao and Roberts. Chapter 9 (payment) is by Hsiao, Chapter 10 (organization) by Roberts and Berman, and Chapter 11 (regulation) by Hsiao and Roberts. Chapter 12 (behavior) is by Reich. Chapter 13 (conclusion) is by Roberts with contributions from all of us. Of course, each of us contributed important ideas to all of the chapters, not adequately reflected in this list.

A project of this complexity and duration required the support of many people. Our greatest debt is to Anne Johansen of the World Bank. As the organizer of and co-teacher in many Flagship courses, she pushed us repeatedly to clarify our ideas and contributed many crucial insights over the years. Paul Shaw, who began this whole effort, and Hadia Karam, also of the World Bank Institute, have likewise been valued critics, commentators, and partners. Others who taught in various Flagship courses and contributed greatly to our thinking include Ricardo Bitran, Alex Preker, Melitta Jakab, Alan Maynard, George Schieber, April Harding, and Jurgen Wassam. We thank our colleague at Harvard, Tom Bossert, whose work on decentralization we drew on extensively, and who provided thoughtful comments on several chapters. Pat Stout, Ted Green, and Lisa Bates provided very helpful comments on Chapter 12 (Behavior). We also appreciate the support from colleagues who taught with us in the regional courses—especially Miklós Szócska and Tamás Evetovits in Budapest, Hungary.

Support for this multiyear effort came in part from a grant to Hsiao from the World Bank for the initial curriculum development, and from a grant to Reich from the Edna McConnell Clark Foundation, through the program directed by Joe Cook. Each of us received support from the World Bank for preparing and teaching in the Flagship course in Washington and in courses offered at partner institutions around the world. We are also grateful for the implicit and explicit support we received from the Harvard School of Public Health, especially from Dean Barry Bloom, the Center for Population and Development Studies, and our departments (Population and International Health, and Health Policy and Management).

Many individuals supported our efforts to write this book. We wish to thank Donald Halstead, who helped improve the style and continuity of the 2001 draft. We appreciate the research assistance and bibliographic help of Karin Lockwood, Iris Boutros, and Andrew Mitchell. Carol Malgitta worked with us to design and produce the figures throughout the book. Those who helped with typing and revisions include Katrina Meyer, Betsy Barker, Vanessa Bingham, Margaret Ou, Terri Saint-Amour, and Stephanie Baldock. For the last round of revisions, Arthur Stokes provided superb word-processing services in deciphering and entering our lengthy hand-scrawled edits. We also wish to recognize the special contributions of one co-author (Reich), who facilitated the group process at critical junctions and pushed the project (and his co-authors) forward with grace and persistence. Without his efforts, who knows when, or if, this book would have been finished.

Finally, we want to thank the literally hundreds of participants in Flagship courses in Washington, at Harvard, and around the world. Their energy, ideas, suggestions, and responses were invaluable, as they (and we) struggled with the evolving versions of this book. We hope that our efforts will help them with the vital work they do every day, seeking to improve the performance and equity of health-care systems around the world.

Boston	Marc J. Roberts
Cambridge	William C. Hsiao
Boston	Peter Berman
Cambridge	Michael R. Reich

Contents

I

HEALTH SYSTEM ANALYSIS

1

Introduction

Setting the Scene

Throughout the world, governments are engaged in health-sector reform (Mills et al. 2001, OECD 1996, Berman 1995). The transitional economies of Eastern Europe are full of new social insurance schemes. Nations in South America are experimenting with ways to extend health insurance coverage to both the rural and urban poor. In Africa experiments with fiscal decentralization have produced additional revenues for hospitals, but also more inequality between rich and poor regions. To improve efficiency, many nations have also experimented with both new payment systems and new ways to organize health-care delivery.

Too often, however, conflicting political calculations, economic implications, and ethical concerns have led to a confused national debate: How should we deal with doctors' demands for more money? What strategies exist to reduce costs for medical care while expanding social insurance to cover the poor? Should we expand the system of publicly provided health centers, or move more to private-practice family physicians? Should we ask patients to pay more out of pocket, or make more use of general tax revenues? Is the answer more new technology or less? More doctors or fewer medical schools? Building new hospitals or spending more on anti-smoking campaigns?

Our approach to such questions is based on looking at the health-care system as a *means to an end*. In order to know whether the health-care system is working well or badly, and to identify promising reforms, it is crucial to keep this perspective in mind. Our method focuses on the need to identify goals explicitly, diagnose causes of poor performance systematically, and devise reforms that will produce real changes in performance. We will argue that reform must be strategic, based on honest means–ends analyses of what is likely to happen in a particular national context. Reforms need to be judged, not on reformers' intentions, but by the changes they actually produce.

Advocates of particular health-sector reform ideas do not always offer arguments that meet this standard. Instead, they sometimes urge adoption of their favorite idea, be it decentralization or family medicine, primary care or private insurance, without critical analysis or reflection (Sen and Koivusalo 1998, Hearst and Blas 2001). Too often, reform advocates do not identify the performance problems they want to improve, or say how the reform they propose will lead to that improvement.

We know from experience that health-sector reform is a difficult process (Berman 1995, Wilsford 1995). As we discuss below (Chapter 4), existing institutions and interest groups often have both the reasons and the resources to vigorously oppose change. As a result, it often takes some sort of political or economic shock to begin the health-sector reform process: a budget crisis, a change in the government coalition, a public scandal, a strike by providers or some combination of these and other similar events. This means that major changes in a country's health sector are infrequent. Hence, reformers have to be prepared to energetically seize the opportunity for major change when the time arises.

We are not so naïve, however, as to believe that a crisis always produces unity about what needs to be done. Differences in values, interests, political philosophy, and institutional responsibility will all make themselves felt. The Ministry of Finance is not likely to agree with the Ministry of Health. The doctors will not necessarily see eye to eye with the hospital administrators; nor will local government leaders agree with pharmaceutical company executives. For this reason we stress the importance of being clear about underlying values—and the ways these values lead to different goals and different reform priorities. Only by clarifying goals and values is it possible to devise a policy that has a hope of achieving the changes that reformers desire.

Experience has also taught us that, because of its complexity, the behavior of a health-care system is not easy to control. Change payment schemes, and doctors and hospitals are likely to modify their behavior to defend their incomes (Gilman 2000, Dowling 1977). Impose regulations on hospitals, and reports may be adjusted to show more compliance than actually occurs. Create new payroll taxes, and some businesses will seek to avoid them (Ron et al. 1990). Furthermore, the causal relationships in the system are complex. Change incentives to hospitals to foster efficiency, but not the authority of hospital managers, and the new scheme may produce little change. Institute competitive bidding in situations where there are few competitors, and the hoped-for decline in prices and costs may not occur.

These characteristics of the health system—its complexity, its resistance to change, and the diversity of perspectives within it—give health-sector reform an episodic and cyclical character. When some internal or external shock does focus national attention on health-sector reform, a specific feature of the system is often identified as critical, and this then becomes a target for major reform efforts. But the initial reform steps often lead to further, unanticipated problems. And additional rounds of reform (often less dramatic) can be expected. As a result, the initial changes are adapted, perfected, and modified (or even dismantled) by subsequent actions. We discuss the health-reform cycle in detail in Chapter 2.

Moreover, because we focus on consequences, we will insist throughout this book that matters of practicality and implementation be kept in mind. While international experience is a valuable source of ideas and guidance, we urge the reader to remember that policies that have worked well in other countries always need to be evaluated in your particular context. Every nation is different, and simple imitation is seldom advisable. Reformers have many questions to ask themselves: How good are our data systems? How respected are our courts? How energetic are our administrators? As we noted above, policy needs to be developed in a realistic and self-critical manner. Such skepticism and self-examination can help lead to plans that have a reasonable prospect of success in a reformer's own national context.

The Evolving Context for Health-Sector Reform

When we began work on this book several years ago, health-sector reform was promoted as a way to solve the problems of the health systems of countries in widely diverging circumstances. In the interim, international discussions about development have come to place even greater emphasis on health—both as a central goal of development and as an instrument to enhance other welfare outcomes (Commission on Macroeconomics and Health 2001). From a philosophical perspective, Amartya Sen has argued that health is an essential element of the human capabilities needed for development (Sen 1999). From an economic perspective, population health has been identified as a cause of economic growth at the national level (Bloom and Canning 2000). In addition, poor health has been connected to household poverty, by studies showing that acute episodes of avoidable illness are a major cause of households falling into poverty and distress (Liu et al. 2003). In sum, a consensus has emerged that health care is important both to improved health status and to general development goals.

Historically, public health scientists have attributed the major gains in population health to such improvements as better nutrition, sanitation, housing, and the healthier behaviors stemming from education (Preston 1975). More recent

dicates that health care also accounts for a significant share of health
ents in poor countries (WHO 1999) and that delivering the right pack-
sic health-care services can achieve important reductions in mortality
idity (World Bank 1993, Gwatkin et al. 1980). These causal connections suggest that health-sector reform has a crucial role to play in health and
development.

In 2003, as this book goes to press, international development policy debates
are focused on achieving the Millennium Development Goals (MDGs), which are
specific targets for poverty reduction, including a number of particular health outcomes such as controlling infectious diseases and managing childhood illnesses
(IMF et al. 2000). With prompting from international agencies, countries are developing Poverty Reduction Strategy Papers (PRSPs) as comprehensive guides to
development investments, including for the health sector (World Bank 2001). In
addition, the Global Fund to Fight AIDS, Tuberculosis, and Malaria has been
established to mobilize new financial resources for these three diseases. Because
these new campaigns focus on poverty reduction and disease control, however,
the language of health-sector reform and the perspective of health system analysis
have received less attention—an unfortunate development.

While the policy debate has evolved, the underlying problems remain. Addressing the urgent health problems that now are the focus of international concern will
generally require effective health-care systems of the sort that do not yet exist in
many countries. For example, the prevention and treatment of HIV/AIDS or the
integrated management of care for sick and malnourished children will require
health-care systems that can provide accessible high-quality services, especially
to the poor and disadvantaged. It is broadly agreed that the health sector in many
developing countries cannot meet these challenges today without substantial
reform. Even huge increases in funding will not suffice, unless and until nations
have in place the institutions and infrastructure to use such funds effectively. In
short, the subject matter of this book remains both timely and urgent.

Concepts and Perspectives

Our approach to the health-sector reform process brings together six important
elements that we consider systematically in the chapters that follow. The first five
points are discussed in Chapters 2 to 7, with a focus on methods. The sixth set of
concepts provides a framework for analyzing health-care systems and reform options in Chapters 8 to 12. These six elements are as follows:

- A description of the *policy cycle* and an identification of the key tasks a reformer
  should be prepared to tackle at each stage of the process (Chapter 2).
- A guide to *ethical theory* to help think through the moral bases for the policy
  goals and priorities that help define the reform agenda (Chapter 3).

- An introduction to *systematic political analysis*, because politics matters at each step of the health-reform cycle. Political analysis should be done early and often throughout the policy cycle (Chapter 4).
- A set of *core health system performance goals and intermediate performance measures* which can serve as guides for evaluating performance. We link these goals to ethical theory (Chapters 5 and 6).
- A *systematic approach to health system diagnosis* that can be taught and practiced effectively. It is based on the idea of working backwards from identified performance problems to their causes and the causes of causes, using a technique we call a "diagnostic tree" (Chapter 7).
- A framework of *five health system "control knobs"* to summarize the options available to reformers (payment, financing, organization, regulation, and behavior) for influencing health system performance. These categories provide the focus for both conducting the diagnostic process and developing substantive policies to achieve better performance (Chapters 8 to 12).

By combining these ideas and techniques, practitioners have a better chance of producing workable reforms to achieve the intended objectives. In our conclusion (Chapter 13) we draw together the key lessons from the methods chapters in Part I and the substantive discussions in Part II. We do *not* seek, however, to present a single set of preferred solutions, because countries are too varied for one approach to be universally applicable. Countries differ widely in their levels of economic development, social conditions, political values, disease patterns, and institutional arrangements. Nations range in per capita income from several hundred dollars per year to twenty thousand and more. In some countries, half the children born alive die before the age of five; in others, child death is a rare event. There are many countries where physicians are as rare as one per 10,000 or 20,000 people, and not a few where there may be one per several hundred (WHO 2000, 79).

Other differences in national conditions are equally striking. In some countries, the civil service is reliable and energetic; in others, it is corrupt and ineffective (Hodess et al. 2001). Some countries are blessed with mineral or agricultural resources; others have a difficult climate or poor soils (Sachs 1999, Bloom and Sachs 1998). Some suffer from endemic infectious diseases or the AIDS epidemic; others struggle with increasing chronic disease; and many countries confront large burdens of both infectious and noncommunicable diseases. Some countries have relatively stable political conditions with good governance; others have experienced years of political terror and instability. These factors affect both how the problems of health-sector reform are defined and the kinds of solutions that are most likely to work.

In addition, countries seek different goals within their health-care systems. Countries have serious and legitimate differences over whether they attempt to provide equal care to rich and poor, urban and rural, productive and unproductive people. They differ over which health conditions they seek to address as high priorities: the burden of maternal and infant mortality, for example, versus chronic conditions such as cardiovascular disease in working adults. Countries also differ in their views about how forcefully citizens can be pushed to change their personal habits or their culture, when these support unhealthy behaviors. In short, not only do problems vary from country to country, but so do values, goals, and ethics (Hollander 2002). We believe, therefore, that developing a plan for health reform requires a direct engagement with philosophy and social values.

Finally, nations differ in their political systems. Some are elected democracies, others are one-party systems, while others are ruled by hereditary monarchs. Among the democracies, some constitutions centralize power, while others decentralize it. Some electoral systems encourage fringe parties, while others discourage them. Some political systems encourage the activities of non-governmental organizations, while others suppress any groups that might challenge the dominant power structure. In addition, different groups within a country vary in power and position, depending on their leadership and history. These differences in political structures, political practices, and political freedom affect the processes of health reform, including how problems and solutions are defined and the kinds of policies that are politically feasible.

The analysis of health reform that we offer is thus resolutely contextual—both problems and solutions depend on the particular situation. Our goal is to illuminate that dependence by presenting conceptual tools for analyzing problems and solutions in specific contexts.

Some Basic Definitions

Before we proceed, we need to address some definitional issues. Our approach to definitions is pragmatic. We want to use terms in ways that are most helpful to our analysis and our readers. For example, no sharp line distinguishes what is and what is not part of the health-care system, nor is it worth much time and energy debating over the system's boundary. We will argue that a pragmatic analysis must focus on the *consequences* of this system for the *well-being* of the target population. The analytical net must be cast wide enough to include all forces and factors that reformers might want to influence in seeking to improve the lives of that population.

What is "The Health Sector"?

Bearing our goals in mind, we use the terms "the health sector" and "the health-care system" interchangeably in this book to include the following:

- All those who deliver health care—public or private, Western or traditional, licensed or unlicensed, including doctors, nurses, hospitals, clinics, pharmacies, village health workers, and traditional healers.

- The money flows that finance such care—official or unofficial, through intermediaries or directly out of patients' pockets.
- The activities of those who provide the specialized inputs into the health-care process—including medical and nursing schools and drug and device manufacturers.
- The financial intermediaries, planners, and regulators who control, fund, and influence those who provide care—encompassing ministries of health, finance, and planning, social and private insurance institutions, and regulatory bodies.
- The activities of organizations that deliver preventive services—such as immunization, family planning, infectious-disease control, and education on nutrition, smoking, and substance abuse. These may be public or private, local, national or international.

What is "Health-Sector Reform"?

We take a similarly pragmatic view of what we mean by "reform." For us, "reform" involves *a significant, purposeful effort to improve the performance of the health-care system*. Reforms differ along at least two dimensions: *(1)* the number of aspects of the health-care system that are changed, and *(2)* how radically the changes depart from past practice. But as we will stress repeatedly (especially when discussing particular options in Chapters 8 to 12), successful reform often involves introducing a set of interdependent and mutually supporting interventions—especially if a major departure from past practice is made in one piece of the system.

What is a "Control Knob"?

We use the term "control knob" as a metaphor. Think of changing the performance of some complex system to produce a specific result. Consider, for example, the pilots of a large aircraft adjusting different controls to achieve the desired altitude, speed, and fuel economy to reach a destination safely and quickly. Or consider the operators in the control room of a steel mill, adjusting the controls on different steps in the production process: the temperature of the blast furnaces, the mix of raw materials being processed, and other key parameters. In each case, system managers select the settings that determine how the system operates and what the system produces.

In similar ways, we conceive of a health system "control knob" as something that *can be adjusted* by government action. Furthermore, adjustments or changes in the control knob must be *significant causal determinants of health system performance*. In other words, our control knobs describe discrete areas of health system structure and function that matter significantly for health system performance and are subject to change as part of health reform. Given this formulation, factors in health system performance that cannot be changed as part of health reform are not part of a "control knob." Conversely, neither is everything that health reform *can* change. Only factors that significantly determine how the health system affects the target population are aspects of a "control knob."

The control-knob approach, of course, is not the only method for understanding health systems. For decades, experts have dissected, analyzed, evaluated and compared health systems around the world, for both rich and poor nations. To provide a context for our approach, we briefly review some alternative modes of health system analysis.

One recent approach is the World Health Organization's analysis of health system performance around the world (WHO 2000). The WHO ranked national health systems according to a series of indicators, using a complex formula to combine the different measures. But while the WHO report did discuss the "functions" of health-care systems, it did not include an extended analysis of the causes and cures for inadequate performance.

A second approach is that adopted by sociologists (Roemer 1993, Raffel 1984). They have typically used capacity indicators (the number of hospital beds, physicians, and nurses), descriptions of government programs, and certain health indicators (infant mortality rate and life expectancy) to describe and compare national health systems. These analyses often provide much descriptive detail, but again, rarely provide guidance on how to change a health system to produce performance gains.

A third approach has focused on resource flows. In the early 1990s, Jeremy Hurst examined health systems in terms of fund flows and payment methods between population groups and institutions (Hurst 1992). Recent developments of this approach, in the form of National Health Accounts, often provide a helpful picture of money flows from revenue sources through intermediaries to providers. Again, however, there is no explanatory model linking policy changes to performance outcomes.

Finally, economics provides another conceptual framework for understanding the health sector—albeit one which has enjoyed only limited success (Jack 1999, Feldstein 1993). Partly this is because a nation's health sector is actually composed of many distinct markets—for different services in different geographic areas. Yet these individual markets are seldom studied in detail; nor is their interaction well understood (Yett et al. 1975, Feldstein 1974). Moreover, economics utilizes the paradigm of supply and demand—where prices signal consumers how much to buy and producers how much to sell. In many countries, however, a large part of the health-care system is not organized on market principles. Moreover, even where there are markets, they are often imperfectly competitive, and physicians can determine much in the way of patient behavior. Given these departures from the competitive ideal, it is not surprising that microeconomic theory has offered few explanations for macro-level health outcomes or for the rate of growth of national health expenditures (Gerdtham and Jonsson 2000).

The Forces Driving Health Reform

With these definitions in mind, we can now explore some of the common patterns in health-sector reform among nations. Four forces are driving health reform in countries around the world. Their relative roles vary from place to place, but these four forces have led to certain widespread dilemmas that now confront many nations in our increasingly globalized world.

The first force is the *rising cost* of health care. In nearly every country, increases are forcing governments to rethink their policies and approaches to the health system. Second, there are *rising expectations*, as citizens demand more, both from government in general and from the health-care system in particular. Third, increases in both costs and expectations are occurring at a time when governments confront *limits on their capacity to pay* the costs of health care. Finally, the current debate is also influenced by growing *skepticism about conventional approaches* to the health sector. For reformers, these pressures create both a challenge and an opportunity: a challenge because more is being demanded and more options must be analyzed, and an opportunity because the resulting crisis often leads to more openness to change and innovation.

These four forces work themselves out in significantly different ways in different countries. The world's poorest nations are especially dependent on international financial institutions, so that health system changes may be requested or imposed as a condition of external assistance. In addition, the HIV/AIDS pandemic is placing immense strains on some of the world's nations that have the least resources to meet that challenge (World Bank 1997). In other middle- and low-income nations, citizens' demands for financial protection from high health-care costs have led governments to seek financing strategies that will be sustainable as development proceeds. Regardless of how the drama unfolds, governments struggle to resolve the conflict between what they are willing and able to spend, and what they or their citizens want, as they try to cope with what has become a common set of challenges to health-care systems around the world.

Force #1: Rising Costs

Almost everywhere, health-care costs are rising steadily. In the world's wealthier countries, health spending rose from an average of 5% of national income in 1970 to 8.1% in 1997—even as per capita income grew steadily (Huber 1999). While data in poorer countries are less reliable, similar patterns can be found in these nations as well.

One force driving costs upward is the aging of the population. For example, the percentage of the population aged 65 years and older is expected to increase from 6% to 18% in Asia between 2000 and 2050, and from 5.5% to 18% in Latin America over the same period. This is due not only to a rise in life expectancy but also because birthrates have declined in many nations (Casterline 2001). More-over, some poorer countries where birthrates remain high now confront a dual burden of disease (WHO 1999, Murray and Lopez 1996). With both younger and older age cohorts growing, such nations have to cope with everything from child-hood diarrheal disease to rising coronary artery disease rates.

To some extent, these developments reflect the success of the health-care sys-tem: more citizens now live long enough to develop chronic diseases. As we age, our arteries harden, our joints grow stiff, our livers and kidneys work less effi-ciently, our hearts get tired, and our minds become cloudy. If more people died be-fore developing such conditions, per capita health-care costs would be lower. Such "failures of success" are reflected in the *rising levels of disability* in many coun-tries (Murray and Lopez 1996). Ironically, countries with successful population-stabilization policies and health-care systems move along this path farther and faster. Indeed, the success of health-care systems in lowering childhood mortality also increases the demand for services from that age group.

Worldwide, life expectancy at birth has increased from 50.2 years in 1960 (UNDP 1997, 167), to an estimated 66.7 years in the period 1995–2000 (UNDP 2000, 189) and is still rising in much of the world. Declining mortality rates are due to many factors, including improved nutrition and housing, expanding clean water supply, and better sewage disposal. Basic health services, including immu-nization and infectious disease control, have also played a role. But whatever the cause, lower mortality increases the number of people who need medical care.

The effects of aging on health-care costs are complex (Mahal and Berman 2001). Especially in high-income countries with extensive and expensive hospital systems, much of the high cost of care among the oldest age groups is associated with termi-nal illnesses. When life expectancy goes up and those illnesses occur later in life, health-care costs in some old-but-not-the-oldest age groups can actually fall. Still, especially in low- and middle-income countries, aging seriously complicates the problem of health sector finance. This is especially so in payroll-tax systems, be-cause aging lowers the percentage of the population who pay such taxes.

Other epidemiological developments, most notably AIDS, are also contributing to cost increases, especially in severely affected countries (UNAIDS 2001). In Eastern Europe, increases in alcoholism and suicide have produced serious sys-temic problems. In Russia and several republics of the former Soviet Union, male life expectancy actually fell five to ten years in the post-Soviet period (McKee and Shkolnikov 2001, Shkolnikov et al. 2001). Despite successes against smallpox and polio, other infectious diseases (from tuberculosis to dengue fever) are on the in-crease in various parts of the world, posing grave challenges to health reformers.

The sellers of health-care goods and services also contribute to rising costs. Many poor countries have large, private, fee-for-service primary-care sectors— a situation that tends to produce significantly higher expenditures (Bennett et al. 1997, Hanson and Berman 1998). Pharmaceutical companies also seek to take advantage of the market and now offer drugs for every organ system—to regrow your hair, cure your depression, lower your cholesterol and blood pressure, combat your ulcers, and improve your sexual functioning. Efforts to market these compounds worldwide go forward every day. In poor countries, even traditional medicine is now becoming commodified and patented by private companies, with modern packaging, marketing, and prices.

New technology is a particularly important force driving up health-care costs. The largest gains from innovation, economically and professionally, come from developing high-priced solutions to previously unsolved problems for an audience that can pay. In contrast, there is not much scientific prestige or profit associated with developing cost-saving changes to existing technology. Even when technological progress lowers unit costs, total costs can still rise if the change unleashes a large unmet demand (Roberts and Clyde 1993). For example, the recent drastic reduction in prices for antiretroviral drugs for HIV/AIDS in Africa will surely not reduce *total spending* on those pharmaceuticals.

The increasing prevalence of chronic disease also disrupts health insurance markets. In a world of chronic disease, many of those who will be sick in the future are already sick today. Since sellers of insurance will try not to sell to sick people, or do so only at a very high price, those who most need coverage, the sick, will often not be able to purchase insurance. Conversely, if insurance costs reflect average risks, then the healthiest have an incentive not to purchase insurance, disproportionately leaving only the sick in any insurance scheme and decreasing the amount of "risk pooling" in the system (Phelps 1997).

Force #2: Rising Expectations

A second worldwide force—rising expectations—derives from three sources: economic, social, and political. As nations develop, their citizens want to spend more on health. These rising expenditures imply the use of more, and costlier, services for both care and cure. In some regions of the world, like East Asia, which until recently had seen years of steady growth, the rise in expectations has been considerable.

Typically, national health-care demand rises as quickly as, and in some cases more quickly than, national income. We now realize that health-care spending has historically been underestimated in the poorest countries because of the failure to fully count the substantial private, out-of-pocket expenditures that are common in such systems (Berman 1997). As a result of recent household surveys, many scholars now accept a lower estimate of the effect of national income on national health spending than formerly. Yet even if health-care spending only rises in proportion to income, the absolute amount of additional money that nations are under pressure to mobilize for health care, as incomes increase, is substantial. Moreover, the share of such spending that goes through the public sector (e.g., through new social insurance schemes) often rises, putting additional pressure on public finances.

Global social developments are reinforcing these demands. Films, television, and the Internet—along with travel and immigration—have given the citizens of many countries an image of life in the world's high-income nations. Such exposure has contributed to a rising materialism and loss of traditional values. Increasingly, people around the world accept that it is desirable to stay young and healthy as long as possible, and to consume as much as possible. And the health systems in many countries are under increasing pressure to deliver on these goals.

Rising expectations lead patients to want the latest and best care, the fanciest technology, and the newest drugs. Knowing what is available elsewhere, they become skeptical (perhaps rightly) of the quality of care in their own local health centers or smaller hospitals. Consequently, they overwhelm regional centers and academic facilities. In many low-income nations, growing urban, middle, and upper classes pressure governments to provide expensive high-technology care (from CT scanners to organ transplants) and to spend a large share of the national health budget on a few elite institutions (Barnum and Kutzin 1993).

Increasing democracy can reinforce these pressures. The subjects of a highly organized authoritarian state are likely to accept whatever health care their government finds it expedient to provide. The active, self-seeking citizens of an open political order are less likely to be satisfied with such arrangements. Moreover, political leaders in a competitive political order are more likely to respond to such popular concerns, and contribute to rising expectations, by making promises about the potential gains from health sector reform.

Force #3: Limited Capacity to Pay

Recent changes in the world economic order have created both problems and opportunities for many nations, but many governments are hard-pressed to meet the demands created by rising costs and expectations.

Worldwide, the second half of the twentieth century passed by much better than the first half. There were some locally very destructive wars and significant regional economic collapses, but nothing to match the two world wars and the worldwide Great Depression of the century's first fifty years. Such peace and prosperity has given many individuals and corporations the opportunity and the funds to invest abroad. At the same time, national governments find their fiscal and monetary policies increasingly constrained by international capital flows and financial institutions. International investors will not buy your government's bonds if you try to pay for social and health services by running too large a deficit. Nor will they invest in private-sector projects if they fear fiscal instability. And loans from the International Monetary Fund (IMF) or the World Bank require a country to reduce its deficits, control public-sector spending, and repay on time (Weil et al. 1990).

Recent economic growth in many countries would seem to mean more funds are available for health care. But often cost and demand in the health sector have grown even faster. And economic growth has been extremely uneven. Until the mid-1990s, some Asian countries routinely achieved economic growth rates greater than 5% annually, while many African countries experienced negative or only marginally positive growth (Commission on Macroeconomics and Health 2001).

Many governments find their fiscal capacities severely constrained. First, for most low-income nations, the ability to raise funds domestically is very limited. Low-income countries raise only about 20% of (a much lower) gross domestic product in taxes, compared with 42% of GDP in high-income countries (Schieber and Maeda 1997). And there are many competing uses for such funds. Citizens want better roads, housing, and education. Infrastructure investments are needed to support economic development. Meanwhile, multinational corporations demand tax concessions from national governments and threaten to relocate if these are not forthcoming. And domestic firms claim the need for protection against international competitors. As a result, often only 1% or 2% of the GDP is available for publicly financed health care apart from international aid (Commission on Macroeconomics and Health 2001).

Moreover, the linkages in the current international economic order can hold significant dangers. When world coffee prices fall, budget deficits in Kenya and Ethiopia skyrocket. If Brazil devalues its currency, then Argentinean exports to third countries suffer, because Brazilian goods are now cheaper than Argentina's. If the property market collapses in Kuala Lumpur, then Malaysia imports less, and its industries cut their prices to try to export more—actions that can cause serious economic problems for Malaysia's neighbors. If one currency falls, international speculative pressure shifts to another.

The increasing sophistication of the economies in poor countries only ties them ever more tightly into such interdependency. Countries that used to make inexpensive radios now assemble advanced computers. Factories that once produced textiles now make the chips for those same computers. Brazil sells jet aircraft in the United States and U.S. computer companies depend on programming offices in India.

These economic processes intersect with political pressures, affecting the amount of money that a country decides to spend on health. In a number of countries, politicians have made election promises they cannot keep concerning social programs, including pension funds. As those programs either go bankrupt or devour extra tax revenues, all other spending (including health) comes under pressure. In response, health-sector advocates often seek to remove health-care financing from the general budget (e.g., by creating new social insurance programs) in order to give it protected status.

At the same time, providers inside the health-care system struggle to preserve their incomes and protect their interests. In Eastern Europe, the large health-care delivery systems created under communism have been difficult to maintain, as governments work to restart economic growth and regain international competitiveness (Goldstein et al. 1996, Healy and McKee 2001). As governments try to control expenditures and prevent inflation, they are tempted to hold down healthcare spending by limiting compensation to doctors, nurses, and other health personnel. These groups, in turn, work desperately inside the political system to increase their falling incomes.

These political developments and economic constraints occur in the context of major social and intellectual changes inside and outside the health system. These broad changes represent the fourth force that is driving health reform.

Force #4: Skepticism of Conventional Ideas

The global turn to the market has brought a trend toward diminished social solidarity and a parallel turn against government action in many countries. In Eastern Europe and the former Soviet Union, the old model of centrally planned, state-owned enterprise has been widely discredited (even as older citizens remember the security it provided with nostalgia and regret). In many low-income countries, bad governance, poor policies, and outright corruption have produced a squandering of limited resources and widespread skepticism about the public sector.

Since the 1980s, advocates of an antigovernment message have aggressively promoted their views around the world. Consultants, entrepreneurs, and experts from private foundations and international agencies have all participated. In the health sector, political leaders have found themselves faced with the argument that the pro-market approach is the solution to all their problems (Griffin 1989).

This discussion extends well beyond the health sector. Poorly run government bureaucracies and inefficient state-owned companies have proliferated, in part because of their political advantages. Using the public sector to provide patronage rather than service, employment rather than output, allows government to build up a political base. Workers are identifiable, easy to organize, and often grateful to political leaders for their employment. Customers, on the other hand, are harder to identify and organize and are likely to have less at stake. These factors often lead to an overstaffed, poorly managed, high-cost public sector, with unhelpful staff, crumbling facilities, and poor service.

With countries increasingly short of money, there has been rising criticism of such arrangements. To break the politics-to-employment link, many institutional reforms have been attempted, ranging from the creation of quasi-autonomous public boards that supervise government activities, to outright privatization. Ideas like "reinventing government" pervade the debates over health reform throughout the world today (Osborne and Gaebler 1992, Saltman and von Otter 1995).

Because this intellectual movement is so widespread, we want to let readers know our view of such matters. Whether new arrangements will perform better than current practice is a complex empirical question. As we argue throughout this book, in predicting outcomes, the devil is often in the details—especially when it comes to how organizations are managed and governed (see Chapter 10). In our view, the applicability of the market model to health care varies with specific circumstances: Is a given market large enough to support a reasonable number of efficient, independent competitors? Do customers know enough, or can they be given enough information, to choose intelligently? Will the savings that result from the competitive pressures be greater than the resources used up through higher transaction costs (i.e., the costs of arranging all the buying and selling)? In our view, health reformers should answer such questions before deciding on policy. This book is designed to equip reformers with the analytical tools they need to conduct the required analyses—in ways that are both open-minded and effective.

Summary

Let us summarize the main points of this introductory chapter:

- Economic, social, and political forces, both inside and outside the health-care system, are causing widespread pressures to spend more on health care.
- New technology (including new drugs), as well as changes in population structure and disease patterns, are continuing to push up per capita health-care costs.
- The evolving international economic system often limits the capacity of governments and the private sector to meet these higher costs, especially in poor countries, because of short-term crises and longer-term competitive pressures.
- Broad shifts in intellectual beliefs about the state and the market have led to widespread promotion of market competition and privatization as solutions for all economic problems, including policies for the health sector.

Many countries today face a gap between what they can pay for and what they would like to provide in the health sector. Expectations continue to rise as economies improve, countries become more democratic, and media-based images spread around the globe. In almost all countries, health-care costs are increasing, due to changing demographics, evolving disease patterns, and new technology. The implications of these changes are fought out in increasingly diverse, open, and egalitarian political and social processes, in countries with severe budget deficits and limited economic resources for health.

At the same time, there is a global move toward new ideas for health reform, combined with an emerging recognition that getting health reform right is a complex social phenomenon indeed. However complex it is, we believe that the ideas in this book can help analysts and decision-makers understand and manage the swirling processes of health reform. We begin our analysis with the health-reform cycle.

References

Barnum, Howard; and Joseph Kutzin. 1993. *Public Hospitals in Developing Countries: Resource Use, Cost, Financing*. Baltimore, MD: Johns Hopkins University Press.

Bennett, Sara; Barbara McPake; and Anne Mills, eds. 1997. *Private Health Providers in Developing Countries: Serving the Public Interest?* Atlantic Highlands, NJ: Zed Books.

Berman, Peter, ed. 1995. *Health Sector Reform in Developing Countries: Making Health Development Sustainable*. Cambridge, MA: Harvard University Press.

Berman, Peter. 1997. "National Health Accounts in Developing Countries: Appropriate Methods and Recent Applications." *Health Economics* 6(1): 11–30.

Bloom, David E.; and David Canning. 2000. "The Health and Wealth of Nations." *Science* 287: 1207, 1209.

Bloom, David; and Jeffrey Sachs. 1998. "Geography, Demography, and Economic Growth in Africa." *Brookings Papers on Economic Activity* 2: 207 95.

Casterline, John B., ed. 2001. *Diffusion Processes and Fertility Transition: Selected Perspectives*. Washington, DC: National Academy Press.

Commission on Macroeconomics and Health. 2001. *Macroeconomics and Health: Investing in Health for Economic Development*. Geneva: World Health Organization.

Dowling, William L. 1977. "Perspective Reimbursement of Hospitals." In Lewis E. Weeks and Howard J. Berman, eds., *Economics in Health Care*. Germantown, MD: Aspen Publishing.

Feldstein, Martin S. 1974. "Econometric Studies of Health Economics." In: M. Intriligator and D. Kendrick, eds. *Frontiers of Quantitative Economics,* Vol. 2. Amsterdam: North-Holland Publishing Company.

Feldstein, Paul J. 1993. *Health Care Economics*. Fourth edition. Albany: Delmar Publishers.

Gerdtham, U. G.; and B. Jonsson. 2000. "International Comparisons of Health Expenditure." In: Anthony J. Culyer and Joseph P. Newhouse, eds. *Handbook of Health Economics*. Amsterdam: Elsevier.

Gilman, Boyd H. 2000. "Hospital Response to DRG Refinements: The Impact of Multiple Reimbursement Incentives on Inpatient Length of Stay." *Health Economics* 9(4): 277–94.

Goldstein, Ellen; Alexander S. Preker; Olusoji Adeyi; and Gnanaraj Chellaraj. 1996. *Trends in Health Status, Services, and Finance: The Transition in Central and Eastern Europe*. World Bank Technical Paper No. 341, Social Challenges of Transition Series, Vol. 1. Washington, DC: World Bank.

Griffin, Charles. 1989. *Strengthening Health Services in Developing Countries Through the Private Sector*. Discussion Paper No. 4. Washington, DC: World Bank, International Finance Corporation.

Gwatkin, Davidson R.; Janet R. Wilcox; and Joe D. Wray. 1980. *Can Health and Nutrition Interventions Make a Difference?* ODC Monograph No. 13. Washington, DC: Overseas Development Council.

Hanson, Kara; and Peter Berman. 1998. "Private Health Care Provision in Developing Countries: A Preliminary Analysis of Levels and Composition." *Health Policy and Planning* 13(3): 195–211.

Healy, Judith; and Martin McKee. 2001. "Reforming Hospital Systems in Turbulent Times." *Eurohealth* Special Issue 2001, 7(3): 2–7.

Hearst, Norman; and Erik Blas. 2001. "Learning from Experience: Research on Health Sector Reform in the Developing World." *Health Policy and Planning* 16(Suppl): 1–3.

Hodess, Robin; Jessie Banfield; and Toby Wolfe. 2001. *Global Corruption Report 2001*. Berlin: Transparency International. Available from www.transparency.org. Accessed June 2002.

Hollander, Christopher, ed. 2002. "Five-Nation Survey: U.S. Adults Least Satisfied with Health System." *The Commonwealth Fund Quarterly* 8(1): 1–3.

Huber, Manfred. 1999. "Health Care Expenditure Trends in OECD Countries, 1970–1997." *Health Care Financing Review* 21(2): 99–117.

Hurst, Jeremy. 1992. *The Reform of Health Care: A Comparative Analysis of Seven OECD Countries*. Paris: OECD.

IMF, OECD, United Nations, and World Bank. 2000. *A Better World For All: Progress Towards the International Development Goals*. New York: United Nations. Available from www.paris21.org/betterworld/. Accessed June 2002.

Jack, William. 1999. *Principles of Health Economics for Developing Countries*. Washington, DC: World Bank.

Liu, Yuanli; William C. Hsiao; and Keqin Rao. 2003. "Medical Spending and Rural Impoverishment in China." *Health Policy and Planning*, forthcoming.

Mahal, Ajay; Peter Berman. 2001. *Health Expenditures and the Elderly: A Survey of Issues in Forecasting, Methods Used, and Relevance for Developing Countries*. The Global Burden of Disease 2000 in Aging Populations, Research Paper No. 01.23. Cambridge, MA: Harvard Burden of Disease Unit, December.

McKee, Martin; and Vladmir Shkolnikov. 2001. "Understanding the Toll of Premature Death among Men in Eastern Europe." *British Medical Journal* 323: 1051–5.

Mills, Anne; Sara Bennett; and Steven Russell. 2001. *The Challenge of Health Sector Reform: What Must Governments Do?* Basingstoke, England: Palgrave.

Murray, Christopher J.; and Alan D. Lopez, eds. 1996. *The Global Burden of Disease: A Comprehensive Assessment of Mortality and Disability from Diseases, Injuries, and Risk Factors in 1990 and Projected to 2020 (Global Burden of Disease and Injury Series, Vol. 1)*. Cambridge, MA: Harvard School of Public Health on behalf of the World Health Organization and World Bank.

OECD. 1996. *Health Care Reform: The Will to Change*. Health Policy Studies No. 8. Paris: OECD, Directorate of Education, Employment, Labour, and Social Affairs.

Osborne, David; and Ted A. Gaebler. 1992. *Reinventing Government: How the Entrepreneurial Spirit Is Transforming the Public Sector*. Reading, MA: Addison-Wesley.

Phelps, Charles E. 1997. *Health Economics*. 2nd ed. Reading, MA: Addison-Wesley. (See Chapters 10, 11, and 12).

Preston, Samuel. 1975. "The Changing Relation Between Mortality and Level of Economic Development." *Population Studies* 29(2): 231–48.

Raffel, Marshall W., ed. 1984. *Comparative Health Systems: Descriptive Analyses of Fourteen National Health Systems*. University Park, PA: Pennsylvania State University Press.

Roberts, Marc J.; with Alexandra T. Clyde. 1993. *Your Money or Your Life: The Health Care Crisis Explained*. New York: Doubleday.

Roemer, Milton I. 1993. *National Health Systems of the World*. New York: Oxford University Press.

Ron, Aviva; Brian Abel-Smith; and Giovanni Tamburi. 1990. *Health Insurance in Developing Countries: The Social Security Approach*. Geneva: International Labor Organization.

Sachs, Jeffrey. 1999. "Helping the World's Poorest." *The Economist* 14 August, 17–20.

Saltman, Richard B.; and Casten von Otter, eds. 1995. *Implementing Planned Markets in Health Care: Balancing Social and Economic Responsibility*. Philadelphia, PA: Open University Press.

Schieber, George; and Akiko Maeda. 1997. "A Curmudgeon's Guide to Financing Health Care in Developing Countries." In: George Schieber, ed., *Innovations in Health Care Financing: Proceedings of a World Bank Conference, March 10–11, 1997*. World Bank Discussion Paper No. 365. Washington, DC: World Bank.

Sen, Amartya. 1999. *Development as Freedom*. New York: Knopf.

Sen, Kasturi; and Meri Koivusalo. 1998. "Health Care Reforms and Developing Countries: A Critical Overview." *International Journal of Health Planning and Management* 13: 199–215.

Shklolnikov, Vladimir; Martin McKee; and David A. Leon. 2001. "Changes in Life Expectancy in Russia in the Mid-1990s." *The Lancet* 357(9260): 917–21.

UNAIDS. 2001. *AIDS Epidemic Update, December 2001*. Available from www.unaids.org. Accessed June 2002.

UNDP. 1997. *Human Development Report 1997*. New York: Oxford University Press.

———. 2000. *Human Development Report 2000*. New York: Oxford University Press.

Weil, Diana E. C.; Adelaida P. Alicbusan; John F. Wilson; Michael R. Reich; and David J. Bradley. 1990. *The Impact of Development Policies on Health: A Review of the Literature*. Geneva: World Health Organization, 5–38.

Wilsford, David. 1995. "States Facing Interests: Struggles over Health Care Policy in Advanced, Industrial Democracies." *Journal of Health Politics, Policy, and Law* 20(3): 571–613.

World Health Organization. 1999. "The Double Burden: Emerging Epidemics and Persistent Problems." In *World Health Report 1999: Making a Difference*. Geneva: World Health Organization.

———. 2000. *World Health Report 2000, Health Systems: Improving Performance*. Geneva: World Health Organization.

World Bank. 1993. *World Development Report 1993: Investing in Health*. New York: Oxford University Press.

———. 1997. *Confronting AIDS: Public Priorities in a Global Epidemic*. New York: Oxford University Press.

———. 2001. *Poverty Reduction Strategy Sourcebook*. Washington, DC: World Bank. Available from www.worldbank.org/poverty/strategies/index.htm. Accessed June 2002.

Yett, Donald; Leonard Drabek; Michael D. Intriligator; and Larry J. Kimbell. 1979. *A Forecasting and Policy Simulation Model of the Health Care Sector: The Human Resources Research Center (HRRC) Prototype Micro-Econometric Model*. Lexington, MA: Lexington Books.

2

The Health-Reform Cycle

In Chapter 1 we introduced the idea that health-sector reform can be viewed as a cycle. Now we want to analyze that process in more detail. In idealized form, the process of policy change moves through a cycle of six stages—problems are defined, a causal diagnosis is made, plans are developed, a political decision is made on reform initiatives, those reforms are then implemented, and their consequences are evaluated. The cycle then begins again, as new problems arise that must be addressed by policymakers (Figure 2.1).

Of course, in the real world reform rarely takes place in such a simple fashion. Instead, reform efforts begin in different places and skip stages, or several stages may occur at the same time. For example, health reformers might begin with a *diagnosis*, declaring, "The cause of all our problems is that public clinics and hospitals do not have enough resources to provide good service." Or reform advocates might start with their favorite *solution:* "What our country needs is a new national social insurance scheme." Yet, however the reform process unfolds, the policy cycle offers a useful way of analyzing that experience and reminding practitioners about the tasks they need to address as part of the reform process.

We have designed Figure 2.1 to highlight some major themes of this book. In particular, the "ethics" and "politics" components remind us that decision-makers confront ethical and political issues throughout the reform cycle. Questions like

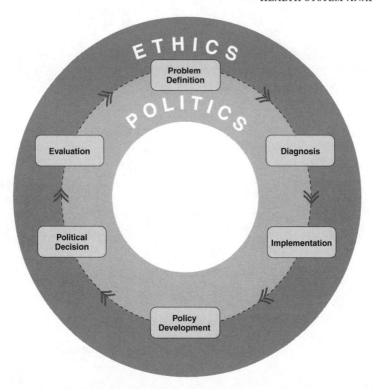

FIGURE 2.1. The policy cycle.

"What are the right priorities?" and "How can political pressures be managed?" pervade efforts at health-sector reform. Our approach calls for an explicit examination of the ethical bases of health policies and rejects the notion that the values of all health systems are, or should be, the same. Because we believe that all policy positions (including our own) involve ethical dimensions, this book seeks to make our own values and goals explicit. Readers can then determine how useful our perspective is to them. We also reject the view that the health-sector reform process is exclusively technical. Instead, we call for direct and extensive consideration of political factors at all stages of the reform process.

While we identify six stages in Figure 2.1, we focus most on the first four: problem definition, diagnosis, policy development, and political decision. This chapter, however, presents an overview of all six stages, and shows how these relate to our approach. The first four stages are then examined in more detail in Chapters 3 to 7, followed, in Part II by a chapter for each "control knob." While we do not have a chapter on implementation, we have provided practical guidance on that point in each control knob chapter, based on experience from around the world. In our view, purely theoretical discussions of health-reform options are not very valuable. To move health reform forward, reformers must realistically consider the difficulties of implementing a policy in their particular national context. And we try to help them do that throughout the book.

Finally, the cyclical nature of Figure 2.1 emphasizes a point we made earlier: The problems of a health-care system are seldom, if ever, resolved once and for all. As countries evolve, their health-care systems have to respond to new challenges. Moreover, successful reform often raises popular expectations and thereby raises demands for further reform. But the process of reform is also imperfect. Reformers often encounter unintended consequences or discover defects in their plans that were not apparent initially. For these reasons, the cycle of reform typically occurs again and again. Let us now look at each step of the health-reform cycle in more detail and at the critical tasks each requires.

The Policy Cycle

Step #1: Problem Definition

The most overlooked, yet one of the most important steps in health-sector reform is defining the problem. Health-care systems give rise to hundreds of statistics on their performance. But which are an appropriate focus for public attention? When is performance "problematic" and thus an appropriate target for reform? As we discussed in Chapter 1, some sort of shock or crisis often initiates the reform process. But even then, competing interests typically have different views about how to define the problem and what constitutes an appropriate solution.

Consider the following hypothetical example: Imagine a middle-income country suffering from a region-wide economic downturn. The Ministry of Finance argues that the health sector is consuming too much of the government's limited budget, while the medical association argues that "the problem" is that quality of health care is suffering because physicians' salaries are not keeping up with inflation. Meanwhile, the managers of the social insurance fund claim that "the problem" is the failure of the government to pay its share of the premiums for retirees, while the association of hospital directors argues that the failure to provide capital for new technology is "the real problem." The group that succeeds in having its problem definition accepted as the basis for discussion about reform will have a great effect on the solutions pursued and the policies adopted.

In thinking about problem definition we can ask two kinds of questions. The first kind is *normative* or *prescriptive*: What makes for a *good* problem definition? What makes one area of poor performance a more appropriate priority than another? Answering this question involves ethics and philosophy. We introduce this topic briefly below, and then provide a more detailed discussion of the ethical aspects of health-sector reform in Chapter 3.

The second kind of question is *empirical* or *descriptive*: What social processes shape how problems are perceived? What factors determine the problem definition that reformers confront? We discuss how problem definition happens and how to manage the political dimensions of health-sector reform in Chapter 4.

As stated previously, our normative approach to problem definition is based on the view that the health sector should be seen as a *means*, not an *end*, that problems should be defined in terms of *outcomes*. As explained in the next chapter, different ethical theories offer different perspectives on which outcomes matter most. Nonetheless, in Chapter 5 we will argue for a particular set of performance goals that we believe reflect the major ethical perspectives that are relevant to health-sector reform (Hsiao 1999). One such concern is the *health status* of the population: How long do people live, what disabilities do they have, and how do these vary across various population groups? A second set of outcomes is the degree of *satisfaction* that health care produces among the citizens of a society. A third set of outcomes involves *financial risk protection*: the capacity of a health-care system to protect individuals against the serious financial burden that disease can produce. We will explain and defend these suggestions in detail below.

This focus on consequences can be difficult for health reformers to adopt. Advocates with strong commitments to a particular policy often begin the reform process with their favorite solution. As the saying goes, "To a man with a hammer, everything looks like a nail." They advocate adopting competitive health insurance funds, or more family medicine, or autonomous hospitals, without explaining how that policy would improve the performance of the health system. Moreover, many in government are not used to being performance-oriented. They focus instead on spending budgets, meeting production targets, or following rules. For them, problems are defined in terms of the failure to fulfill particular norms or rules, not in terms of the *consequences* of what is done or not done (Barzelay and Armajani 1992).

From our experience around the world, we understand that old habits of mind die hard. As the historian of science T.S. Kuhn explained, basic framing assumptions, which he called "paradigms," generally shape our thinking about a particular problem (Kuhn 1962). Our emphasis on explicit means–ends analysis and critical strategic thinking represents something of a "paradigm shift"—a new way of thinking about health-sector reform. We are convinced of the value of this focus on consequences, however awkward it may seem at first. This perspective forces reformers to identify goals and link their proposed reforms to those goals. As a result, reformers are more likely to be explicit and self-critical about their goals in ways that increase the chances of achieving their objectives, whatever they may be.

This perspective helps clarify the role of data in defining problems and setting priorities. Some health-sector planners seem to argue that all one needs to identify problems are good data. But this is not how the world operates. Many reforms move ahead without good data. Many well-documented problems are ignored in reform programs. For example, the financial hardships suffered by Chinese peasants who get seriously ill are well known, but this has not been enough to mobilize that nation's policymakers (Liu et al. 1996).

Moreover, from a normative point of view, data alone cannot completely define problems and priorities for health reform. Any policy decision must rely, implicitly or explicitly, on both science and ethics. For example, in most countries women live longer than men (UNDP 2000). Whether this represents an unfairness to men that public policy should seek to correct cannot be settled by data alone.

Yet data do have a vital role to play. Information alone cannot reconcile conflicting positions based on genuine value differences, but scientific understanding can help define options and clarify consequences. Data can help move the debate to a more honest and consensual understanding of the choices available. For that reason, we believe that experts have a particular responsibility for helping the political process understand what is at stake in health reform. Otherwise, myth, ideology, and group interests will dominate and drive the debate.

One important use of data in the process of problem definition is through a process called "benchmarking," a term we borrow from the quality-management literature (Deming 1982, Juran and Gyrna 1980). In an industrial context, managers use benchmarking when they look at the costs, defect rates, or productivity of competitive businesses to determine the levels of performance they can reasonably aspire to achieve. In health-sector reform, benchmarking means looking at countries similar to one's own in income and spending levels, whose health system performance is particularly effective. Thus, reformers in Thailand might wonder why Sri Lanka has longer life expectancy while spending less on health care, and use that fact to focus their own problem definition. Similarly, Latin American countries could look at health statistics from Cuba or Costa Rica for setting their own objectives (PAHO 2001). Despite the differences among countries, international benchmarks can serve as a useful starting point for a discussion of performance problems. (There are other forms of benchmarking as well, and we discuss these more extensively at the end of Chapter 6.)

Step #2: Diagnosing the Causes of Health-Sector Problems

Just as a physician proceeds from symptoms to causes, a health-sector reformer also has to undertake a *diagnostic journey* (see Chapter 7). After defining problems based on health system outcomes, the next task is to work backwards to identify the causes of unsatisfactory results. Physicians explore anatomy and physiology. Health-sector reformers have to examine the causes of problems by exploring what we call the *five control knobs of the health sector*.

This is not a simple task. One prominent Japanese quality-improvement expert argues that the diagnostic process requires someone to "Ask 'why' five times," to look for causes behind, beyond, and beneath the obvious (Ishikawa 1988). The challenge is to dig deeper and deeper in order to understand why the system behaves as it does.

For example, researchers interested in explaining the problem of higher-than-expected costs of health care in urban areas in China discovered that there was unusually high use of certain pharmaceuticals (World Bank 1997). Going on a diagnostic journey revealed the following:

- In response to budget pressures, the Chinese government had substantially decreased payments to hospitals.
- The hospitals were then forced to rely either on payments from the insurance funds that covered government and industrial workers, or on patient payments.
- The fee schedule for insurance reimbursement made high-tech imaging and dispensing the newest pharmaceuticals particularly profitable.
- Based on traditional Chinese herbal medicine practice, the hospitals directly sold to patients the pharmaceuticals their doctors prescribed. They also provided much of the country's outpatient care.
- To influence their physicians, hospitals had begun compensating them based on the profits to the hospital that the physicians' prescriptions produced.

As a result, prescription rates for the most profitable pharmaceuticals rose dramatically (Dai 1993, Gao 1996). Understanding this process does not by itself determine the "treatment" to prescribe for this "illness"—one could change hospital funding, the insurance system, the price list, physician compensation schemes, or drug regulations. But diagnosing the causes of the problem is a necessary step toward devising an effective response.

The Five Control Knobs for Health-Sector Reform

To facilitate the diagnostic and policy development processes of health-sector reform, we refer throughout this book to five "control knobs." These five categories cover the mechanisms and processes that reformers can adjust to improve system performance. As we noted, not every important cause is part of one of the control knobs, because it may not be changeable by health-sector reform (Figure 2.2). Our choice of five critical categories for health-system reform—the five control knobs—reflects our considered judgment about the most important factors that determine a health system's outcomes and that can be used deliberately to change those outcomes. Below we briefly present the five control knobs, which are examined in more detail in Chapters 8 to 12. Here is a list of the control knobs we have identified, with a brief description of each:

Financing refers to all mechanisms for raising the money that pays for activities in the health sector. These mechanisms include taxes, insurance premiums, and direct payments by patients. The design of the institutions that collect the money (e.g., insurance companies, social insurance funds) is also part of this control knob, as is the allocation of resources to different priorities (Chapter 8).

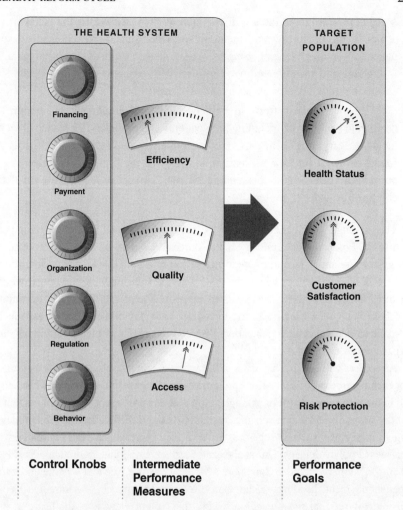

FIGURE 2.2. The five control knobs for health-sector reform.

Payment refers to the methods for transferring money to health-care providers (doctors, hospitals, and public health workers), such as fees, capitation, and budgets. These methods in turn create incentives, which influence how providers behave. Money paid directly by patients is also included in this control knob (Chapter 9).

Organization refers to the mechanisms reformers use to affect the mix of providers in health-care markets, their roles and functions, and how the providers operate internally. These mechanisms typically include measures affecting competition, decentralization, and direct control of providers making up government service delivery. It includes who does what and who competes with whom, as well as the managerial aspects of how providers work internally, such as how managers are chosen and how employees are rewarded (Chapter 10).

Regulation refers to the use of coercion by the state to alter the behavior of actors in the health system, including providers, insurance companies, and patients. We note that just because a regulation is on the books does not mean it is implemented and enforced. We consider what reformers must bear in mind to ensure that regulation works as intended (Chapter 11).

Behavior includes efforts to influence how individuals act in relation to health and health care, including both patients and providers. This control knob includes everything from mass media campaigns on smoking, to changes in sexual behavior for HIV prevention, to using the medical society to influence physicians' behavior, to persuading citizens to accept restrictions on their choice of provider (Chapter 12).

The "settings" on these control knobs explain many aspects of health system performance. *Financing* determines what resources are available. *Payment* determines on what terms those resources are available to providers. *Organization* determines the kinds of provider organizations that exist and their internal structures, which in turn shapes how these organizations perform. *Regulation* imposes constraints on those behaviors. Finally, efforts to change *behavior* influence how individuals respond to health-sector organizations, which in turn shapes the opportunities that organizations confront.

As readers will see in Chapters 8 to 12, we have identified the different "settings" for each control knob (i.e., various policy options) in ways that we hope will be helpful in the reform process. For example, even though some economists lump together all tax-supported financing schemes, we have distinguished general revenue financing from social insurance schemes, because they represent distinct alternatives in real-world policy debates. Our analysis also reflects important theoretical ideas. For example, we have included Singapore's Medical Savings Account scheme under the "patient payment" heading—rather than as a form of insurance—because it lacks the theoretically critical risk-spreading feature that, in our view, is at the heart of any insurance arrangement. Similarly, because we are concerned with consequences, we do not make much use of the distinction in the literature between "remuneration" (internal payments) and "reimbursement" (external payments). Instead, we classify payment systems (in either context) based on their likely incentive effects.

In thinking about the use of these control knobs, three themes emerge. First, significant reform generally requires the use of more than one control knob. For instance, many countries are now considering new social insurance schemes. Yet new regulation is also likely to be required to ensure the solvency of such schemes and to enhance access and risk-sharing. Social marketing efforts to get patients to change their behavior may also be needed to encourage appropriate use of care and to discourage abuse by both patients and providers. Similarly, hospital organization may need to be changed to enable providers to respond to the incentives created by the new financing system.

A second point is that changing one control knob often produces changes in other control knobs. For instance, establishing a new social insurance system is likely to change the payment methods to providers. Similarly, quality regulation through tougher physician licensing can eliminate some providers, altering the organization of the delivery system. Reformers should consider using such interactions to produce complementary or reinforcing policy changes.

Third, governments act in different ways to change control knob settings. In particular, governments often raise much of the revenue for the health system through taxes and directly operate a large part of the health-care delivery system. In such cases, governments can use their direct authority to influence what occurs—for example, by changing hospital governance or by introducing a new financing scheme. In other cases, government acts indirectly, to change the behavior of those outside government, through payment, purchasing, or regulatory policies. Thus, governments undertake both *steering roles* (through policy) and *rowing roles* (through provision) in the health system (Osborne and Gaebler 1993).

But the control knobs do not explain everything. Other cultural and structural factors also influence the outcomes of the health sector. For example, understanding why a country's regulatory agencies do not function effectively might require us to understand a nation's political institutions and cultural traditions—including its social capital (Putnam 1993)—factors that are not easily changed by health reformers.

Forces in other sectors also affect the health status of a population, as shown in WHO's work on intersectoral action for health (WHO 1986). Health status, for instance, is strongly influenced by the educational system, especially the education of girls and women. Research shows that an educated mother in South India is more likely to recognize a child's sickness and to take action within the family and in health clinics (Caldwell et al. 1983). Development policies for agriculture and industry also affect health status through multiple pathways, both positive and negative, including pesticide exposure, income generation, food availability, and nutritional effects (Weil et al. 1990). Water resource development projects influence the health of populations through environmental changes that affect the habitats of vectors for tropical diseases. The impact of new dams on increasing the spread of schistosomiasis, for example, is well recognized through international experience in Egypt, Sudan, Tanzania, Zimbabwe, and other countries (WHO 1986, 115). Macroeconomic policy also has multiple effects on health status in developing countries, as shown by the debate over structural adjustment policies in the 1980s (Bell and Reich 1988).

We agree with those who argue that a comprehensive approach to health improvement requires intersectoral cooperation and coordination. We have had to draw the line somewhere, however, and so have chosen not to consider here the role of factors outside the health sector. Yet understanding the role of such factors can help health reformers understand the problems they confront. Engineers designing automobiles cannot change gravity, but they have to work with its effects in mind.

Step #3: Policy Development

Once the causes of a problem have been diagnosed, the next question is what to do. What is the right therapy for the problem? What is an appropriate policy to address the causes? The process of policy development is more difficult than it might seem. In this section, we first consider why new policy ideas are difficult to develop and where such ideas come from. We also want to explain why it is important to look *forward* in the policy cycle to matters of politics, implementation, and evaluation when designing policy. Finally, we consider how the *process* of option development influences what happens at later stages of the policy cycle.

New ideas

Human thinking is heavily ruled by assumption and habit. We have already mentioned how dominant paradigms shape how questions are posed, what kind of evidence is acceptable, and what kinds of answers are viewed as legitimate. Professions typically educate their members in a particular paradigm and reinforce these ways of thinking through practice and experience (Goode 1969). Economists, for example, tend to view everything in terms of prices and markets, just as public health specialists largely focus on epidemiology and prevention. When powerful organizations adopt and promote a particular paradigm within a certain field, change is even more difficult. For example, the World Health Organization promoted the concept of "primary health care" for several decades, which significantly decreased the attention given to alternative policy approaches (Tarimo and Webster 1997, WHO 1978).

Where, then, can reformers look for new ideas? International learning is one helpful approach. For example, if your country wants to develop urban health clinics, it would be sensible to examine the experience with such clinics in other countries and the lessons learned from their failures and successes. Of course, because economic circumstances and political institutions vary, ideas from other nations need to be adapted for local conditions. But since the volume of policy experimentation around the world has been substantial in recent years, international experience is a useful place for reformers to start their work.

Policy innovations outside the health sector are another source of new ideas. In Bangladesh, for example, the nongovernmental development agency the Bangladesh Rural Advancement Committee (BRAC) has implemented a program for microfinance, which provides loans to small groups who want to initiate income-generating activities. The monies are provided at the community level through a revolving loan fund, which is managed by a village organization of mostly women members (BRAC 2000). This idea of a community-managed revolving fund is now being considered as an approach for community financing of health insurance, as explored in Chapter 8. Similarly, in our discussion of social marketing in Chapter 12, we review how ideas developed in a commercial context have health-sector applications.

A third source of ideas is theory. We have already expressed our skepticism about arguments not rooted in real-life examples. Yet theory can be a useful source of provocation and inspiration, as long as implementation issues are adequately considered. For example, the arguments for so-called quasi-markets and purchaser–provider separation have their roots in economic theory (Enthoven 1988).

Looking forward

To develop an effective plan for health-sector reform, reformers have to think ahead to political decisions and implementation—and design policy with those tasks in mind (as we discuss more fully in Chapter 7 on diagnosis).

The first kind of forward thinking involves politics (see Chapter 4). Sensible reformers begin to think about the political acceptability of their policies as they are developing them. Why devise an ideal plan that has little chance of being adopted?

Similar considerations apply to implementation. We have noted how countries vary in administrative capacity and in the attitudes that citizens have toward government. For example, Hungary began paying hospitals a fixed fee for each type of admission. To raise their reimbursement, however, many hospitals reported nearly all baby deliveries as "complicated" (Evetovits 2002). A country where providers are likely to game the system, therefore, must anticipate those responses in policy design. Similarly, some clinics in Thailand only establish medical records for seriously ill patients, as one of us observed during a site visit. Given manpower shortages, this may be a sensible use of their limited resources, but it means that certain kinds of regulatory options, which would require more extensive data, are not available to health reformers.

Another implementation issue is whether to proceed immediately to full-scale nationwide implementation or take a more limited demonstration project approach. We have noted that reform often occurs in the context of a crisis, which creates a window of opportunity for change. In such situations, it is tempting to move directly to a bold initiative, while public attention is focused on the problem and supporting forces are mobilized. On the other hand, an experimental or demonstration project approach allows for learning. Why not try out a new idea in a few cities or regions first, to reveal difficulties in implementation and flaws in the plan's logic, before it is adopted nationwide?

Viewing policy innovation as an experiment allows reformers to evaluate competing proposals. For example, in recent health insurance reform efforts in China, first two, and then twenty municipalities were involved in various experimental programs, before the national scheme was finalized (Yip and Hsiao 2001). On the other hand, experimental programs can attract energy and enthusiasm that lead to a degree of success that is hard to emulate when a program is "scaled up" for system-wide adoption. And in some cases, the demonstration project is never scaled up, so that the project ends as a limited experiment with little impact on the broader health system.

The design process

The task of designing reform plans is as much political as analytical. This refers to both the *content* of the reform ideas and the *process* of developing the ideas. This design process can be a key step in mobilizing support for reform. Thus, the process of policy development should produce a plan that is both technically sound and politically feasible.

A classic example of how *not* to do policy design in this regard is the failed health-reform plan in the United States under President Bill Clinton (Skocpol 1996). Technical experts developed the plan behind closed doors, with limited consultation with either the major interest groups or political leaders in Congress. As a result, even groups that stood to benefit from the reforms, such as hospitals that would have received additional revenue from previously uninsured patients, were slow to support the scheme and never did so enthusiastically. Similarly, legislative leaders who were excluded from the process never felt responsible for the plan. As a result, none of the committees in Congress (all controlled by Democrats) ever produced draft legislation that embodied the main ideas of the Clinton plan.

Involving groups with diverse perspectives in policy development can serve both political and technical ends, as we discuss in Chapter 7. Giving potential supporters a role in the design process can help transform them into actual supporters. The process can also provide a testing ground for new ideas, and help protect experts from becoming prisoners of their own enthusiasm. Involving those who actually work in the system can result in substantive changes that improve the chances of effective implementation. Of course, too much "participation" can limit reformers' ability to get what they want and need from the process. Reformers therefore need to oversee the day-to-day operation of the reform group, designing the terms of reference for members and staff of the task force or committee that is created to do detailed policy development. Carefully managing the policy design process requires a good deal of skill and experience and may be key to reform success in the long run.

Step #4: Political Decision

As shown in Figure 2.1, each stage in the policy cycle is affected by politics, including problem definition, policy development, and implementation. The adoption of a reform proposal, however, provides a focus for political decision-making, often by the executive and legislative branches of government. As Chapter 4 examines the politics of health reform in greater detail, we will only address these processes briefly in this section.

Health reform typically confronts difficult political challenges. Organized interest groups with a large stake in the current system (e.g., physicians, hospital owners, and the pharmaceutical industry) are likely to oppose reform. On the other hand, the intended beneficiaries of health reform (e.g., sick patients, the poor, and the underserved) are often less powerful and less well organized. Some potential beneficiaries within the health system (e.g., new family doctors yet to be trained) may not exist, and so cannot play an effective role. As always in the pull and tug of political decision-making, the future tends to be underrepresented compared with the past (Banfield and Wilson 1972).

Getting health-sector reform adopted is not just a matter of political commitment and risk-taking (*political will*); it is also a matter of effective political strategy and coalition building (*political skill*). Like other skills, political skills can be analyzed and understood, taught and learned—and for health reformers, political skills are essential. Whether a proposed reform is adopted will depend on the skill, commitment, and resources of its proponents (and opponents) and on the political strategies they employ.

There is nothing dishonorable in being politically astute in the service of health-sector reform. Politics is how governments do their work and how societies make decisions. In democratic states, electoral and legislative politics may be key. In one-party systems, bureaucratic politics plays a comparable role. Decisions are made through struggles within the state apparatus, as agencies and factions fight for control. Someone who truly cares about results in health reform thus must learn to think politically and act strategically, no matter what kind of system they operate within.

A key political task in all situations is building a strong support coalition. As we discuss in Chapter 4, this means identifying groups and individuals with enough collective political power to get the proposed policy accepted. The political strategist for health reform needs to map the power and position of key groups and to devise strategies that will produce the required support. These strategies also must take into account the country's institutional and political structure. In addition, politics doesn't end once a plan is adopted, but continues to play a significant role in whether a reform is conscientiously implemented—which brings us to the next stage in the cycle.

Step #5: Implementation

The American political scientist Aaron Wildavsky argued that good ideas are not worth much if they cannot be implemented (Pressman and Wildavsky 1973). Many allegedly good health-reform ideas have failed because, *in practice*, they were *not* good ideas—exactly because they could not be implemented.

Health-sector reform *always* requires organizations and individuals to behave differently. Without such changes, nothing new would be accomplished. Yet change is almost always resisted. One reason is psychological. New procedures and structures are strange and unfamiliar. For many, the mere fact of newness creates anxiety and resistance. The old adage "Better the devil you know than the devil you don't," embodies this idea. Resistance to change also arises because change can bring costs to specific groups and individuals. New procedures and arrangements take time and effort to learn. Existing hierarchies can be upset. Those who benefited from the old system can lose a lot. Moreover, those most successful under the old system have the most to lose; hence, the currently powerful are often the most opposed to reform.

Another force that inhibits change is the difficulty we all have in giving up familiar ways of thinking. Ingrained patterns of thought and behavior, which have evolved slowly and served well in the past, can have a strong hold over us. Moreover, established patterns of interaction are often strongly supported by a network of mutual expectations (influenced by culture, class, position, and gender, for example). If a doctor wants to treat a nurse differently, or a patient wants to relate to a doctor differently, they can encounter all sorts of pressures to conform to expected behavior. To most of us, these assumptions—like many features of our culture—are invisible. Yet implementation of health reform can depend on changing some of these same cultural patterns, a process that can be very difficult.

Overcoming the resistance to change requires sophisticated leadership. Yet such leadership is often in short supply. Health-sector reformers (including ministers of health or finance) are often physicians, politicians, or economists. Few have had experience as the chief executive of a large organization, and they rarely fully grasp the importance of management skills. Senior academic physicians can be particularly deficient in this regard, given the hierarchical nature of academic medicine in many countries. They often do not realize that giving instructions is not sufficient; that reforming a health system differs from performing surgery in an operating room. Implementing health reform involves many basic organizational tasks: developing an implementation plan, assembling a team to carry out the plan and assigning tasks to them, devising and coordinating schedules, and motivating and giving feedback to those involved. Given that ministers often serve less than one year, and frequently less than two, it is not surprising that inadequate attention is paid to implementation. But when that occurs, results are likely to be commensurately disappointing.

To bring about real change, health-sector reform efforts must be continuously and closely monitored, so that problems can be identified and corrective measures instituted. An appropriate reporting system is therefore key to successful policy implementation (Behn 2001). But many problems can arise in collecting the relevant information. The incentives for providers to misrepresent, even lie, can be substantial. The data that are easily available may not exactly measure the performance that reformers care about—and that can lead to incentives that distort behavior. Thus, a key task for reformers is to design a monitoring system that balances costs against data quality, and ease of operation against resistance to fraud. Such a system is critical to effective implementation, and also to the evaluation of health reform.

Step #6: Evaluation

Experienced evaluators know that successful evaluation has to begin well before a new program is implemented. Determining the effects of a new policy in a changing world is inherently difficult. The question often arises of whether what happens is the result of the reform or would have occurred anyway. Since data gathering consumes scarce administrative and organizational resources, a series of strategic decisions must be made if the evaluation process is to be both effective and sustainable.

The simplest evaluation approach is a before-and-after comparison. This involves examining how outcomes change over time as reforms are implemented. But this approach does not allow evaluators to detect the role played by other events or circumstances. For example, improvements in health status could be due to a surge in economic growth, rather than to the introduction of a new financing or physician-payment scheme.

The classic solution to this problem is to establish a "control group," a population *not* subject to a new program or policy, but that is studied in the same way as the experimental group. This allows a "difference in differences" approach, which compares the before-and-after differences between the experimental and control groups. This approach works best in conjunction with a demonstration project strategy, since a nationwide reform leaves no room for a control group for comparison purposes (Smith and Morrow 1996, Rossi et al. 1998).

When no control group is available, an evaluator has several fallback options. Perhaps different regions of the country vary in the extent to which potentially confounding variables influence outcomes. Alternatively, a similar neighboring country could provide something of a baseline. These issues need to be thought through carefully in designing the evaluation process. But even the simplest before-and-after comparison for a new policy cannot be made unless there are good "before" data. Health reformers, therefore, need to collect baseline data well before a new policy or program is instituted.

While we cannot explore the many issues relevant to evaluation in health-sector reform in this book, reformers should keep in mind a few key lessons about the role of data in evidence-based evaluation. First, data collection is not free, and better data typically cost more to collect. A good scheme for evaluation must balance cost against usefulness. Second, the cost of data collection typically falls on the people doing the reporting. If the costs to them of providing good data are too high, they will provide poor data. For example, a study of maternity ward data in a district in northern Ghana found multiple problems with data quality, so that much of the information collected was of "questionable accuracy" (Allotey and Reidpath 2000). Midwives reported that recordkeeping was time consuming for them, the figures were not analyzed beyond the annual report, and the effort therefore seemed of little value. The authors concluded that exhorting the midwives to do a better job at data collection was unlikely to succeed, since the information had neither negative nor positive consequences for the nurses involved. In short, the nurses had no reason to take the time and effort to obtain better information.

Third, it is possible to collect too much data. Over-collection can produce "data cemeteries," in which piles of "dead" data accumulate, too massive for anyone to analyze. A key question for any manager to ask of a proposed data collection effort is, "How will I use these data once I have them?" Data that are not linked to actual decisions are likely to be buried in an early grave by those too busy to look at them.

One strategy for getting reliable information is to use data that organizations collect for their own purposes. Such data are more likely to be collected and recorded accurately since managers need them to run the organization. In some countries, payroll data, personnel records, or hospital discharge records may be relatively accurate. When such records exist, reports to government agencies are potentially verifiable against the underlying sources, and this process can increase reporting accuracy.

In sum, evaluation has to be an early concern for health reformers. It cannot wait until after a new program has been implemented. Baseline data have to be collected before implementation, and administrative systems have to be designed with evaluation in mind. Unintended consequences are frequent in health-sector reform. To make a difference, health reformers must take evaluation seriously, so that such consequences can be detected and addressed. Ironically, reformers will know that evaluation has been done well when the data collected reveal new problems that start the policy cycle all over again.

Summary

This chapter has provided an introduction to the policy cycle for health-sector reform. In subsequent chapters, we will explore selected aspects of the cycle in greater detail with attention to five main themes.

Step #1: Problem Definition

Health systems are social responses to social problems. Problem definition and health-reform priorities are always based on value choices. We believe these choices should be explicitly stated and examined. Our approach to these choices includes a guide to *ethical theory*, which we address in Chapter 3.

For sound policy development, problems should be defined in terms of *health-system performance goals*. Although health reformers often hold multiple objectives, we believe that a short list of health-system goals—those that in our experience are the most relevant to health reform—can be identified. We present these in Chapter 5, and link them to the ideas of ethical theory presented in Chapter 3.

Step #2: Diagnosis

In order to identify potential solutions to improve performance, the assessment of health system performance requires a diagnosis of the causes of poor performance. We have designed a method of diagnosis that is systematic, can be taught, and can be practiced. We elaborate this approach to health system diagnosis in Chapter 7.

Step #3: Policy Development

Health systems are complex, with many steps that link broad policy strategies with final outcomes. We propose a conceptual framework of five control knobs that include the causal factors that meet two essential criteria: they are significant determinants of health-system performance, and they can be manipulated through policy reform and effective implementation. In Chapters 8 through 12, we provide detailed discussion of these mechanisms and processes. For each control knob, we provide practical guidance on the design and implementation of interventions and on the expected impact of different reform strategies.

Step #4: Political Decision

In health reform, politics matters throughout the policy cycle, and we have integrated our concern with politics in each chapter of this book. As it is presented in Chapter 4, systematic *political analysis* and the use of that analysis to develop *political strategies* are essential for effective reform. The emphasis on political analysis in this book reflects our view that it should be done early and often throughout the policy cycle.

These five elements—the importance of ethical theory, explicitly identified health system performance objectives, a systematic approach to health-system diagnosis, use of the health system control knobs, and political analysis—are the core of what is new and useful in this book. These points are developed in detail in subsequent chapters, where we provide the substance of our approach for getting health reform right.

References

Allotey, A. Pascale; and Daniel Reidpath. 2000. "Information Quality in a Remote Rural Maternity Unit in Ghana." *Health Policy and Planning* 15(2): 170–76.

Banfield, Edward C.; and James Q. Wilson. 1972. "Power Structure and Civic Leadership."
    In: Fred M. Cox, John L. Erlich, Jack Rothman, and John Tropman, eds., *Strategies of
    Community Organization*. Itasca, IL: Peacock, 112–22.
Barzelay, Michael; with the collaboration of Babak J. Armajani. 1992. *Breaking Through
    Bureaucracy: A New Vision for Managing in Government*. Berkeley, CA: University
    of California Press.
Behn, Robert D. 2001. *Rethinking Democratic Accountability*. Washington, DC: Brook-
    ings Institution Press.
Bell, David E.; and Michael R. Reich, eds. 1988. *Health, Nutrition, and Economic Crises:
    Approaches to Policy in the Third World*. Dover, MA: Auburn House.
BRAC. 2000. *Annual Report 2000*. Dhaka, Bangladesh: BRAC. Available from www.brac.
    net. Accessed June 2002.
Caldwell, John C.; P. H. Reddy; and Pat Caldwell. 1983. "The Social Component of
    Mortality Decline: An Investigation in South India Employing Alternative Method-
    ologies." *Population Studies* 37(2): 185–205.
Dai, D. 1993. "A Review of the Health Care Reform." *Chinese Journal of Health Econom-
    ics* 4: 28–30.
Deming, W. Edwards. 1982. *Quality, Productivity, and Competitive Position*. Cambridge,
    MA: MIT Press.
Enthoven, Alain C. 1988. *Theory and Practice of Managed Competition in Health Care
    Finance*. Amsterdam: Elsevier.
Evetovits, Tamás. 2002. Health Services Management Training Center, Semmelweis Uni-
    versity, personal communication.
Gao, F. W. 1996. "The Simple Methods of Prediction for Pharmaceutical Market." *Chinese
    Pharmaceutical Information* 2(1): 15–21.
Goode, William J. 1969. "The Theoretical Limits of Professionalization." In: Amitai Etzioni,
    ed., *The Semi-Professions and Their Organization*. New York: The Free Press, 266–313.
Hsiao, William C. 1999. *Primer on Health Care Policy for Macroeconomists*. Preliminary
    draft. Washington, DC: International Monetary Fund.
Ishikawa, Kaoru. 1988. *What Is Total Quality Control? The Japanese Way*. Translated by
    David J. Lu. Englewood Cliffs, NJ: Prentice Hall.
Juran, Joseph M.; and Frank M. Gryna, Jr. 1980. *Quality Planning and Analysis*. New
    York: McGraw-Hill.
Kuhn, Thomas S. 1962. *The Structure of Scientific Revolutions*. Chicago: University of
    Chicago Press.
Liu, Yuanli; Shanlian Hu; Wei Fu; and Wiliam C. Hsiao. 1996. "Is Community Financing
    Necessary and Feasible for Rural China?" *Health Policy* 38(3): 155–71.
Osborne, David; and Ted Gaebler. 1993. *Reinventing Government: How the Entrepreneur-
    ial Spirit Is Transforming the Public Sector*. New York: Plume.
PAHO. 2001. *Health Systems Performance Assessment and Improvement in the Region of
    the Americas*. Washington, DC: Pan American Health Organization.
Pressman, Jeffrey L.; and Aaron Wildavsky. 1973. *Implementation: How Great Expecta-
    tions in Washington Are Dashed in Oakland*. Berkeley, CA: University of California
    Press.
Putnam, Robert D. 1993. "Social Capital and Institutional Success." In: Robert D. Putnam,
    with Robert Leonardi and Rafaella Y. Nanetti, *Making Democracy Work: Civic Tradi-
    tions in Modern Italy*. Princeton, NJ: Princeton University Press.
Rossi, Peter; Howard Freeman; and Mark Lipsey. 1998. *Evaluation: A Systematic Approach*.
    6th edition. Thousand Oaks, CA: Sage.

Skocpol, Theda. 1996. *Boomerang: Clinton's Health Security Effort and the Turn Against Government in U.S. Politics*. New York: W.W. Norton.

Smith, Peter G.; and Richard H. Morrow, eds. 1996. *Field Trials of Health Interventions in Developing Countries*. London: MacMillan.

Tarimo, Eleuther; and E. G. Webster. 1997. *Primary Health Care: Concepts and Challenges in a Changing World—Alma-Ata Revisited*. Geneva: World Health Organization.

UNDP. 2000. *Human Development Report 2000*. New York: Oxford University Press.

Weil, Diana E.C.; Adelaida Alicbusan; John F. Wilson; Michael R. Reich; and David J. Bradley. 1990. *The Impact of Development Policies on Health: A Review of the Literature*. Geneva: World Health Organization.

WHO. 1978. *Primary Health Care—Report of the International Conference on Primary Health Care, Alma-Ata*. Health for All series, No. 1. Geneva: World Health Organization.

———. 1986. *Intersectoral Action for Health: The Role of Intersectoral Cooperation in National Strategies for Health for All*. Geneva: World Health Organization.

———. 2000. *World Health Report 2000, Health Systems: Improving Performance*. Geneva: World Health Organization.

World Bank. 1997. *Financing Health Care: Issues and Options for China*. Washington, DC: World Bank.

Yip, Winnie; and William C. Hsiao. 2001. "Economic Transition and Urban Health Care in China: Impacts and Prospects." Prepared for the Conference on Financial Sector Reform in China, Cambridge, MA, September 11–13, 2001, sponsored by the Center for Business and Government, John F. Kennedy School of Government.

3

Judging Health-Sector Performance: Ethical Theory

Arguments about what society *ought* to do always involve ethics. This is so even when someone asserts that the claim they are making is purely technical and does not involve values. Economists, for example, often argue that they are not concerned with ethics, only with economic efficiency. Public-health experts often take similar positions, asserting that they do not deal with ethics, they only protect the public's health. But how do we know that efficiency or health is the goal that society should try to achieve? Suppose that efficiency conflicts with fairness, or that efforts to improve health lead to restrictions on individual liberty? Why value health or efficiency over these other objectives?

This book is based on our deep conviction that judging health-sector performance requires ethical analysis. In this chapter, we introduce three major ethical perspectives as a basis for making such judgments: *utilitarianism, liberalism,* and *communitarianism.* Our purpose throughout is not to explore moral philosophy for its own sake, but rather to use it as a tool for making decisions about health-sector reform. Understanding the larger ethical perspectives that lie behind debates on health reform can help policy analysts and policymakers do their jobs more effectively. They can better explain and defend their own positions, and can better understand and respond to the positions of others.

The first doctrine we discuss, *utilitarianism*, says that we should judge a policy by its consequences. Utilitarianism evaluates consequences by examining the effects of a decision on the sum total of individual well-being in a society. This perspective motivates many health reform efforts around the world.

The second doctrine, *liberalism*, focuses on rights and opportunities, on where people start, not on where they end up. This view also has an important role in health-sector reform debates. The frequent claim that citizens have rights to health care—or even to health itself—reflects liberal concerns.

The third perspective, *communitarianism*, states that what matters is the kind of society that public policy helps create and the kind of individuals who live in it. In this view, communities have an obligation to raise their members to share the community's notions of virtue and good behavior. Communitarianism can conflict with both consequence-based and rights-based thinking, since inculcating virtue can involve actions that do not maximize well-being or that constrain individual liberty.

In this chapter, we discuss these three ethical theories and explore their implications for health-sector reform. We also explore some of the variations in points of view within each of these broad approaches. In Chapters 5 and 6, we will describe how these theories relate to various criteria used to judge health reform and discuss how ethical analysis can help a reformer think about setting priorities in the reform process.

Ethical Theory #1: Utilitarianism

The most widespread approach to the problem of making ethical judgments about the performance of the health sector is based on consequences. This approach generally assumes that "the end justifies the means." It says we should judge a policy by asking how it affects the individuals in a society and pick the option that most improves the sum total of their well-being. To be helpful in making decisions about health reform, several more-specific questions need to be answered. Whose well-being counts, and for how much? Also, how can well-being be measured in a practical way for the purpose of health reform? There are two major intellectual traditions about how to answer these questions: subjective utilitarianism and objective utilitarianism. Both approaches seek to use resources efficiently to produce the most "good"—but there are important differences in their methods and implications.

Subjective Utilitarianism

The first position derives from the work of the English philosopher Jeremy Bentham (1748–1832), who believed that individuals could best judge for themselves what makes them happy. He argued that people experience different levels of "utility" in various situations, depending on their particular tastes and prefer-ences. By "utility" he meant the internal feelings of happiness people had, and his doctrine came to be known as *utilitarianism*. He proposed that the rightness of an action is determined by the "hedonic calculus" of adding up the pleasure and pain it produces. The right action is the one that produces "the greatest happiness of the greatest number" (Bentham 1789). According to this philosophy the way to evaluate the performance of the health-care system is to determine how happy it makes everyone, and add those measurements up to reveal the utility that the sys-tem produces.

Bentham argued that all tastes are equally valid. This viewpoint decentralizes evaluation, since all individuals judge their own happiness for themselves. We call Bentham's position *subjective utilitarianism*. In certain ways, this is a very non-hierarchical concept. It posits that all individuals matter and matter equally. Judging a policy requires us to add up everyone's utility level for each policy op-tion and then choose the policy that leads to the most happiness or utility.

Economists take this analytical framework one step further. They advocate the use of *cost–benefit analysis* to determine which action produces the greatest total utility. This involves finding out how much all potential beneficiaries of a policy or program would be *willing to pay* for its benefits. If the estimated benefits are greater than the costs, then the policy would advance the greatest good for the greatest number and should be adopted. This analysis thus evaluates both costs and benefits in monetary terms (Mishan 1988, Culyer and Newhouse 2000).

Economists compare benefits with costs because the costs of a program actu-ally represent the benefits we give up elsewhere in the economy in order to implement the program. These foregone benefits are called *opportunity costs*. Economists argue that in a competitive economy, the price for an input—like labor or equipment—will be set by the value of the outputs that the input can produce. A worker can earn $10 an hour, if the worker, by working an additional hour, can produce goods that can be sold for $10. If a program costs $100,000, then its inputs could have produced goods worth $100,000 elsewhere in the econ-omy. Thus, cost–benefit analysis is really benefit–benefit analysis. Subjective util-itarians tell us to choose those activities where the benefits we gain are greater than the benefits we give up.

Evaluating proposed health reforms by using formal cost–benefit analysis is not easy. One reason is the difficulty in determining what people would be willing to pay for services. Often, we cannot use what they do pay as a guideline, since they may not pay anything (e.g., for free services in a public clinic). If we use sur-veys to assess willingness to pay, will people answer questionnaires honestly? Do they even know what they would pay for a hypothetical benefit?

Nevertheless, subjective utilitarianism has been very influential in debates about health reform. Policymakers are often urged (especially by economists) to use markets to allocate health care. The basic idea behind subjective utilitarians' enthusiasm for markets is that when markets work well, consumers only buy those goods and services for which their willingness to pay exceeds the costs of production. Such recommendations are based on economic models in which consumers have complete knowledge and markets are perfectly competitive. This kind of market system has desirable properties from a subjective utilitarian perspective. In particular, it leads to a situation in which there are no unexploited gains left in the economy, so that the only way to increase one person's utility is to decrease someone else's. Such a set of markets is then considered efficient in its allocation of resources (Graaf 1967). This situation is called "Pareto Optimal" in honor of the Italian economist who first defined the concept.

Unfortunately, most real health-care markets are far from satisfying the preconditions for perfect competition and hence far from Pareto Optimal (Arrow 1963). First, patients typically rely on doctors to tell them what care they should receive. This makes it possible for doctors, as the patients' "agents," to influence care decisions in ways that suit the doctors' interests. For example, doctors paid by fee-for-service have every reason to encourage unnecessary or inappropriate care (which is called "supplier-induced demand"; Folland et al. 2001, Feldstein 1993). Buyers also have great difficulty in judging the clinical quality of the services they receive. They cannot tell if the chemical composition of the drugs they buy is as advertised or if the surgeon has performed the operation skillfully. Add in strong elements of monopoly power and we can see that health-care markets are often characterized by what economists call "market failure." For these reasons, as we discuss in Chapter 11, health-care markets are often heavily regulated to counteract these deficiencies.

The enthusiasm for markets in health care also ignores important equity issues. In a market, each person's consumption is based on the individual's income. Even if the situation is "Pareto Optimal", the poor will typically get less, often very much less than the rich. Indeed, the poorest of the poor often cannot even afford basic services. As a result, those concerned with maintaining equitable access (a concern we share) have to think carefully about how and where to use markets, and how to counteract their adverse effects when markets are employed. Nonetheless, market-based arguments have gained substantial political influence in recent years, providing an avenue for subjective utilitarian thinking to enter the health-reform debate.

Another way to highlight the equity issues raised by a subjective utilitarian viewpoint is to see that this approach can easily lead to the conclusion that we should not provide costly services to the poor, since they would be unable to pay for them. Such services would not pass the test of willingness-to-pay for benefits in excess of costs that subjective utilitarians would impose. A subjective utilitarian might argue in response that if we want to make the poor as well off as possible, we should give them money and let them spend it as they choose. If other things are more valuable to the poor than health care, that should be their choice.

This line of reasoning reflects the view of subjective utilitarians that health is not a special good, but is just one more commodity that citizens buy or not, as they choose. Since only each person really knows what will make them happy, their choices should be respected. The optimism of this view about individual choice seems unwarranted to many critics, however (Dworkin 1993). They are not prepared to base social policy entirely on individuals' wants and decisions. Instead, they are attracted to the objective utilitarian approach as an alternative.

Objective Utilitarianism

What if you believe that health reform ought to be judged by its consequences, but doubt that individuals always make good choices about actions that affect their health? For example, should governments act to promote markets that provide cigarette smokers with what they want? If patients want dangerous or ineffective medicines, or want to patronize unqualified doctors, should government allow people to make these choices?

Reformers who want to promote individual well-being, but are skeptical of the reliability and validity of individual choices, argue for basing decisions on individual well-being defined in objective terms by a group of experts. These experts develop an index that embodies the "rationally knowable" components of well-being, and that index is then used to evaluate everyone's circumstances. This position is known as *objective utilitarianism* (Griffin 1986).

Objective utilitarianism has a long history in public health. In the nineteenth century, Florence Nightingale showed that it was less costly for the British Army to care for the wounded than to let them die and then train new recruits (Nightingale 1858). There were various attempts to construct health-status indices both before and after World War II. Objective utilitarian approaches have also been widely employed in clinical research, where measures of "quality of life" have been developed to evaluate the results of alternative treatments (McDowell and Newell 1987). It is also the philosophical position behind the analysis of disease burdens through such measures as Disability-Adjusted Life Years (DALYs) or Quality-Adjusted Life Years (QALYs), as conducted by the World Bank (1993) and the WHO (2000). This approach tells us to pick policies with the "biggest bang for the buck," with "bang" measured in health gains. Notably, this approach does not translate health gains into monetary terms as occurs with cost–benefit analysis.

In the broader world of policy analysis, objective utilitarianism provides the basis for *cost-effectiveness analysis*. This approach has been widely used beyond the health sector, under various labels. During World War II, British mathematicians used such methods to calculate the best way to conduct military operations (e.g., searching for a flyer downed in the English Channel) giving rise to the term *operations research*. In the 1950s, similar techniques were applied at the Rand Corporation in the United States to evaluate the comparative efficiency of different weapons systems, in what came to be called *systems analysis* (Quade and Miser 1985).

Objective utilitarians centralize what Bentham sought to decentralize. Using a single index to measure well-being disregards individual variations in preferences. One individual may want to avoid physical disability or chronic pain, even if this means a shorter life span; another may seek the longest possible life, whatever suffering that life entails. Such variations have no place in an objective utilitarian calculation.

The practical measurement of health gains confronts many technical problems. One critical question is how to combine extensions in the length of life with improvements in the quality of life. The QALYs and DALYs methods use a similar (and controversial) solution. Health status is described on a scale from zero (for death) to one (for perfect health). Experts assign each disease or disability state a particular quality-of-life score somewhere on this scale. A year of life in good health counts as one unit of gain. A year while suffering some disability counts as a fraction of this, say seven-tenths of a unit. The value of life extension is then counted as the quality of life of the person saved, multiplied by the number of years provided. An improvement in quality is measured by the fractional gain in quality times the number of years it persists. Thus, adding five years of life to a person at 0.8 quality level is calculated to produce 4 QALYs, since $5 \times 0.8 = 4\,\text{QALYs}$. A major problem with this approach is that many people seem to value the saving of life more than the alleviation of disability, which raises fundamental questions about the method's assumptions and calculations.

One example of this approach was the Oregon Health Plan in the United States. In 1994, that state conducted a study to rank all medical treatments covered by the Medicaid program (an insurance plan for low-income individuals) in terms of QALYs produced per dollar spent, and then proposed to restrict coverage to only the most cost-effective interventions (Bodenheimer 1997). The plan was later drastically modified, because of public dissatisfaction with the results of the analysis, because it seemed to them to undervalue life-saving interventions (Hardon 1991).

A health-status index inevitably embodies value judgments about the relative desirability of different kinds of health gains. For example, how serious is mental disability compared to physical disability? Are years of life lost at different ages to be counted equally or unequally? The DALY index, for example, values years of life in middle age more highly than years lost by younger or older citizens (Murray 1994). This differential assessment reflects a particular productivity-oriented perspective that would be inconsistent with social values in a society where, for example, the old are viewed as a source of special wisdom. Users of this approach must contend, therefore, with the objection that not all societies or individuals value health outcomes the same way (Anand and Hanson 1997). In practice, advocates of this approach have convened panels of experts and used consensus-building methods to select a single set of weights for evaluating health gains and losses for specific ill-health conditions (Murray 1994).

Objective utilitarian health reformers also can proceed without using a comprehensive measure of health gain. For example, many health ministries use measures like the infant mortality rate (IMR) to identify high-priority target areas, or analyze policies in terms of the expected number of lives saved by a proposed policy intervention. These more limited indexes require less data and analysis than comprehensive scales like DALYs. Their disadvantage is that, because they are not comprehensive, they can give a distorted picture of the situation. For example, the development of a neonatal intensive care unit in a local hospital can have the effect of *increasing* the area's observed IMR, as sick newborns live long enough to be counted as neonatal deaths rather than as stillbirths. Thus, any partial index ought to be employed carefully.

A number of practical problems also arise in interpreting any health statistics. In some countries, for example, differences in the reported IMR reflect variations in local customs about when babies are considered truly "born" or differences in bureaucratic competence in collecting data from remote villages, rather than variations in actual mortality rates.

Another practical difficulty is the assessment of causation. To use consequence-based analysis, one must evaluate the results of past policies and predict the impact of future policies. Making reliable predictions is often complicated. Suppose a country is considering a shift from a "vertical" immunization program to a system in which immunization is integrated into the primary care system. For an objective utilitarian, the expected cost savings of this change need to be balanced against an estimate of the health consequences that might result from a decline in immunization coverage. Estimating the impacts on immunization coverage requires an assessment of how the new program will be implemented. How will the changes affect the follow-up of missing cases, the preservation of the cold chain to keep vaccines effective, and the tendency to use expired vaccines? And then, how will those changes combine over time to affect health status? These predictions are not easy to make, yet an objective utilitarian must undertake this kind of analysis for each proposed policy change.

Some Utilitarian Complications: Uncertainty and Time

Two technical problems with utilitarian analysis deserve brief additional consideration: uncertainty and time. The consequences of health reform are always uncertain to some extent, and some will not occur until quite a few years into the future (Weinstein and Stason 1977, Wenz 1986).

For subjective utilitarians, valuing uncertain gains is straightforward, at least in theory. Uncertain benefits and costs are evaluated by asking the affected persons how much the uncertainty changes the value of the gains or costs to them. Uncertainty is incorporated directly into each person's willingness to pay.

This approach, however, introduces a complex set of assumptions and implications. In particular, it requires us to assume that people know, not only whether they prefer outcome A to outcome B, but also *how much more* they value one over the other. Whether individuals have consistent and stable evaluations of such outcomes has been a subject of substantial debate and empirical research. These evaluations become especially important when the *gain* in impact depends on a change in probability, such as a change in the probability of death from a particular disease.

The problem of benefits that occur in the future raises similar issues. Here the debate focuses on what is called the *discount rate*. In financial markets, the relative value of returns this year versus returns next year is expressed by the interest rate. For example, a rate of 7% implies that next year, a borrower has to give a lender 1.07 times what was borrowed today. In such markets, dollars next year are worth *less* than dollars this year. This process is repeated for gains that occur farther in the future. The procedure for computing the decrease in value of future gains is called *discounting*, and the interest rate used in the calculations is called the *discount rate*. This rate allows analysts to compute the present value of future benefits, so that they can be compared to current costs in the same monetary terms (Parsonage and Neuburger 1992, Folland et al. 2001, Olsen 1993).

When evaluating health reform, should future health benefits be discounted, and if so, at what rate? Some analysts argue that, as a matter of social policy, future gains should be valued the same as current ones, since discounting effectively discriminates against the future. Others believe that if we don't use discounting, we then encounter what is called the "investment paradox," as the following example illustrates: Suppose we take $100,000 from current health spending and put it in the bank. Since science is always advancing, and we can earn interest on the investment over time, the $100,000 will produce more health gain in ten years than today. Thus, without discounting, we would defer far too much spending to the future.

The discount rate can have a major impact on the relative attractiveness of policies that produce short-run versus long-run gains. At a 7% discount rate, gains ten years from now are worth half of what they are today—and gains forty years from now are worth less than 6% of their current value. Lower discount rates give greater relative value to future benefits (long-run gains), and will be more favorable to projects that promise long-run gains over those that promise more short-run gains (Keeler and Cretin 1983).

There are two major arguments on how to set the discount rate. One school of thought argues for market-based interest rates. This school proposes using rates similar to those in a nation's financial markets or the rates of return earned by private-sector entrepreneurs. They argue that *market discount rates* reflect the actual opportunities open to investors—and hence, the opportunity cost of withdrawing resources from the private sector and spending them in the public sector (Marglin 1967).

Other analysts believe that private capital markets do not function well and that society should make an independent judgment about the value of gains that occur at different times. They argue for using a *social discount rate* based on this separate valuation (which represents more of an objective utilitarian position). Whether a market rate or social rate is used in analysis can have a major impact on priority setting, since some policies (e.g., hepatitis B vaccination) produce benefits quite far in the future. These policies look much less attractive (compared to, say, the immediate gains from flu vaccinations) when a high discount rate is used.

A final problem for health reformers who consider the utilitarian approach is the ruthlessness implicit in the position's commitment to producing the largest gain for the available resources—regardless of the fairness or equity of the result. Negative consequences for particular individuals or specific groups are acceptable, as long as the total results are beneficial in the aggregate. Utilitarian policymakers can disregard patients who are too expensive to save, and can sacrifice the few for the sake of the many. Following utilitarian logic, passengers who are starving on a lifeboat could kill and eat a few of their fellows, provided the gains exceed the losses. Many health reformers—including ourselves—find this lack of focus on equity a serious objection; an intuition that leads to a different approach for deciding priorities for health reform.

Ethical Theory #2: Liberalism

In the language of philosophy, utilitarians are willing to treat some individuals as means and others as ends—to sacrifice some for the sake of others. But to many reformers, this attitude does not take the interests of those being sacrificed seriously enough. Don't those individuals have rights and aren't they entitled to as much respect as those we wind up healing? If we are going to take such ideas seriously, how can we ground them philosophically, and what would they imply for health-sector reform?

The most influential philosopher associated with conceptions of individual respect and autonomy is the eighteenth-century German philosopher Immanuel Kant. According to Kant, all human beings have the capacity for *moral action* (Kant 1788), the power to know what is morally correct, and to decide whether to follow the dictates of morality. Modern Kantians argue that since human beings have the capacity to develop and implement their own decisions about how to live—what philosophers call "life plans"—they have the right to do so. Because these rights derive from each person's status as a human being, they are seen as universal, and all political systems are obliged to honor them (O'Neill 1989). This view, based on mutual respect, directly opposes utilitarianism's willingness to treat some people as a means. The philosophical descendents of Kant's approach, now called "liberals," have developed arguments about how states should operate and how policies should be determined (Rawls 1971).

The critical concept for liberals is *rights*—claims that all individuals can make on each other by virtue of their humanity. The rights implied by the principle of mutual respect are interpreted by liberals in two different ways. *Libertarians* believe that only *negative rights* deserve protection (Nozick 1974). These rights guarantee individual freedom, so that people can do what they want without state infringement on personal choice. Extended to the political realm, this formulation leads to fundamental political and civil rights, like freedom of speech, assembly, and political participation. Libertarians want the state to have only the limited role of protecting individual property rights and personal liberty. They typically oppose restrictions on drug use, limits on abortion, or even the licensing of physicians, since these actions restrict individual freedom of choice.

In contrast, *egalitarian liberals* argue that the right to choose is meaningless without adequate resources. They argue that genuinely respecting others as moral actors requires us to provide them with the preconditions that make meaningful choice possible. Therefore, everyone has a *positive right* to the minimum level of services and resources needed to assure fair equality of opportunity (Daniels 1985). Someone who is starving, homeless, uneducated, and ill does not have much opportunity for meaningful choice. The question is, what does the principle of mutual respect require that the state provide in order to ensure positive rights? In particular, is there is a right to health care or to health itself? This question has important implications for health-sector reformers.

Positive-rights arguments generally lead to a *redistributive* perspective that favors those people who are worst off from a lifetime perspective. That is, the health-care system should place priority on averting premature death and disability versus extending the life of the aged, who have already had the chance to develop and implement their life plans. John Rawls (1971) called this perspective "justice as fairness."

Egalitarian liberals disagree among themselves over exactly how positive rights should be addressed in the health-care system. Some assert that the best way to respect everyone's moral capacity is to distribute income fairly, and let individuals buy the health care (or health insurance) they want (Dworkin 1993). For these liberals, health is no different from other goods and services that people are free to purchase, like food and clothes. They believe there are no special rights to health or health care.

Other egalitarian liberals believe that society has a special obligation with regard to health (Daniels 1985). But here again there is division. Some think that the key is providing a minimum level of *health care* for all, while others think that the critical issue is individuals' actual *health status*. In other words, if citizens have health rights, should we judge whether those rights are satisfied by the availability of clinics or by citizens' average life expectancy? The latter view holds that if society is to provide everyone with a certain range of opportunities, access to care is not enough. This positive-rights perspective makes government responsible for a minimum quantity and quality of life for all, and to provide the health care needed to guarantee that minimum.

The disagreement over whether government should be responsible for a level of health status or for access to health care has important implications for the relationship between the state and the individual. Much ill health today depends on each individual's own behavior. Smoking, diet, substance abuse, exercise, and risk-taking of various kinds all have significant health consequences. To say that government is responsible for everyone's health means that society is responsible for influencing individual choices about such matters.

On the other hand, if society is only responsible for providing services, and not for whether people use them, then individuals have much greater responsibility for their own health. Health status then becomes a result of individual choice, not an inherent right. This perspective is consistent with Amartya Sen's argument that society should be responsible for creating opportunities (which he calls "capabilities") among which citizens can choose, not for the choices that individuals make (Sen 1999).

Asserting a right to health still leaves many questions unanswered. If individuals have a right to a minimum health status, what should the minimum level be? Are there limits to society's obligation to very ill people, who require high-cost services to improve their health status even a little? After all, society's resources are limited, and the money to provide for such care comes from other citizens, in ways that effectively diminish their opportunities. Moreover, what care should people receive if their ill health results from their own behavior? In practice, any society committed to egalitarian goals in the process of health-sector reform will have to find politically and economically viable answers to these questions. And those answers will depend, in part, on the nation's level of economic development.

Liberalism and Health-Care Financing

In deciding how much to spend on health (or health care), a critical issue for liberals is the legitimacy of taxation. For libertarians, the negative right to be left alone includes a right to enjoy one's own property. For them, therefore, taxation is theft. They might consent to limited taxes to provide minimal state services like defense and police, but taxation that seeks to redistribute resources is fundamentally not legitimate, because it treats one person (the taxpayer) as the means to another's end (the benefit recipient).

Egalitarian liberals, on the other hand, approve of redistributive taxation in part because they believe that much of the existing distribution of wealth in society has arisen in ways that do not deserve to be respected. Aristocrats acquired wealth through force and conquest. Fortunes were made through monopoly or fraud. Some individuals earn high incomes due to superior education or family contacts because they were lucky enough to be born into privileged social groups. Such gains are the result of the *social lottery*, since, according to egalitarian liberals, the people who enjoy such advantages did nothing to deserve them (Rawls 1971, Rawls 1999). The gains they produced can be legitimately taxed to help the poor. Property rights are not violated by taxing away these various illegitimate gains, because the gains themselves were not properly obtained.

Even differences in rewards due to differences in innate talent are not legitimate, since no one deserves their own biological advantages. The gains from such advantages are not the result of individual effort. Income differences due to this *natural lottery*, like those due to the social lottery, can be claimed by the state for redistributive purposes.

In the context of health reform, as we discuss in Chapters 5 and 8, egalitarian liberals argue that it is best to finance health-care services with redistributive taxes. Thus, comprehensive income taxes are better than payroll taxes, especially since the latter exclude investment income. To egalitarian liberals, income from investments is generally non-effort dependent and hence is an appropriate source of funds to finance redistribution.

Many egalitarian liberals—including the authors—view the U.S. health system as particularly objectionable on equity grounds compared to that of other industrialized countries. The United States finances most health care through private, premium-based insurance schemes in which costs are the same for all, regardless of income. As a result, consumption of health care in the United States, like the consumption of expensive consumer goods, such as sailboats, reflects an individual's ability to pay: rich people own large boats, middle-class people own modest boats, and poor people swim (or sink). The same is true when it comes to health care. Most of the uninsured in the United States belong to low-income families.

Any claim about the "unfairness" of the distribution of health or health care in a society is likely, at its root, to be based on egalitarian liberal ethics. For example, in most poor countries, in rural areas health spending is well below that in urban areas, and life expectancy is shorter. Should this problem be a focus for health reform? The answer will depend on the values of those responding to the question. Egalitarian liberals would probably make it a high priority to correct this inequality. They would advocate raising the bottom end of the distribution to ensure that everyone has some minimum level of opportunity. On the other hand, objective utilitarians whose goal is maximizing health status would want to know the cost-effectiveness of different interventions in rural versus urban areas, and would make a decision based on where the greatest impact could be achieved. (We return to attitudes toward equity, from different philosophical perspectives, in more detail in Chapter 5.)

Despite deep differences, there are some basic similarities between liberalism and utilitarianism. Both doctrines are universal; they seek to develop a single moral standard for all human societies. In addition, they focus on the individual— on *individual* well-being and *individual* rights. Both perspectives have therefore been criticized for ignoring the social nature of human life (Sandel 1982). Critics of liberalism argue that important community values are ignored by its individualistic vision. Utilitarianism is faulted for implying that you cannot favor your own family, friends, or fellow citizens over strangers, if helping strangers would yield more utility (Williams 1973). Similarly, utilitarian approaches to improve health status can conflict with a society's views about moral conduct. Consider, for example, the controversies in the United States over distributing clean needles to drug users or contraceptives to high school students (Moss 2000). These criticisms derive from ethical perspectives that are not based on well-being or rights, but focus instead on inculcating virtue and fostering community, which leads to the next category of arguments.

Ethical Theory #3: Communitarianism

The third major approach to ethical theory we want to review argues that what matters in judging public policy is the kind of society and kind of person that state action seeks to create. This perspective focuses on the nature of the community and is called *communitarianism*. This theory argues that the character of a community depends on the character of the individuals who compose it. The state, therefore, should ensure that individuals develop good character and help produce a good society.

Just as we examined two kinds of utilitarians (objective and subjective) and two kinds of liberals (libertarian and egalitarian), we distinguish between two kinds of communitarians. The first are *universal communitarians*, who believe there is a single universal model for the good individual and the good society. There are many examples of this, both secular and religious. The world's proselytizing, monotheistic religions (Islam and Christianity) are forms of universal communitarianism; so, too, is the position of ecological activists who want to transform man's relationship to nature; and that of some in the feminist movement, who want to create a society with a different relationship between men and women. The same can be said of revolutionary Maoists. As these examples show, the substantive moral positions contained under this heading are quite varied— much more so than the differences within either the utilitarian or liberal camps.

A communitarian viewpoint of particular relevance to health-sector reformers in East Asia is the doctrine known as Confucianism. This perspective, articulated through the writings of Confucius (551–479 B.C.) and his followers, prescribes how people should behave, both as individuals and as collectivities, through the "five relationships." Human interaction begins in the family and extends out to the state, providing a distinct Confucian continuity between these two realms of collectivity. The core literature of Confucianism, known collectively as the Four Books, provides a universal view of humanity, based on internal reflection on one's duties and rights, and on understanding one's human interactions within specific collectivities (Bloom 1996).

The Confucian arguments about duty and responsibility and about fulfilling social roles resemble the arguments offered in the Greek philosopher Plato's famous work, *The Republic*, but with important differences. Plato viewed the family as a particularistic distraction from the social obligations of citizenship. Confucius, on the other hand, considered the family as the basic model of human interaction, for ruler and subject and for public and private matters (Bloom 1996, 134). Confucian ethics continue to influence individual and social values in many countries. For example, the willingness of the government of Singapore to use the power of the state to preserve order and instill individual virtue expresses just this perspective (Bell 1997, Wong 1996, Kuah 1990).

The second kind of communitarianism historically was heavily influenced by anthropology and the work of early twentieth-century pioneers in that field, like Boas and Mead (Boas 1932, Mead 1964). This perspective recognizes the wide variety of cultural practices in the world and the extent to which individuals are embedded in those cultures. This form of *relativist communitarianism* emphasizes that each community does and should decide its own norms and mode of social organization. These communitarians see morality as inherently contextual, lacking a universal place outside of society to judge particular cultural traditions.

Certain practices, like female genital cutting, pose the question of the acceptability of local community norms in an acute manner (Obermeyer 1999) . Some relativist communitarians support this practice, arguing that it should be respected by outsiders, because it has deep meaning for people who belong to the culture, and constitutes an integral part of their life. Objective utilitarians oppose this practice on the grounds that it injures the health of women. Liberals consider the practice objectionable, because it is imposed on girls early in their lives without their consent and limits their long-term life opportunities.

Those who believe that each community defines its own norms must decide on the boundaries of the community, and on the representatives for the community. Many ethnic and religious minorities have asserted the right to depart from the norms of the larger community and the right to create their own communities. How should such disagreements be decided? Can Catholic majorities in Latin American countries legitimately impose their views about divorce and abortion on all citizens, based on their interpretation of community values? What rights do religious minorities have in Israel, India, or Iran, if their practices offend the majority? Suppose people of the same sex want to marry or adopt children in a country where the majority considers it immoral? Until twenty years ago, women in Switzerland could not vote, and the Swiss defended this limitation as their traditional practice. Who decides whether a community is legitimate and how much coercion a community can use in promoting its values and assuring compliance? These are critical questions if relativist communitarianism is to guide decisions about health-sector reform.

Communitarian arguments arise in health reform in many ways. For some in public health, living a healthy lifestyle is a matter of virtue, not just a way to improve health status. For example, some public health advocates view tobacco or intra-venous drug use as ethically objectionable forms of self-destructive behavior, not just as unhealthy. Advocates of these views are not persuaded by the fact that some indi-viduals prefer the pleasures of tobacco or reject the joys of exercising—despite the health consequences. These choices would be acceptable to a subjective utilitarian (the smoker is seeking happiness) or to a liberal (the smoker has rights), but are opposed by public health communitarians (as not following the right kind of life).

Communitarians may also have strong views about particular health-care ser-vices. In many countries, religious conservatives oppose the availability of abor-tion or family planning services on communitarian grounds. In some countries (e.g., Japan), the practice of defining death by the end of heart action limits the number of organs available for transplant (Kimura 1998). Should public health professionals, arguing on objective utilitarian grounds, seek to change such com-munity norms? Some countries (e.g., Austria) presume that those who die are or-gan donors unless the family actively opposes it, a practice that has obvious health-status gains but also poses some problems for liberals (Kennedy et al. 1998, Veatch and Pitt 1995). Should other countries follow suit, even if doing so runs counter to local tradition? Questions around traditional medical practices raise similar issues. If a sincere believer visits a religious healer who seeks to ex-pel evil spirits to treat a medical problem, should the healer be required to follow a nation's legal guidelines for medical practitioners? In offering these examples, we seek to illustrate how using community norms to define the agenda for health reform often raises conflicts with other values. Because these issues are so impor-tant, we believe they deserve special attention in the process of setting priorities for health-sector reform, and we discuss them again in Chapter 5.

This chapter has emphasized the normative dimensions of health reform, asking how a society *should* decide what to accomplish in health reform. Ethical analysis can help reformers with this process, by highlighting what is assumed and im-plied in various communitarian positions, and their relationship to consequence-based and rights-based perspectives.

The Problem of Justification

Confronted with these three basic ethical positions, a reformer might well ask which one is correct. What arguments are available to select one ethical view over another? Such questions about justification fall into the realm of meta-ethics, or questions about the nature of ethics itself.

Various approaches exist when it comes to the problem of justifying an ethical po-sition. Religious faith is one such approach. Another is the view that human beings have a special faculty for perceiving morality, so that moral truth is revealed to us by our emotions or intuition. A third view holds that logic or reason can dictate the con-tent of morality (Harman 1977). The most widely accepted modern argument is moral realism (Putnam 1990). This is the position that the content of morality can be learned from our experience, when that is properly understood and processed. Moral realists believe that moral truth exists and can be discovered, and that moral facts can be learned by understanding human nature, analyzing human needs, and assessing the requirements of social life.

Other contemporary thinkers, in the *postmodern* school, argue that ethics is not justifiable in any foundational way (Lyotard 1984). Instead, postmodernists argue, ethics is created, like art or poetry. Criteria for judging moral arguments are based on rules internal to the enterprise, like the stylistic norms that govern an artistic tradition. But those rules cannot be derived from more fundamental principles. They do not and cannot have a deeper justification. The words that human beings use to describe concepts like "justice," "well-being," or "tradition" are just that—words—symbols to express ideas invented by people, just as Gothic architecture and country music were invented by people (Johnson 1993).

A postmodern health reformer must still grapple with the problems of making moral decisions. If there is no fundamental justification, then are all moral views and all courses of action equally compelling? Richard Rorty (1989), a prominent American postmodernist, argues that moral judgments are possible, even though they cannot be justified in a foundational manner. We have no choice, he says, but to act on our own view of the good, and to seek to persuade others to accept our perspective. For example, Rorty still seeks to promote the movement for human rights, even though he cannot prove that this moral position is correct by reference to a higher law or basic principle. Instead, Rorty (1993) urges a modern version of the doctrine of pragmatism, argued by John Dewey (1929). Rorty proposes the acceptance of moral views that work to make the world a better place, as best we know how. Rorty's personal choice is a form of egalitarian liberalism, and he seeks broader acceptance of this moral perspective via poetic or prophetic means, since he recognizes that rational argument alone will not suffice.

Developing an Ethical Position

We have presented these ethical theories as if they were mutually exclusive—as many philosophers have done before us. But such a purist approach is not consistent with how many health reformers see their tasks and do their work. To assist the process of health reform, we believe that the various theories are better viewed as embodying complementary rather than competitive insights. Taking this possibility seriously helps explain why many individuals find it more appealing to take a mixed position, drawing on more than one of the ethical perspectives we have presented above.

How can a serious reformer develop an ethical position that is appropriate for public policy yet compatible with their personal values? One approach is to work both forward and backward—that is, one can start with an appealing theory and explore its implications for practice. One can also do the reverse: begin with intuitions about desirable practice and work back to the theoretical stance that would support the policy position. When theoretical presumptions and policy intuitions conflict, as they often do, the task then is to adjust either or both. In this way, both specific intuitions and more general theoretical ideas can be successfully modified in pursuit of the internal consistency that philosophers call *reflective equilibrium* (Rawls 1971).

This iterative process can reveal the limits of a particular theoretical position. For example, an individual committed to an objective utilitarian view of health maximization may find that she would constrain the level of coercion employed to reach that goal. Perhaps those constraints are rooted in the intuitive appeal to her of liberal ideas of mutual respect. After some self reflection, and the consideration of various cases, she might reach a mixed position that could be called "rights-constrained utilitarianism."

Our attitude toward mixed ethical positions is based on our view of ethical theory more generally. We are acutely aware of the simplified terms in which ethical issues are normally discussed in public policy debates. The words used in most health-sector reform debates—words like "rights" or "well-being" or "community" or "health" itself—map imperfectly to the complex texture of actual problems. Like pictures of the same landscape painted by painters with sharply different styles, different ethical theories capture distinct perspectives on any one scene, calling our attention to different features and patterns. Each rendition can contribute to a fuller appreciation of the overall terrain, depending in part on the viewer's willingness to assimilate each perspective.

We do believe, however, that health reformers should seek consistency and coherence in their own ethical views. That is, we should strive to do more than just pick and choose from various theories as whim moves us, in what could be styled "buffet ethics." If that is all we do, then ethical theory becomes window dressing, a fancy rationale for a previously chosen position, without any analytical force.

Coherence and explicitness are important for several reasons. First, they make one's views more explainable, which is critical for public debate about health-reform proposals. Coherence and explicitness create the potential for agreement and disagreement, allowing others to understand what is at stake and to modify or defend their ethical positions more effectively than an ad hoc maze of disconnected arguments would allow. And explicitness contributes to transparency and accountability. It is far more difficult for reformers to be held accountable for the values behind their policy recommendations if they cannot articulate those values clearly (Roberts and Reich 2002, Gutmann and Thompson 1996).

Advocates of a mixed ethical view, therefore, should be prepared to provide a coherent rationale for their particular choices. Take our earlier example of someone who believes that the pursuit of utility is to be limited by certain rights. This person should be able to offer reasons why the boundary between these two principles is drawn where it is, and explain to others why they should accept this particular mix of utilitarian goals and rights concerns.

It is also important to recognize that the development of an ethical stance for health reform is an ongoing process and not a once-and-for-all activity. The complexity of health-system problems and the limits of ethical-analysis categories help ensure that the process will continue. As reformers move around the cycle of health-sector reform, as presented in Chapter 2, they should seek to learn and grow ethically as well as scientifically and politically.

Summary and Discussion

Each ethical theory we have considered in this chapter has its characteristic questions, which reflect unresolved issues:

- For utilitarians, how should well-being be measured?
- For liberals, which rights do people have?
- For communitarians, what are the boundaries and values of the good community?

Each ethical theory provides important insights that can guide the decisions that must be taken in health reform. Utilitarians focus on consequences—where people end up; liberals focus on rights and opportunities—where people start; and communitarians focus on the kinds of individuals and communities that we seek to create.

The four authors of this book take an ethical point of view that has certain egalitarian commitments at its core. We believe that nations should make it a priority to improve the opportunities available to the least-well-off among their citizens. This implies making a concerted effort to improving the health, economic, and social status of those individuals. This commitment requires governments to ensure both financial risk protection and effective access to basic health-care services for the most disadvantaged groups of their population. We also believe, however, that achieving such goals has to be done in ways that take into account cost-effectiveness and efficiency concerns. With limited resources, no nation, especially a poor nation, can afford to ignore the imperative of reaching its objectives at the lowest possible cost.

We do not believe, however, that all reformers need to share our point of view. On the contrary, we have reviewed a variety of ethical theories exactly because we recognize a degree of pluralism in moral visions. Not everyone will view these issues in the same way. In practice, local culture and politics will assure variation. And it is the responsibility of reformers in each society to take such variations into account as they formulate their national policies.

Indeed, everyone involved in health reform must decide for themselves what their personal values are and how far they are willing to go to advance those values. This process raises difficult questions when political institutions and power structures produce answers that conflict with personal values. If the parliament, or the prime minister, or the minister of health is promoting a policy you disagree with, how far can you legitimately go to discuss, protest, or undermine such decisions? The answer may depend on the quality of the process that produced the decision. The more accountable, open, and democratic the process, the more worthy the answer is of respect, even from dissenters (Applbaum 2000).

The answer may also depend on how important the issue seems to the reformer. Disagreements that involve fundamental principles may seem worth taking farther than those that turn on narrow technical issues. Still, reformers cannot avoid the responsibility that comes with their expertise and their authority. Political leaders often do not know what they want. Legislatures can produce ambiguous or contradictory policies. The political process is a human institution—one that must be understood and managed if health-sector reform is to be undertaken successfully.

Given the centrality of politics to health-reform efforts, we now turn to understanding those processes and how they can be influenced. In subsequent chapters, we return to the problems of setting reform priorities in a context where both ethics and politics play critical roles.

References

Anand, Sudhir; and Kara Hanson. 1997. "Disability-Adjusted Life Years: A Critical Review." *Journal of Health Economics* 16: 685–702.

Applbaum, Arthur I. 2000. *Ethics for Adversaries: The Morality of Roles in Public and Professional Life*. Princeton, NJ: Princeton University Press.

Arrow, Kenneth J. 1963. "Uncertainty and the Welfare Economics of Medical Care." *American Economic Review* 53: 941–73.

Bell, Daniel A. 1997. "A Communitarian Critique of Authoritarianism: The Case of Singapore." *Political Theory* 25(1): 6–32.

Bentham, Jeremy. 1789. *An Introduction to the Principles of Morals and Legislation*. Edited by J. H. Burns and H. L. A. Hart. New York: Oxford University Press, 1996.

Bloom, Irene. 1996. "Confucian Perspectives on the Individual and the Collectivity." In: Irene Bloom, J. Paul Martin, and Wayne L. Proudfoot, eds., *Religious Diversity and Human Rights*. New York: Columbia University Press, 114–51.

Boas, Franz. 1932. *Anthropology and Modern Life*. New York: W. W. Norton.

Bodenheimer, Thomas. 1997. "The Oregon Health Plan—Lessons for the Nation." *New England Journal of Medicine* 337: 651–5, 720–3.

Culyer, Anthony J.; and Joseph P. Newhouse. eds. 2000. *Handbook of Health Economics*. New York: Elsevier.

Daniels, Norman. 1985. *Just Health Care*. New York: Cambridge University Press.

Dewey, John. 1929. *The Quest for Certainty: A Study of the Relation of Knowledge and Action*. New York: Putnam.

Dworkin, Ronald. 1993. "Justice in the Distribution of Health Care." *McGill Law Journal* 38: 883–98.

Feldstein, Paul J. 1993. *Health Care Economics*. Albany, N.Y.: Delmar Publishers.

Folland, Sherman; Allen C. Goodman; and Miron Stano. 2001. *The Economics of Health and Health Care*. Upper Saddle River, NJ: Prentice Hall.

Graaff, J. de V. 1967. *Theoretical Welfare Economics*. New York: Cambridge University Press.

Griffin, James. 1986. *Well Being: Its Meaning, Measurement and Moral Importance*. New York: Oxford University Press.

Gutmann, Amy; and Dennis Thompson. 1996. *Democracy and Disagreement*. Cambridge, MA: Harvard University Press.

Hardon, D. C. 1991. "Setting Health Care Priorities in Oregon: Cost-effectiveness Meets the Rule of Rescue." *Journal of the American Medical Association* 265: 2218–25.

Harman, Gilbert. 1977. *The Nature of Morality: An Introduction to Ethics*. New York: Oxford University Press.

Johnson, Mark. 1993. *Moral Imagination: Implications of Cognitive Science for Ethics*. Chicago: University of Chicago Press.

Kant, Immanuel. 1788. *Critique of Practical Reason*, English trans. by L.W. Beck. New York: Liberal Arts Press, 1956.

Keeler, Emmett B.; and Shan Cretin. 1983. "Discounting of Life-saving and Other Non-monetary Effects." *Management Science* 29: 300–6.

Kennedy, I.; R. A. Sells; A. S. Daar; et al. 1998. "The Case for 'Presumed Consent' in Organ Donation." *The Lancet* 351: 1650–2.

Kimura, Rihito. 1998. "Organ Transplantation and Brain-Death in Japan: Cultural, Legal and Bioethical Background." *Annals of Transplantation* 3(3): 55–8.

Kuah, Khun E. 1990. "Confucian Ideology and Social Engineering in Singapore." *Journal of Contemporary Asia* 20(3): 371–83.

Lyotard, Jean Francois. 1984. *The Postmodern Condition: A Report on Knowledge*. Trans. by Geoff Bennington and Brian Massumi. Minneapolis, MN: University of Minneapolis Press.

Marglin, Stephen A. 1967. *Public Investment Criteria: Benefit-Cost Analysis for Planned Economic Growth*. Cambridge, MA: MIT Press.

McDowell, Ian; and Newell Claire. 1987. *Measuring Health: A Guide to Rating Scales and Questionnaires*. New York: Oxford University Press.

Mead, Margaret. 1964. *Continuities in Cultural Evolution*. New Haven, CT: Yale University Press.

Mishan, Edward J. 1988. *Cost-Benefit Analysis*. London: George Allen and Unwin.

Moss, A. R. 2000. "Epidemiology and the Politics of Needle Exchange." *American Journal of Public Health* 90: 1385–7.

Murray, Christopher J. L. 1994. "Quantifying the Burden of Disease: The Technical Basis for Disability-Adjusted Life Years." *Bulletin of the World Health Organization* 72(3): 495–509.

Nightingale, Florence. 1858. *Notes on Matters Affecting the Health, Efficiency, and Hospital Administration of the British Army*. London: Harrison and Sons.

Nozick, Robert. 1974. *Anarchy, State and Utopia*. New York: Basic Books.

Obermeyer, Carla Makhlouf. 1999. "Female Genital Surgeries, the Known, the Unknown and the Unknowable." *Medieval Anthropology Quarterly* 13: 79–106.

Olsen, J. A. 1993. "On What Basis Should Health Be Discounted?" *Journal of Health Economics* 12: 39–53.

O'Neill, Onora. 1989. *Constructions of Reason: Explorations of Kant's Practical Philosophy*. New York: Cambridge University Press.

Parsonage, M.; and H. Neuburger. 1992. "Discounting and Health Benefits." *Health Economics* 1: 71–6.

Putnam, Hilary. 1990. *Realism with a Human Face*. Cambridge, MA: Harvard University Press.

Quade, Edward S.; and Hugh J. Miser, eds. 1985. *Handbook of Systems Analysis: Overview of Uses, Procedures, Applications, and Practice*. New York: North-Holland.

Rawls, John. 1971. *A Theory of Justice*. Cambridge, MA: Harvard University Press.

———(Samuel Freeman, ed.). 1999. *Collected Papers: John Rawls*. Cambridge, MA: Harvard University Press. See in particular "Distributional Justice" and "Distributional Justice: Some Addenda."

Roberts, Marc J.; and Michael R. Reich. 2002. "Ethical Analysis in Public Health." *The Lancet* 359: 1055–9.

Rorty, Richard. 1989. *Contingency, Irony, and Social Solidarity*. New York: Cambridge University Press.

Sandel, Michael J. 1982. *Liberalism and the Limits of Justice*. New York: Cambridge University Press.

Sen, Amartya. 1999. *Development as Freedom*. New York: Knopf.

Veatch R. M.; and J. B. Pitt. 1995. "The Myth of Presumed Consent: Ethical Problems in New Organ Procurement Strategies." *Transplant Proceedings* 27: 1888–91.

Weinstein, Milton C.; and William B. Stason. 1977. "Foundations of Cost-Effectiveness Analysis for Health and Medical Practices." *New England Journal of Medicine* 296: 716–21.

Wenz, Peter S. 1986. "CBA, Utilitarianism and Reliance Upon Intuitions." In: George J. Agich and Charles C. Beyley, eds., *The Price of Health*. Boston, MA: D. Reichel Publishing Co.

Williams, Bernard. 1973. "A Critique of Utilitarianism." In: J. J. C. Smart and Bernard Williams, eds., *Utilitarianism For and Against*. New York: Cambridge University Press.

Wong, J. 1996. "Promoting Confucianism for Socioeconomic Development: The Singapore Experience." In: Tu Wei-ming, ed., *Confucian Traditions in East Asian Modernity*. Cambridge, MA: Harvard University Press.

World Bank. 1993. *World Development Report: Investing in Health*. New York: Oxford University Press.

World Health Organization. 2000. *World Health Report 2000. Health Systems: Improving Performance*. Geneva: World Health Organization.

4

Political Analysis and Strategies

Health-sector reform, like all policy reform, is a profoundly political process. As we stressed in Chapter 2, astute policy developers begin political analysis early in the policy cycle; they do not delay political analysis until after the policy has been developed. Waiting to assess the political implications of a policy can lead to proposals that are not likely to be adopted. The technical work of policy development and the political work of feasibility assessment need to occur *at the same time*. Political analysis and political strategies are required at each stage in the policy cycle, and are not confined to the box of "political decision" as shown in Figure 2.1.

Advocates of health reform in developing countries have not always recognized the political challenges they confront or developed the political strategies they need. One example of limited political analysis of major health reforms is the *World Development Report* of 1993 (World Bank 1993). This report provided seven chapters on what countries should do to improve the efficiency of investments in health in poor countries, but only five paragraphs on the process of health-sector reform (Reich 1997). Furthermore, the report provided few concrete or specific ideas about how to manage what it called the "continuous and complex struggle" of health-sector reform. It simply observed that "Broad reforms in the health sector are possible when there is sufficient political will and when changes to the health sector are designed and implemented by capable planners and managers" (World Bank 1993, 15). *The World Health Report* of 2000, on the topic of health-system performance, gave greater attention to the role of politics, including a paragraph on the importance of mobilizing stakeholders (WHO 2000, 134). But this report subsumed politics within the broader function of "stewardship," meaning government's responsibility for social welfare and concern about trust and legitimacy (p. 119). The WHO report gave very limited attention to political analysis or political strategies, which we consider essential components of efforts to improve health system performance.

How then should health reformers develop and carry out political strategies in order to improve the chances that their plan will be adopted and put into action? Our approach emphasizes the importance of systematic and continuous political analysis. We first examine how the agenda is set for public policy in general and for health-sector reform in particular. Next, we discuss how to manage this process of agenda-setting, through the use of stakeholder analysis. This is a systematic way of analyzing the relevant groups and individuals inside and outside government who might influence the process of policy choice. We then present four basic political strategies for improving the chances that a policy reform will be adopted, concluding with lessons from negotiation theory about how to build a winning political coalition. Finally, we discuss some of the ethical dimensions of political strategizing, including the personal decisions faced by health reformers.

Agenda-Setting for Health Reform

What determines the health-reform agenda in a given country? A naïve response might be, "Public attention focuses on areas where the performance of the health-care system is unsatisfactory." But the problems defined by policymakers as issues for public attention may not be those that experts identify as unsatisfactory or as high-priority—a pattern we discussed in Chapter 2. For example, in Ghana, the disease burden of cervical cancer greatly exceeds that of breast cancer, but policy attention has focused more on breast cancer than on cervical cancer because of various social and political processes (Reichenbach 1999). As this example suggests, the "facts" do not simply speak for themselves in setting priorities for health-sector reform. More broadly, the issues selected for public policy attention do not necessarily correspond to the choices one would make based on ethical analysis or an assessment of performance goals (as discussed in Chapters 3 and 5).

In practice, health-sector problems get defined as public issues through larger social and political processes (Reich 1995). Issues come and go in political life as a matter of public attention, in what has been called the "issue-attention cycle" (Downs 1972). Let us consider some of the important factors that determine public attention to issues in the agenda-setting process.

The mass media play an important role in shaping this cycle of issues for public debate, in both developed and developing countries. The media can transform private troubles into public issues, create awareness among the public and political elites, and shape the boundaries and symbols of public debate. The issue cycle is influenced in part by economic incentives. Newspapers, magazines, radio, and television stations depend on revenues from circulation, either from direct sales or advertising. Readers, listeners, and viewers consume the news in part as entertainment. As stories become worn out and boring over time, the media have every reason to find new, interesting topics to attract viewers and readers. The interest of the media in specific issues can also be driven by their ownership or their relationship to specific political parties, and can be limited by the state's lack of tolerance for public criticism and its respect for basic freedoms (such as freedom of the press).

The availability of proposed solutions also affects the definition of an issue. As we noted in Chapter 2, the definition of a "problem" can be driven by the availability of a "solution." This is usually an active process and depends on the existence of a committed individual or organization working to promote the solution. For example, international agencies have sometimes played a key role in focusing attention on specific solutions that fit with their missions and in setting the policy agenda within countries (Reich 1995). In the 1970s and 1980s, for instance, UNICEF made major efforts to promote Growth monitoring, Oral rehydration, Breast-feeding, and Immunization (GOBI) as its solution to high infant mortality rates (UNICEF 1985). International agencies use various means to promote their policy solutions, including powerful incentives and diplomatic pressure. These means include targeted loans and gifts, and the practice of putting various conditions on their aid. In these situations, international agencies become *policy entrepreneurs*—actors who seek to promote a particular issue and a particular solution (Kingdon 1995).

Policy entrepreneurs also exist within national contexts. Consider, for example, the efforts of a group of Japanese women parliamentarians who successfully focused legislative action on child pornography (Strom 1999), or efforts by physicians in Eastern Europe who are trying to define their own falling incomes as a problem for health reform (Bossert and Wlodarczyk 2000). The ability of a group to focus political and social attention on a particular aspect of the health system depends on many factors, including their own resources, features of the broader environment, and political timing. The advocates of health reform, at both national and international levels, often function as policy entrepreneurs. In this role, they need to understand the policy cycle (presented in Chapter 2) and how they can most effectively influence the policy agenda to support reform at each stage in the cycle.

A crisis can provide an opportunity to put an issue on the policy agenda (Rochefort and Cobb 1994). The crisis can be a natural disaster, such as an earthquake, which can highlight problems in the health system that need attention; or it can be a human-caused disaster, such as an economic crisis, which can focus

attention on costly imported pharmaceuticals and provide the impetus for introducing an essential-drugs policy. In some cases, policy entrepreneurs seek for
years to introduce a particular policy reform, and achieve success only when the
right combination of crisis and political circumstances come together, as occurred
with pharmaceutical policy reform in Bangladesh in 1983 when a military dictator took power (Reich 1994b).

Political cycles and timing also affect which issues get on a country's policy
agenda (Heclo 1974). By focusing attention on specific issues, different groups
and individuals fight for political advantage, especially during elections, seeking
recognition for their concerns on the policy agenda. Once an issue has become
salient, one policy suggestion tends to generate alternative proposals, as competing groups claim ownership for the issue in ways that will work to each group's
advantage. Once an issue is on the policy agenda, it tends to push other issues off;
a country can only consider a limited number of major social-reform problems at
a time. Policy entrepreneurs not only must make their definition of the problem
more attractive than alternative ones, but they also have to make it more attractive
than competing issues. Political timing therefore is critical, since the window of
opportunity for policy change is often limited and subject to unanticipated events
(Kingdon 1995). Policy entrepreneurs need to develop an understanding of when
the window is open, how long it is likely to remain open, and how to squeeze their
policy changes through the window quickly—before it slams shut again.

Changes in the policy agenda can also occur when new actors enter the political system. A new minister of health, for example, often seeks to define a new
policy agenda shortly after entering office. Such proposals are not only intended
to solve social problems, but also to create a political legacy for posterity and to
demonstrate that the minister deserves to stay in office and receive rewards when
the term is over—while recognizing that their time as minister is likely to be
short, averaging six months to a year in many developing countries.

How the minister defines the policy agenda will be shaped by broader political
incentives and the perceived costs and benefits of specific policies, including the
views held by the head of state. This process of agenda-setting by a minister of
health is illustrated by the decision in Egypt to design a new policy for health insurance of school-aged children in 1983 (Nandakumar et al. 2000). In Colombia,
the minister of health worked with senators and developed alliances with key legislators in order to assure passage of his law for health reform (González-Rossetti
and Ramírez 2000). This example shows how a policy entrepreneur needs to consider the political circumstances of the specific policy arena in developing a strategy for agenda-setting.

Policy entrepreneurs also act on the basis of their beliefs about what would
make the system better—beliefs and values that are often shaped by personal experiences and by a sense of moral leadership (Coles 2000). Advocates of better
care for the mentally ill may have a mentally ill family member and therefore

have personal experience with poor service and its impact on the family. A politician who has experienced a personal loss from a traffic accident may respond by pushing for legislation requiring seatbelts to enhance safety. Ideology and professional training can also influence the issues that a policy entrepreneur selects. For example, public-health professionals generally believe in the value of prevention, and these beliefs influence their selection and definition of problems to address.

Sudden changes in government can provide an opportunity for health-sector reform; for example, when a military dictator comes to power in a coup. But even authoritarian rulers must design political strategies for dealing with powerful interest groups and opposition to new policies. In Bangladesh, the new military government in 1983 quickly introduced and implemented a new pharmaceutical policy at the start of its term, but was unable to push through a new health policy seven years later because of persistent opposition from the physicians' association (Reich 1994b). In Chile, the Pinochet regime overcame substantial opposition to its health reform from medical and public-health groups in 1979, but the reforms still required five to ten years for implementation because of resistance both inside and outside the military government (Jimenez de la Jara and Bossert 1999).

The general culture of a society also influences the agenda-setting process, by making some topics easy to raise in public and blocking other topics as taboo (Douglas and Wildavsky 1982). These values and beliefs tend to be specific to a particular country's culture and traditions (or to a community within the country), at a particular moment in time. For example, in some countries, it is taboo to discuss higher infant mortality rates for female children, or the existence of a free market for kidneys being sold to rich foreigners.

It is important to remember that cultural beliefs are not static but change over time, so that topics once considered out of bounds for public debate can become defined as problems and as public issues. For instance, female genital cutting was considered taboo in many countries, until after the International Conference on Population and Development in Cairo in 1994, which opened the issue up for debate in Egypt and throughout the world (Seif El Dawla 1999). This case shows how once-taboo topics can become public issues for health-reform debate, with wide-ranging political and cultural consequences. Understanding the role of cultural values in the definition and selection of topics for public consideration can help health reformers plan which problems to address and how, as we discuss below.

Of course, agenda-setting processes can be unpredictable. A determined, skilled, and powerful leader can make the unthinkable become thinkable. A crisis can focus attention and alter political calculations about a problem, creating an unanticipated opportunity for policy change. Political scientist John Kingdon (1995) has argued that the best chances for successful policy change occur when three streams of events come together: *1)* the objective situation—the problem stream, *2)* the availability of a possible solution—the policy stream, and *3)* the flow of political events—the political stream. When these three streams converge, according to Kingdon, some policy response is likely to result—although the response may not resolve the problem.

Health reformers therefore require the ability to assess and manage the flow of political events (skills in which they are rarely trained) as well as the capacity to analyze the objective situation and design possible solutions (skills in which they usually do receive training). Health reformers need to understand how agendas for public policy are set, and how they can modify the agenda-setting processes for health reform. In short, health reformers do not have to accept the problem as defined by the agenda-setting processes in their country. Health reformers can use ethical theory (presented in Chapter 3) and the performance goals (described in Chapter 5) to define the problems they think should be addressed. They then must use political processes to expand public acceptance of these problem definitions, in order to shape the policy agenda.

Health reformers thus must be centrally concerned with the *political feasibility* of a given policy proposal. Can the proposal be adopted, and can it be implemented? But the concept of feasibility is not a dichotomous, yes/no variable: feasibility involves probabilities that can vary from zero to one. The likelihood of getting a policy adopted depends on the situation, and the skill and commitment of its advocates (and opponents). What political resources does each group have at their disposal and how much is each prepared to commit to this particular battle? How clever and effective are they at such diverse tasks as assessing the political consequences of technical proposals, making emotional public appeals, and negotiating private deals with key political actors? Are they able to persuade individuals and organizations to commit their limited political resources and capital for this particular reform effort?

Leadership here is critical. Talented political leaders, like talented generals, can win battles and campaigns that would overwhelm those less able or less energetic (Heifetz 1994). So, asking if a policy is *feasible* is, in part, asking a question about the advocates of reform, especially their creativity, commitment, and skills—and about their opponents. Passing health-care reform often means overcoming or deflecting powerful interests that will vigorously defend their positions.

Constructing health reform so that it is politically feasible thus demands political skills, political analysis, and political strategies—rather than some vague notion of "political will," as was called for by the World Bank in its 1993 *World Development Report*. Players involved in health reform make their own calculations of the likely political costs and benefits of reform, and take positions and spend resources accordingly. Advocates of health reform need to understand these calculations from each player's perspective, and then construct strategies that will influence these calculations and tip the probabilities in favor of reform. This process requires the collection and analysis of political data, including subjective judgments about how different players are likely to respond to different reform proposals. It therefore requires a good understanding of the politics of health-sector reform.

Politics of Health-Sector Reform

Four factors are particularly important in understanding how to manage the politics of health-sector reform. These factors affect the origins of health reform as an issue, the content of reform policies, and the implementation of adopted programs. The four factors are:

- *Players*: the set of individuals and groups who are involved in the reform process, or who might enter the debate over the policy's fate;
- *Power*: the relative power of each player in the political game (based on the political resources available to each player);
- *Position*: the position taken by each player, including whether the player supports or opposes the policy, and the intensity of commitment for or against the policy for each player (i.e., the proportion of resources that the player is willing to expend on promoting or resisting the policy);
- *Perception*: the public perception of the policy, including the definition of the problem and the solution, and the material and symbolic consequences for particular players.

These four factors—players, power, position, and perception—can be influenced through the political strategies adopted by health reformers. A central purpose of this chapter is to provide guidance on how to design effective political strategies.

Of course, the political feasibility of a proposed policy is affected by other factors beyond these four. Changing the content of a policy can affect the distribution of political costs and benefits among players, and thereby alter the calculus of political feasibility. In addition, the strategies adopted by some key players can alter the behavior of others. One player can also take actions that alter the power and position of other players. Sometimes those decisions change the rules of the game itself. Other important factors are difficult or impossible for health reformers to modify or manipulate, including deep-rooted cultural beliefs, the structure of political institutions, the incentives presented by international agencies, and the occurrence of natural or economic disasters.

What would be an appropriate metaphor for policymaking and for thinking about political feasibility? First, policymaking is not like a game of checkers, where all players are equal and can only move in predetermined ways. It is more like a game of chess, with different moves for different players, and where pawns can become kings if they reach the other side. But there is a major difference: in policymaking, the rules of the game are not stable, and they can change (imperceptibly or suddenly) as the game proceeds. A policy's feasibility can be determined by the rules and who controls them; and no player is assured that the rules will continue unchanged.

In addition, the politics of health-sector reform has certain *systematic characteristics* that make it a difficult process—perhaps even more so than other kinds of policy reform. These include:

- *Technical complexity/difficulty*: Fixing the health sector is not easy. Many parts and pieces are interrelated, and many consequences (both intended and unintended) occur. Designing a comprehensive health reform is a complex technical process, as health reformers turn the five control knobs in various directions. Reformers often seek to improve many parts of the system at the same time, making both the details and the overall impact of the program difficult for non-experts to grasp. These technical challenges create political challenges through their impact on players and the potential for public confusion.
- *Concentrated costs to well-organized groups*: Health-sector reform efforts commonly entail concentrated new costs for well-mobilized, powerful groups, such as physicians (often well organized in a national medical association), or the pharmaceutical industry (often well organized in an industry association). This problem of concentrated costs can create significant political obstacles to reform, if the high-power groups mobilize to oppose the reform in order to protect their interests.
- *Dispersed benefits to nonorganized groups*: Health-sector reform often seeks to make new benefits available to previously disadvantaged groups; for example, the poor, or rural residents. Such groups often are not well organized or politically well connected. In addition, these changes may only result in modest benefits for each individual. Dispersed benefits among low-power groups make it more difficult to mobilize significant political support for reform.

The combination of concentrated costs to well-organized groups and dispersed benefits to nonorganized groups constitutes what Mancur Olson (1965) called a collective action dilemma. Overcoming the politics of this collective action dilemma is a major challenge for health reformers. Together, the three characteristics of health-sector reform described above create considerable political challenges. Yet they also allow common approaches to the politics of health reform, especially in conducting stakeholder analysis and designing political strategies.

Political Analysis

A basic building block in designing political strategies for reform is stakeholder analysis (Reich 1996). This takes place in three stages. First, identify the relevant groups and individuals. Second, assess their political resources and their roles in the political structure to determine their relative power over the policy question at hand. Third, evaluate their current position on the proposed policy (including the

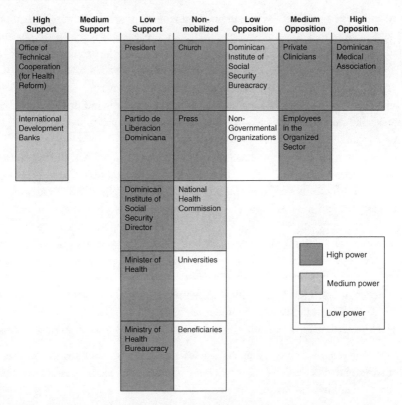

FIGURE 4.1. Position map for major players in health reform in the Dominican Republic in 1995.

intensity of their commitment) and their underlying interests. This analysis can be presented visually, as shown in Figure 4.1 for the case of health reform in the Dominican Republic (Glassman et al. 1999). Once the stakeholder analysis is completed, with a clear understanding of the relevant groups and their power and positions, a health reformer can proceed to the next stage—designing political strategies to enhance the chances that the reform will be adopted. These analytical tasks of conducting a stakeholder analysis and designing political strategies can be assisted by a computer software program, *PolicyMaker* (Reich and Cooper 1996), which has been widely used for training policy analysts how to think strategically about politics.

Obtaining reliable information for the stakeholder analysis—about the positions and power of different players—can be quite difficult. Sophisticated political players may purposefully mislead others in order to gain advantages in the negotiations over a critical policy issues, for example by masking or exaggerating their power. Sometimes they play both sides in such a debate. Even if you can assess a player's power with some accuracy, it can be difficult to know how much effort they will exert on a given issue. Public statements may reveal the public positions of key players, but these positions may not represent the actual positions that players ultimately take when pressed for a decision. The most important task for analysts is to determine the *core* position and power of stakeholders—what they are not willing to give up, and the amount of resources they can mobilize to assure their goals are met. Finding out this information requires multiple sources and careful judgment about specific players—questions usefully considered by a team of analysts with differing perspectives.

Stakeholder analysis combines two distinct modes of analysis. One is interest group analysis (Lindblom 1965). This consists of understanding the social groups that are seeking to move the government in a particular direction, including private business and nongovernmental organizations. The second mode of analysis examines bureaucratic politics and is focused on the competition among agencies and individuals within government (Downs 1967). The stakeholders relevant to health-sector reform include both kinds of players: those outside government and those inside government. For health-sector reform in developing countries, one also needs to consider the activities of international agencies, such as the World Bank, UNICEF, or the World Health Organization.

Health-sector reform typically involves the following kinds of interest groups:

- *Producer groups*: doctors, dentists, nurses, pharmacists, other health-sector employees and their unions, domestic and international pharmaceutical companies, and equipment manufacturers;
- *Consumer groups*: disease-based organizations, local and regional consumer groups, women's organizations, unions representing insured workers, retirees, and military groups;
- *Economic groups*: businesses with health insurance schemes, industries affected by health policies (e.g., tobacco farmers, drug sellers), and workers who gain or lose jobs;
- *Ideological groups*: political parties, reform organizations, single-issue advocates (e.g., environmentalists, anti-abortion activists);
- *Health-development groups*: multilateral development banks, bilateral aid agencies, international health organizations, nongovernmental development organizations.

This list of interest groups is illustrative. Health reformers need to adapt the list to the specific political circumstances for the policy at hand, and focus attention on the most critical groups and individuals. Deciding on the list of interest-group players for analysis requires judgment about the groups most likely to be mobilized or those that could be mobilized to affect the balance of power in the policy debate.

Similarly, when examining bureaucratic groups, a political analyst must decide which actors to consider and where to draw various lines. Is the ministry of health a single player, or are different parts, such as the minister and his immediate staff, best thought of as separate groups? There is no one correct answer to such questions. Carrying out a good political analysis is an art as well as a science. The goal is to identify the important players who can act independently and can control significant political resources. But considering too many separate players makes the analysis unwieldy and frustrating.

In addition to the ministry of health (MOH), the following government actors often play important roles in health-sector reform debates and decisions:

- *Ministry of Finance*: especially if the reform involves changes in the financing of health services or changes in the MOH's budget;
- *Social Security Institute*: particularly if the reform proposal involves changes in the provision of health care and a reorganization of government health facilities;
- *Economic and/or Planning Ministries*: very likely if the reform proposal involves calculations about overall economic growth or decisions about debt forgiveness;
- *Local and/or Regional Governments*: expected if the reform proposal involves decentralization;
- *Ministry of Education*: for school health policies or for policies that affect medical schools;
- *Ministry of Agriculture, Trade, and Industry*: for policies on alcohol, tobacco, pharmaceuticals, or medical equipment.

In compiling the list of stakeholders, the analyst needs to consider the implications of the proposed policy for each player: Who cares about the policy? Who is likely to act—or could be convinced to act? Who has the potential to influence the outcome? Who is likely to be affected by the reform's consequences, in positive and negative ways?

The analyst also must consider critical political actors: individuals or groups who have special power over the policy in question. In some cases, a powerful individual may have veto power over the adoption of a policy reform; in many cases, a particular group can determine whether a policy is implemented at all. Leaders deserve particular attention. The prime minister or president, specific senators or governors, heads of important parliamentary factions and political parties: all may well matter. Media outlets also should be examined, especially those identified with particular points of view, parties, or factions. The editors or managers of media organizations often have their own political agendas, and these actors need to be considered in the political analysis of health-sector reform.

Sources of Power and Influence

Having identified a list of players (the groups and individuals who are relevant to the policy proposal), the next step is to estimate the power and influence of each player. This requires an assessment of the following for each player:

- The player's political resources and place in the political system, which determine their potential capacity to influence policy decisions;
- The player's interests, position, and commitment, which will influence how the player's resources—and how much of those resources—will be used in the policy debate.

Political resources come in two forms: tangible and intangible (see Table 4.1). Tangible resources include money, organization, people, votes, equipment, and offices, all of which affect a group's ability to influence the policy process. Money can provide political contributions and purchase other resources such as expertise, media access, and organizational support. People can distribute literature, participate in rallies and demonstrations, and help with lobbying government officials on particular policy issues. Votes can matter, depending on whether a decision is to be made through an electoral process, in a legislature or committee or a popular election. The underlying level of organization also affects a group's influence. Groups with existing infrastructure (offices, staff, electricity, telephone services, fax machines, and computers) have a substantial advantage in the policy process. These groups have already paid the transaction costs of organizing themselves and can use that investment to influence the issue at hand. A new group, on the other hand, first has to pay the costs of getting organized: it has to recruit members, arrange a staff, develop materials, and construct systems. These costs reinforce the anti-change bias and inertia of political systems, because new groups (which could arise with a new policy) are not yet organized to express and defend their interests.

The second set of political resources is intangible. These resources include information on the policy and the problem, as well as relevant expertise, which allow the group to develop a position. Two important intangible resources are the group's expertise and legitimacy. Groups whose members have access to key decision-makers, whether from personal contacts or past favors, do better than those without connections to powerholders. Health reformers also require the political skills to manage the lobbying process. Knowing where to go, whom

TABLE 4.1. Sources of Political Power

TANGIBLE	INTANGIBLE
Money	Information
Organization	Access to leaders
People	Access to media
Votes	Expertise
Equipment	Legitimacy
Offices	Skills

to talk to, and how to get the press interested—all enhance a group's policy impact.

This analysis of political resources helps explain why particular groups play the roles they do in shaping health-sector reform. Physicians tend to be influential because they are usually well organized, wealthy, skillful, expert, and seen as legitimate by other players; moreover, every top decision-maker has a personal physician. Consequently, the medical association is often well positioned to place its issues on the political agenda for consideration and to influence policies in the health sector, especially on matters that directly affect their interests, such as provider payment (Marmor and Thomas 1972). International pharmaceutical companies often have significant influence because of their financial resources and political connections, but they also tend to have limited grassroots organization and limited social legitimacy, which can constrain their power on particular issues. Groups that are not wealthy or well organized (such as the rural poor) confront major obstacles before they can begin to defend their interests in an effective way. In short, political power and political resources are not equally distributed in society—and that distribution affects the politics of health reform. The result is often some form of the collective-action dilemma mentioned above, which leads to fundamental political obstacles to reform.

The value of different kinds of political resources depends partly on the nature of the political system. The degree of democracy in a country, as expressed in freedom of speech and freedom of association, can affect group activities in fundamental ways. These factors shape the distribution of power in society and the kinds of participation that occur in the policy process. In many developing countries, interest groups are not well organized, and policy elites in government dominate the process of decision-making (Grindle and Thomas 1991). Still, for health policy, the physicians' association, trade unions, and the pharmaceutical manufacturers' association often exert significant influence on policies that affect their interests. Moreover, the role of nongovernmental organizations in policy debates is growing both within developing countries and at international levels, for all kinds of economic and social policy reforms (Matthews 1997). For these reasons, it is important to consider how the existing health system distributes both economic and political benefits to certain interest groups, and restricts benefits to other groups (Reich 1994a).

As part of their political analysis of the policy debate, health reformers are well advised to conduct an inventory of political resources held by different players. Differentiating tangible from intangible resources is useful because players build their strategies based on their resources. This means that players weak in material resources (for example, with limited money and equipment) will often rely on political strategies that depend on intangible resources (for example, protest actions or challenges to legitimacy). You should know your own political resources, and build your strategies accordingly. Even if you lack material resources, you can still design political strategies that may give you substantial leverage in a policy debate, by wisely using symbols that connect to broad social values. On the other hand, powerful political actors can use symbolic strategies to prevent the serious consideration of a new policy issue, by linking their position on a policy to strongly held cultural worldviews in ways that control the policy agenda (Cobb and Ross 1997).

Elements of political structure also influence the leverage of different social groups. For example, in some developed countries media-based electoral and policy campaigns are essential. This increases the influence of those with money, as money is vital for television advertising in public debates. In countries without competitive elections, or where the state controls radio and television broadcasting, money is less important for purchasing air time to promote a particular policy position. In a corrupt political system, however, money is often important for purchasing access to decision-makers or for purchasing a specific policy decision. In parliamentary systems, proportional representation can force political leaders to give more attention to minorities than occurs in legislatures with winner-take-all single-member constituencies. On the other hand, single-member constituency systems give an advantage to geographically concentrated groups that might control swing seats. But those systems also create obstacles to the influence of dispersed groups of committed believers (who have more impact under proportional representation).

A group's role in the existing pattern of political competition can affect the group's influence. An important distinction is between *swing* and *base* groups. A swing group is one that might vote for either party in an election, or a legislative bloc that might be for or against the government. A base group, in contrast, is a firm member of a party's core support.

For many interest groups, the strategic question is how to persuade the ruling coalition to pay attention to the group's views. In some cases, an interest group may seek to keep its loyalty uncertain, in order to induce competing parties to bid for the group's support. For example, powerful health-care interests may decide to contribute heavily to both political parties. Political leaders, on the other hand, seek to expand their political support by relying on the loyal support of their base groups while trying to attract the conditional loyalty of swing groups. Reaching out too far to attract support from a swing group, however, can threaten the ongoing support of a base group, and persuade a politician to pull back. One example is the efforts of Prime Minister Atal Behari Vajpayee of India, in March 2002, to placate Hindu nationalists who are the base of his Bharatiya Janata Party over the issue of building a Hindu temple on the site of a former mosque in Ayodhya, while simultaneously trying to appeal to swing groups that include secular allies for his government and Muslim voters (Duggin 2002).

Interest groups thus use their role in the political system as a resource for seeking concessions from politicians in either the ruling coalition or the opposition.

During elections, groups may be able to obtain concessions or promises on policies that may be difficult to elicit under normal circumstances. Elections can therefore provide opportunities for relatively powerless groups to expand their influence on health policy issues, such as the distribution of health facilities or access to health services. Furthermore, an ongoing political struggle within a country, or an economic crisis, can change the distribution of power and present opportunities for interest groups and bureaucratic actors to shape policy decisions in the health sector.

Position and Commitment

Knowing a group's political resources does not enable one to predict whether or how those resources will be used. Stakeholder analysis therefore needs to assess how each group views the policy issue, and what its position is.

A first step is to assess the group's interests. These may not be clear, even to the group itself, nor does a group necessarily pursue its own interests. But in many cases, interests do shape policy positions. For example, knowing that physicians' incomes will decrease under a proposed payment plan strongly suggests that the medical association is likely to oppose the plan. Anticipated economic consequences of a policy often determine political positions on that policy.

It is also important to examine the positions that the players have taken publicly. Do the positions correspond with their interests as you understand them? If not, how can the discrepancy be explained? Is it because some groups are confused, because they are proceeding tactically, or because they know something that you do not? Differences can also arise between public positions and private positions, between what a group says it will do and what a group will actually do. In some cases, political ideology is a good predictor of a player's position on health sector reform. For example, the Pinochet regime in Chile adopted major changes in health policy that were consistent with its market-oriented approach to public policy (Jimenez de la Jara and Bossert 1995). In other cases, ideology may not be a good predictor of position, since political action often involves both interests and willingness to bargain and compromise as well as values. For example, in Costa Rica the trade unions and the Communists were willing to support some efforts to privatize social security, in order to introduce competition and make the bureaucracy more interested in efficiency and quality (Ramírez et al. 1998).

As part of this analysis, we also need to describe the intensity of each group's current position on an issue. How much of their available resources is the group willing to use to promote its position? For example, how much time is the group's leader spending on the issue? Is the group expending a significant portion of its financial resources on the issue? Is this an issue that the group is totally committed to fight for, as part of its mission, or is the commitment tepid, less resource-intensive, more "just going through the motions"?

Developing effective political strategies requires an understanding of why the key groups are taking their positions. Here are two hypothetical examples. First, suppose the ministry of finance is opposing an increase in the tobacco tax that is intended to support rural health care. Is that a result of a general bureaucratic reflex, or because the minister has a different, specific use for the money in mind? If the latter, then how important is that alternative to the minister? A minister acting out of a general desire to protect his turf poses a different political problem than someone strongly committed to an alternative program. In a second example, suppose the medical association is vigorously opposing the new fee schedule in the national health insurance plan. Is that because most of its members genuinely understand and oppose the new system, or is a small group of high-income specialists driving that position? If the latter, then the association's leaders might be willing to make a symbolic protest to satisfy an internal constituency, and they might accept a deal if most association members could be protected from adverse effects. On the other hand, if the association's president is driving the opposition to the policy, it may be difficult to change the official position as long as that individual remains in charge, or unless the individual has a specific request that can be met.

The intensity of group mobilization thus depends in part on how the policy is expected to affect the group's interests and how those likely consequences are perceived. Decisions that are clearly recognized as affecting a well-organized group (especially those with a small number of highly committed members) often result in high mobilization. For example, a government policy to restrict imports of high-cost medicines through an essential-drugs policy would probably result in strong opposition from multinational pharmaceutical companies and their industry association. On the other hand, decisions that are perceived as having marginal impacts on the members of poorly organized groups may not result in much mobilization. For example, a policy to increase user fees for patients at rural clinics may not result in protests by patients from rural areas.

The positions of the major political parties can be critical to health-sector reform. Because parties are coalitions, bargaining is a core part of the process of developing programs and positions. If a party has already embraced health-sector reform as a priority issue for its agenda, then much of the work for reform advocates has already been accomplished. Using parties to help manage the political issue of health reform is always an option to be considered in the development of political strategies, the topic that we discuss next.

Political Strategies for Reform

How can a health reformer develop political strategies that will help forge a winning coalition? We noted above that the political feasibility of health-sector reform (and policy reform more generally) is shaped by the *position* of the players, the *power* of each player, the number of *players* mobilized, and the *perception* of the problem and the solution. Reform advocates need political strategies to manage each of these factors in order to increase the probability that their reform plan will be adopted and implemented. Below we consider four sets of political strategies for reform.

Position Strategies: Bargain to Change the Position of Players

The first set of political strategies involves bargaining within the existing distribution of power to change the position of players. This can involve deals, promises, trades, and threats.

One approach is to change a specific element of the policy to move various key actors to be more in favor, to switch sides, or to be less opposed. Perhaps the minister of finance will agree not to oppose the proposal for higher cigarette taxes for rural health care, if part of the revenue is used for health care and the rest is left for other government purposes (possibly including the minister's personal projects). Or, in another example, suppose that a country proposes changing from per-day to per-admission payments for hospitals. Perhaps the owners of private hospitals will not oppose the new payment system if, for the first three years, there is a hold-harmless rule that guarantees that no institution will lose revenue for that time period.

A second kind of bargaining involves inter-issue exchanges, in which cooperation on one issue is sought in return for some concession on a different issue. Such "logrolling" is normal in many political contexts. If the medical association accepts the new fee schedule, perhaps the ministry will agree to accept new limits on the number of doctors who can practice in crowded (i.e., desirable) areas. Or suppose that provincial governments ask the central government to take on responsibility for financially troubled provincial hospitals—in return, they might offer to accept a different formula for dividing the national tax revenue so that more goes to the central government. While the trades in these examples are on related issues, that does not have to be the case. Maybe the unions will accept an increase in payroll taxes to support the health insurance scheme, if the government promises some other efforts to increase overall employment.

Bargains can involve threats as well as promises: doctors may threaten a strike if their salaries are not raised; consumers can threaten demonstrations if their health benefits are reduced; pharmaceutical companies can threaten to close their plants if the country implements a price-control scheme. Sometimes the threat is to stop cooperating. For instance, small-business owners might say they will refuse to report earnings and will stop paying taxes on those earnings for the new health insurance scheme unless their overall contribution ceiling is lowered.

Constructing an effective bargain to change the positions of key players requires intelligence, skill, and trial-and-error experimentation. Skills in negotiation and conflict resolution are particularly important for these strategies. Finding out what it takes to change a player's position may require an actual offer or threat. The bargain could involve modifying the policy's content; in that case, the health reformer should determine how the change influences the policy's expected effectiveness. A compromise that produces a supportive coalition but undermines the reform's overall goals could create a reform that is politically feasible but technically ineffective or even counterproductive. For someone who cares about consequences (such as our performance goals), that kind of compromise would not be a good deal.

Power Strategies: Distribute Power Resources to Strengthen Friends and Weaken Enemies

The second set of political strategies is designed to change the distribution of power among key players. Since a group's impact on the policy process depends partly on its resources, reform advocates can adopt strategies to enhance the tangible and intangible political resources of supporters and decrease those resources of opponents. Here are some examples:

- Give or lend money, staff, or facilities to groups that support the reform;
- Provide information and education to supporters in order to increase their expertise;
- Give allies expanded access to lobby key decision-makers;
- Provide allies with media time and attention in order to enhance their legitimacy; focus attention on their expertise, impartiality, national loyalty, and other positive social values.

A tough political strategist can also do the same—in reverse—to opponents:

- Decrease opponents' resources by inducing people not to contribute and not to work for them; do this by attacking the group's legitimacy, honesty, or motives;
- Refuse to cooperate with opponents, for example, by not providing information; keep them uninformed and out of the loop;
- Reduce opponents' access to key decision-makers;
- Urge the media not to cover opponents; characterize them as inexpert, self-serving, disloyal, etc.

These power strategies may not be effective, or ethical, in all cases. The list above illustrates some examples of the kinds of power-oriented moves that a strategist might consider, rather than an inclusive list of what should always be done. Deciding on which power strategies to select requires an assessment of the players involved in health reform (both for and against), the kinds of power resources available to health-reform advocates, and judgments about the likely impact of different power strategies on specific players.

Player Strategies: *Change the Number of Players by Creating New Friends and Discouraging Foes*

Reform advocates can also consider political strategies that try to change the set of friends and foes. These strategies seek to mobilize players who are not yet organized and demobilize players who are already organized. It means changing the balance of mobilized players by recruiting political actors to the health reform cause and away from the side of the opponents. The number and balance of political actors engaged in a policy debate is a key factor of political feasibility (Schattschneider 1960).

Mobilizing groups requires convincing people that they should pay the non-trivial costs of getting involved in an issue they have so far ignored, or the substantial costs of organizing a new group. Sometimes, mobilizing a previously uninvolved group may simply require bringing the issue to the group's attention—once the group knows what is going on, it may decide to take a position. If the nation's medical students have not begun to protest a proposed tuition increase, it may be because they have not yet heard of the proposal. Informing the student group (or its leaders) about the proposal and its consequences may be sufficient to mobilize students as a support group. But, competing factions within a group may have different views on the group's interests and values and on the policy's consequences, and they therefore may take different positions on the policy, making it difficult to mobilize the group as a whole.

Mobilizing the unorganized is more complicated, because it often requires substantial resources (time and money) to create an organization that can then join the policy debate. For instance, workers may be concerned about the consequences of a new competitive private-health-insurance scheme, but if they are not already organized as a union it may be difficult for them to develop a collective view of the proposed policy (and its potential impacts on premiums and co-payments) and difficult for them to take action as a group to protect their interests.

Nor is demobilizing a group that has taken a public position easy, for reasons of "face" and interest. In some cases, a group may shift its position after a discussion of its key interests, in which there may be a chance to explain to the group that its stake in the issue is different from what they thought it was, and that other issues should be of more concern to them.

Health reformers should also consider the potential to mobilize or discourage political leaders. For political leaders, the argument is often a mixture of self-interest and public-interest considerations. Show them how supporting you (or opposing you) will work to their political advantage (or disadvantage), and why this is a good (or a bad) issue for them to get involved in.

Merit-based arguments about the public interest can sometimes be as powerful as arguments based on political interests. Here is a generic example: "Senator, I know your constituents want you to do this, but they are being short-sighted. This policy will adversely affect the nation in the following ways. . . . So, perhaps you need to make a speech or two against this subject for the sake of the people in your district, but at the same time you don't need to actively work against us on this policy."

On the negative side, it is important to consider how to divide or undermine co-alitions that are opposing you. Suppose that the medical association has decided to oppose a new insurance scheme because it will limit reimbursement for high-cost procedures, which would negatively affect the income of some physicians. It may be possible to persuade doctors who provide primary care to switch sides and support the plan, and thereby divide the medical association, if primary-care doctors can be persuaded to see their interests in a different light.

A final way to change the number and balance of mobilized players is to change the arena of decision-making. Moving the policy decision from the executive branch to the legislature, for example, can allow advocates to mobilize new groups of politicians or to bypass certain political obstacles to reform. This occurred in Colombia, when the minister of health was unable to place health reform on the agenda in the executive branch because the president's priority was pension re-form. So he moved the debate to the legislature, which made health reform a con-dition for action on pension reform (González-Rossetti and Ramírez 2000). Shifting the policy arena, however, can also have unanticipated consequences. For example, when 40 pharmaceutical companies challenged a South African medicines law in court, seeking to protect their patent rights for AIDS medicines, activists mobilized nongovernmental groups around the world in opposition to the court case and to U.S. government efforts to change the law (Bond 1999). The companies eventually retracted the case, and the U.S. government changed its position on the policy. In this instance, the companies miscalculated, not in terms of legal argument, but in terms of how political mobilization and public opinion would prevent them from resolving the issue in a purely legal arena.

Political strategies can thus be used to alter the number of mobilized players and thereby influence the political feasibility of health reform. New players can enter the policy debate and take controlling positions, and current players can leave, change their positions, become inactive, or wait on the sidelines. Advocates of health-sector reform need to consider these possibilities and select strategies that change the balance of mobilized players in favor of their agenda.

Perception Strategies: Change the Perception of the Problem and the Solution

So far, we have discussed political strategy with a focus on stakeholders: the play-ers, their power, and their positions. In many contexts, this approach may be the most useful and pragmatic. For example, in a one-party political system, most of the relevant political competition will be among well-organized interest groups and established bureaucratic actors, occurring within limited processes of consultation.

In such situations, direct appeals to the public may not influence political decision-makers. But in open and competitive political systems, a public appeal through the media and to specific targeted groups can change the general perception of an issue. This approach can be an effective political strategy for influencing bureaucratic and political leaders, as well as mass audiences. Even in relatively closed political systems, reframing an issue can change the positions and power of key players and thereby affect the political feasibility of reform.

Political strategies directed at perceptions seek to change how people think and talk about a policy problem, how the issue is defined and framed, and which values are at stake (Majone 1989). The perception of an issue is also affected by how it is connected (or not) to important national symbols or values: Is this reform going to advance the nation's identity in some fundamental way? This connection can influence the priority given to the issue on the country's policy agenda.

Perception strategies relate to how the human mind works. Human beings often have trouble grasping complicated situations and seek simpler ways to make sense of a confusing reality (Simon 1957). This is especially true in situations where reality is complex, outcomes are uncertain, and conflicting goals are involved—all of which apply to health-sector reform. In such cases, health reformers need to manage public perceptions, because these change how problems are defined and which solutions are deemed acceptable. At the center of the political debate is a contest over the meaning of images and words, the symbols for policy reform (Edelman 1977). How is the problem characterized, how are the choices described, and how is the issue framed?

Consider the following example. A country is proposing to introduce private health insurance, which would allow citizens to take their contributions out of the monopoly national insurance scheme. Opponents characterize this proposal as "privatization," a disastrous decline in national solidarity and a loss of protection, since coverage under the new insurance scheme would be decreased for the first time in a generation. On the other side, supporters characterize the change as an increase in choice for individual subscribers and a challenge to the ineffective state bureaucracy. Depending on which formulation becomes widely accepted, the public and key players will view the reform effort in starkly different terms. In short, reframing an issue can change political circumstances in important ways, with significant consequences for the mobilized players, their power, and their positions, and for the feasibility of reform.

How does one alter public perceptions of an issue? There are various possibilities. One can argue facts and values, reframe the issue, or seek to define key symbols associated with the issue. An advocate could, for example, argue that an opponent's problem definition is based on poor data, that the problem is unimportant compared to other national priorities, that the problem is not fixable at a feasible cost, or that the problem should be a matter of private, not public, responsibility. Identifying some citizens as undeserving victims of greedy social forces can also be an effective way of reframing the public debate and altering the political balance. Another technique is to invoke important national symbols (such as a respected political figure or a popular singer), in order to connect the proposed policy to broadly accepted social values. Political mobilization is about emotions as well as data, and values can be used to oppose as well as promote health-sector reform.

Strategies based on eliciting core social values can also be used, as illustrated by the debate over the Clinton health reform plan in the United States in the early 1990s. Opponents to the Clinton reform developed a series of television commercials around "Harry and Louise," a fictional middle-class married couple, who presented the Clinton plan as threatening their lives. Sponsored by the health insurance industry, these commercials raised deep fears that the Clinton plan would limit the freedom of choice for existing health insurance and would produce a "government-run" health system (Johnson and Broder 1996, 16). This campaign connected to deeply felt social values in the American middle class, including anti-government sentiments, and fears of an eroding standard of living.

In contrast, the proponents of the Clinton health reform failed in the arena of public perceptions. The reform proposal was so complicated that it defied simple explanation (Starr 1995). For instance, the proposal included new institutions for managed competition that were first called "health insurance purchasing cooperatives" or HIPCs—an idea that few people could understand, pronounce, or remember. They were renamed "health alliances," which sounded friendlier but still remained obscure to most people. Overall, reform proponents failed to find effective symbols, to explain how the plan would work, what the policy would accomplish, or how it would promote core social values. As one key technocrat later reflected, "Many people couldn't understand what we were proposing. There were too many parts, too many new ideas, even for many policy experts to keep straight" (Starr 1995, 25).

Health reformers, trained in technical skills, are often uneasy about designing political strategies for shaping public perceptions and are often not prepared to implement them. But these perception strategies are an essential part of the overall political strategy for promoting health-sector reform. If the supporters of reform neglect the domain of perception strategies, they are likely to face those strategies wielded by their opponents.

Negotiation and Political Strategies

Many political strategies involve a process of negotiation. In recent years, systematic research on such processes has identified methods for conducting negotiations successfully. Here we briefly review the lessons about negotiation that are relevant to health-sector reform.

The first point is that *negotiations are often successful when the issue is constructed in win–win terms* rather than win–lose terms. A key challenge in negotiation is to seek *value-creating* solutions so that enough participants are willing to support the deal, producing win–win outcomes (Fisher and Ury 1981, 73). The contrasting approach of "I win, you lose" represents a *value-dividing* negotiation, which sharpens differences and makes agreement more difficult. In our discussion of bargaining strategies above, we gave several examples of arrangements in which advocates improved the status quo and potential opponents also gained. For example, if the reform plan created new revenue sources, then potential gains could be divided to enhance the potential of a win–win situation. In Egypt, a new government health insurance plan for school children was financed largely by a new tax on cigarettes, which made the proposal acceptable to key politicians in parliament who were concerned about the equity impacts of premium payments on poor rural families with many children (Nandakumar et al. 2000). Of course, finding new revenue sources is not always possible, and a winning coalition does not have to include everyone. On the other hand, formulating the issue in win–lose terms can push potential supporters into a position of active opposition.

A second lesson about negotiation, in looking for a win-win agreement, is to *respond to the real interests of other parties, not to the positions they happen to take* (Fisher and Ury 1981, 41). After all, a position may well be a stance designed to produce advantage in the negotiations. The hospitals in a country may say they will never accept budget responsibility, but their opposition to this idea may depend on their lack of authority to manage their own costs—for example, with regard to hiring and firing. If a negotiator knows that the combination of expanded autonomy and budget responsibility would be in the interests of hospitals, then offering the hospitals that deal may bring them into the support coalition.

A third lesson is that *some value-dividing conflicts may be inevitable*. For example, no matter how one reframes the issue, physicians may want to be paid more, while the ministry of health wants to pay them less (because of pressure from the ministry of finance). In such situations, one approach is to substitute specific substantive confrontation with *principle-based* negotiation, in which parties try to agree in advance to a set of principles that they will use to settle disagreements before they deal with the problems in detail (Fisher and Ury 1981, 84). For example, they might agree on how much of the national budget should go for health or what the payroll tax rate ought to be, and then decide on what fraction should go toward salaries, before they talk about specific items in the fee schedule. This approach can soften the sharp edge of confrontation and opposition in a constructive manner, since once an agreement on general principles has been reached, some of the details may follow accordingly.

A fourth guiding principle is for negotiators to *cast the emotional tone and energy in a positive instead of a negative direction*—or at least seek to establish a neutral and professional environment. Negotiation is a human process, filled with emotion as well as logic. Negotiators, therefore, need to manage the emotional dimensions as well as the logical content for success (Fisher and Ury 1981, 19).

The tone of negotiations is important because reform rarely is a one-time event. Instead, reform usually is an ongoing process, a series of connected conversations, as policies are designed, adopted, implemented, and modified over time. Moves in one round of bargaining have consequences for subsequent rounds, and can be understood as plays in a long series of games. In this series of negotiations, successful agreements make possible future successful agreements, and the converse is also true. A critical dimension is trust among the players. For example, different industries in different countries show large variations in their climate of labor relations. Some employers and unions are always in conflict with each other, while others resolve problems in a cooperative manner. Through repeated negotiations, they have become engaged in mutually reinforcing cycles of trust or distrust over time. The same can happen between nations. When political commentators discuss "momentum" in the Middle East peace process, they are talking about rising or falling relationships of trust. Similarly, health-sector reformers need to consider the role of trust in making it easier or harder to achieve their goals.

Conducting negotiations also requires an understanding of yourself and others. You cannot make proposals focused on other person's interests unless you know what those interests are; you cannot know what deals you can offer without undermining your own core goals unless you first understand your own objectives; you cannot identify which groups might constitute a winning coalition unless you have made a systematic analysis of all possible supporters and opponents, and their positions and power. You need to understand that initial offers on both sides often represent maximal positions. And you should clearly define your own bottom line, the Best Alternative To a Negotiated Agreement (BATNA) (Fisher and Ury 1981, 104). The better-off any player is without an agreement (the higher their BATNA), the less they need the agreement—and the more they can insist on their interests. Knowing your BATNA—and those of the other parties—is thus essential in knowing how hard to push for your view, which can risk ending the negotiations altogether.

The analysis for negotiation requires a serious investment of time and energy. As we said above, health-sector reform is a profoundly political process. The choice is not whether to negotiate, but rather how to conduct the negotiations. The better prepared a health reformer is to negotiate in terms of intelligence, skills, and stamina, the greater their chances of success in the policy process.

Political Strategies and Ethics

We believe that the politics of health reform should not be approached solely as an instrumental or Machiavellian problem. Health reformers need to consider the ethical dimensions of their political strategies, as well as how to get the policies they want. Values shape not only the substance, but also the process of health reform. How, then, can a health reformer assess the ethics of the political process for reform?

It is our premise that health reformers can be, should be, and almost inevitably will be active participants in the political process that society uses to decide on government policy. Hence, the classic public-administration view of the role of government officials—that politicians make policy and bureaucrats implement policy—does not capture the choices those officials must make in deciding how to conduct themselves.

Reformers themselves will have various kinds of goals, and those goals will not always coincide. People almost always have personal goals for career advancement, financial security, power, and influence. They also generally have broad goals for making society a better place. The ethical perspectives we discussed in Chapter 3 reflect these latter concerns. Between these, people are likely to have goals related to various organizations and groups—loyalty to a political party, identification with colleagues in the ministry, or concern for a professional group, for example.

The easy decisions are when someone's goals all line up. If the nation, the ministry, the medical profession, and a reformer personally will all benefit from a policy, then it is easy to pursue reform aggressively. But what happens when the goals do not line up? Suppose health reform will help the country, but could destroy a reformer's career (or family) if the reformer is committed to fully supporting it? Or suppose the reformer believes that the nation would be better off if many of the functions of the reformer's current agency were privatized or taken over by others? This could be a serious blow not only to the individual reformer, but also to many friends and colleagues.

Once a reform plan is formulated and a set of political strategies designed, advocates might well want to consider the costs and benefits of committing themselves to the necessary efforts. This involves asking, "How likely is it that the effort will succeed? Are the gains of achieving this reform worth the time, effort, money, emotion, and conflict that such an effort would entail?" Making these decisions involves difficult soul-searching, just as evaluating the costs and benefits is fraught with uncertainties and intangibles. To be effective, health reformers, like other leaders who seek to produce policy change, need to be both introspective and outward-reaching to connect their personal challenges with broader social transformation (Heifetz 1994).

Another aspect of the ethics of reform processes derives from our own ethical views about the importance of fostering transparency and public deliberation as obligations for technical experts (Landy et al. 1990). Within the political process, the critical role for public deliberation derives from our belief that there are no easy answers in health reform. The various available analytical and political paradigms typically provide only a limited perspective on health systems. As a result, both problems and solutions tend to be artificially constrained, so that important problems are ignored and alternative solutions are not given serious consideration. In these situations, public deliberation can help identify uncertainties in facts and values, can contribute to a social process of determining and grappling with what matters to a specific community, and can lead to innovative public policy design and democratic decisions.

Technical experts thus have ethical obligations in their consideration of political strategies. First, experts should be aware of the problems inherent in the reform process, particularly the potential for experts to conceal uncertainties of fact and disagreements over value. Second, experts should be aware of how their own values and their personal ethics shape their recommendations for choices about public policy (as we have tried to be, in this book). Third, we believe that experts have an ethical obligation to encourage public transparency and openness in helping societies confront policy decisions that involve uncertain facts and difficult value choices. We do not have evidence to prove that public transparency about these issues results in "better" social choices about health-sector reform, but we do believe that this approach promotes a respect for individuals while building a tolerant, yet supportive, democratic community (Gutmann and Thompson 1996).

Experts and officials also face serious ethical choices in the implementation process, particularly when they do not fully agree with the decisions made or policies chosen. There is always a choice about how hard to struggle to make the best of a policy one believes is technically flawed or ethically misguided. The question is, how far can officials go to use available discretion in implementation to move the policy in directions they believe appropriate—but not intended by policymakers? Here we believe an important distinction must be made between issues of fact and of value.

For matters of value, a critical question is the degree of legitimacy of the process that formulated the policy initially. Applbaum (2000) has argued—and we agree—that the more such processes meet the procedural requirements of democratic representation, the more an administrator should feel bound by the philosophical commitments embodied in the policy. This is not an all-or-nothing judgment, however, but rather a matter of setting variable and imprecise limits on the extent to which officials can deploy their own values in resolving ambiguities or conflicts in legislative or policy language in the course of implementation.

On the other hand, technical experts can and should exercise their expertise and their discretion to improve the functioning of a reform effort. Critical to their responsibilities, however, is again to foster transparency and their own accountability about their decisions. The role of "speaking truth to power" (Wildavsky 1979) and telling the parliament or the minister that their policies will not achieve their intended results is seldom easy. But we believe that conscientious reformers should be expected to play this role throughout the reform cycle.

These challenges make health-sector reform more than just a technical process—it is a testing ground for social values and personal commitments. In constructing a plan for change, health reformers have to confront basic issues of principle, identity, and interest. Health-sector reform can be as complex on a personal level as it is on

POLITICAL ANALYSIS AND STRATEGIES

a technical level. As advocates embark on the health-reform voyage, they need to understand how political challenges and ethical dilemmas intersect with technical issues, and how to address those intersections at both the public and the personal levels.

References

Applbaum, Arthur I. 2000. *Ethics for Adversaries: The Morality of Roles in Public and Professional Life*. Princeton, NJ: Princeton University Press.

Bond, Patrick. 1999. "Globalization, Pharmaceutical Pricing and South African Health Policy: Managing Confrontation with U.S. Firms and Politicians." *International Journal of Health Services* 29(4): 765–92.

Bossert, Thomas; and Cesary Wlodarczyk. 2000. *Unpredictable Politics: Policy Process of Health Reform in Poland*. Data for Decision Making Project Paper No. 74. Boston, MA: Harvard School of Public Health.

Cobb, Roger W.; and Marc Howard Ross, eds. 1997. *Cultural Strategies of Agenda Denial: Avoidance, Attack, and Redefinition*. Lawrence, KS: University Press of Kansas.

Coles, Robert. 2000. *Lives of Moral Leadership: Men and Women Who Have Made a Difference*. New York: Random House.

Douglas, Mary; and Aaron Wildavsky. 1982. *Risk and Culture*. Berkeley, CA: University of California Press.

Downs, Anthony. 1967. *Inside Bureaucracy*. Boston, MA: Little, Brown.

——— 1972. "Up and Down with Ecology—The 'Issue-Attention Cycle.'" *The Public Interest* 28(Summer): 38–50.

Duggin, C. W. 2002. "Court Bars Hindus' Rite Where They Razed Mosque." *The New York Times*, March 14: A9.

Edelman, Murray. 1977. *Political Language, Words That Succeed and Policies That Fail*. New York: Academic Press.

Fisher, Roger; and William Ury. 1981. *Getting to Yes: Negotiating Agreement Without Giving In*. New York: Penguin Books.

Glassman, Amanda; Michael R. Reich; Kayla Laserson; and Fernando Rojas. 1999. "Political Analysis of Health Reform in the Dominican Republic." *Health Policy and Planning* 14: 115–26.

González-Rossetti, Alejandra; and Thoams J. Bossert. 2000. *Enhancing the Political Feasibility of Health Reform: A Comparative Analysis of Chile, Colombia, and Mexico*. Boston, MA: Harvard School of Public Health/Data for Decision Making Project, June.

Grindle, Merilee S.; and John W. Thomas. 1991. *Public Choices and Policy Change: The Political Economy of Reform in Development Countries*. Baltimore, MD: Johns Hopkins University Press.

Gutmann, Amy; and Dennis Thompson. 1996. *Democracy and Disagreement*. Cambridge, MA: Belknap Press of the Harvard University Press.

Heclo, Hugh. 1974. *Modern Social Politics in Britain and Sweden*. New Haven, CT: Yale University Press.

Heifetz, Ronald A. 1994. *Leadership Without Easy Answers*. Cambridge, MA: Belknap Press of Harvard University Press.

Jimenez de la Jara, Jorge; and Thomas T. Bossert. 1999. "Chile's Health Sector Reform: Lessons from Four Reform Periods." In: Peter A. Berman, ed., *Health Sector Reform in Developing Countries: Making Health Development Sustainable*. Boston: Harvard School of Public Health. Distributed by Harvard University Press, 199–214.

Johnson, Haynes; and David S. Broder. 1996. *The System: The American Way of Politics at the Breaking Point*. Boston, MA: Little, Brown.

Kingdon, John W. 1995. *Agendas, Alternatives, and Public Policies*. 2nd edition. New York: HarperCollins.

Kuhn, Thomas S. 1962. *Structure of Scientific Revolutions*. Chicago: University of Chicago Press.

Landy, Marc K.; Marc J. Roberts; and Stephen R. Thomas. 1994. *The Environmental Protection Agency: Asking the Wrong Questions from Nixon to Clinton*. Expanded ed. New York: Oxford University Press.

Lindblom, Charles E. 1965. *The Intelligence of Democracy: Decision Making Through Mutual Adjustment*. New York: Free Press.

Majone, Giandomenico. 1989. *Evidence, Argument and Persuasion in the Policy Process*. New Haven, CT: Yale University Press.

Marmor, Theodore R.; and David Thomas. 1972. "Doctors, Politics and Pay Disputes: 'Pressure Group Politics' Revisited." *British Journal of Political Science* 2: 421–41.

Matthews, Jessica T. 1997. "Power Shift." *Foreign Affairs* 76(1): 50–66.

Nandakumar, A. K.; Michael R. Reich; Mukesh Chawla; Peter Berman; and Winnie Yip. 2000. "Health Reform for Children: The Egyptian Experience with School Health Insurance." *Health Policy* 50: 155–70.

Olson, Mancur. 1965. *The Logic of Collective Action: Public Goods and the Theory of Groups*. Cambridge, MA: Harvard University Press.

Ramírez, Claudio Arce; Julia Li Vargas; Luis Bernardo Sáenz Delgado; Ana Lorena Solís Guevara; María Isabel Solís Ramírez; Thomas Bossert; Alejandra González; and Michael Reich. 1998. *Ejercicio de Mapeo Político de Tres Opciones de Política de Desconcentración de Los Servicios de La Caja Costarricense de Seguro Social*. San Jose, Costa Rica: Caja Costarricense de Seguro Social, December.

Reich, Michael R. 1994a. "The Political Economy of Health Transitions in the Third World." In: Lincoln C. Chen, Arthur Kleinman, and Norma C. Ware, eds., *Health and Social Change in International Perspective*. Boston, MA: Harvard School of Public Health, 413–51.

――― 1994b. "Bangladesh Pharmaceutical Policy and Politics." *Health Policy and Planning* 9(2): 130–43.

――― 1995. "The Politics of Agenda-Setting in International Health: Child Health Versus Adult Health in Developing Countries." *Journal of International Development* 7: 489–502.

――― 1996. "Applied Political Analysis for Health Policy Reform." *Current Issues in Public Health* 2: 186–91.

――― 1997. "Review of *World Development Report: Investing in Health* (New York: Oxford University Press, 1993)." *Economic Development and Cultural Change* 45: 899–903.

Reich, Michael R.; and David M. Cooper. 1996. *PolicyMaker: Computer-Assisted Political Analysis*. Software and Manual. Brookline, MA: PoliMap. (http://www.polimap.com)

Reichenbach, Laura Jean. 1999. *The Politics of Priority Setting: Reproductive Cancers in Ghana*. Doctoral dissertation. Boston, MA: Harvard School of Public Health.

Rochefort, David A.; and Roger W. Cobb, eds. 1995. *The Politics of Problem Definition: Shaping the Policy Agenda*. Lawrence, KS: University Press of Kansas.

Schattschneider, E. E. 1960. *The Semi-Sovereign People: A Realist's View of Democracy in America*. New York: Holt, Rinehart, and Winston.

Seif El Dawla, Aida. 1999. "The Political and Legal Struggle Over Female Genital Mutilation in Egypt: Five Years Since ICPD." *Reproductive Health Matters* 7(13): 128–36.

Simon, Herbert A. 1957. *Models of Man: Social and Rational: Mathematical Essays on Rational Human Behavior in a Social Setting*. New York: Wiley.

Starr, Paul. 1995. "What Happened to Health Care Reform?" *The American Prospect* Winter: 20–31.

Strom, Stephanie. 1999. "Japan's Legislators Tighten the Ban on Under-Age Sex." *The New York Times*, May 19.

UNICEF (United Nations Children's Fund). 1985. *The State of the World's Children 1985*. New York: Oxford University Press.

Wildavsky, Aaron. 1979. *Speaking Truth to Power: The Art and Craft of Policy Analysis*. Boston, MA: Little, Brown.

World Bank. 1993. *World Development Report: Investing in Health*. New York: Oxford University Press.

World Health Organization. 2000. *The World Health Report 2000. Health Systems: Improving Performance*. Geneva: World Health Organization.

5

Goals for Evaluating Health Systems

How can we go from the philosophical discussion of Chapter 3 to judgments about the performance of a health-care system? Adherents of different ethical theories may well endorse different criteria for evaluating that performance—or differ about the importance of achieving various performance goals. Does that mean that all we can say about such judgments is, "It depends?"

While all performance judgments are value-relative, we believe that, as a practical matter, health-sector reformers will generally find it useful to focus on a limited number of performance goals to define problems and to evaluate solutions. In this chapter we propose such a set of *performance goals*; namely, *(1)* the health status of the population, *(2)* the satisfaction citizens derive from the system, and *(3)* the degree to which citizens are protected from the financial risks of ill health (see Figure 2.2). We will discuss how these goals can be measured and how a nation's performance can be evaluated. We also explore how the connections between the health sector and the rest of the society influence performance judgments. In particular, we will argue that cost considerations and social values and political processes both do and should play a role in setting the agenda for health-sector reform.

In what follows we first discuss how to choose performance goals. Next we explain and defend the particular goals we have proposed. Then we explore the fiscal and political connections between the health sector and the larger social and economic arena. We reserve for the next chapter discussion of what we call "intermediate performance measures"—like efficiency and quality—that help determine performance on the ultimate goals we discuss here. Throughout, we assume that someone is thinking about health-sector reform, and our advice is directed at the decisions and choices that such an individual has to make.

Our proposal is, of course, influenced by our personal judgments, experience, and values. Picking performance goals is not a mechanical process. Since we cannot escape the force of our own ethical concerns, we try to acknowledge these as we proceed, so that those with different views can still use our framework to pose evaluative questions clearly and explicitly.

Choosing and Using Performance Goals

To pick performance goals sensibly, an analyst has to know their purpose. For example, the WHO's recent *World Health Report* ranked all countries' health-care systems on a single scale. This required constructing a small number of numerical measures for each country that could then be combined via a simple formula. Our task is different. We want to identify performance problems for priority attention within the process of health-sector reform. This makes numerical scores less useful, and detailed descriptive data more useful, for our purposes.

To reiterate a point made in Chapter 2, performance measures should reflect the *results*, *consequences*, or *outcomes* of the health sector. This insistence on starting with outcomes is one of the distinctive features of our approach. A reformer can then go on a "diagnostic journey" (see Chapter 7) to determine the causes of that inadequate performance and then devise sensible reform strategies to improve that performance. (The same set of criteria can also be used to evaluate policies once they are implemented.)

In using the term *"problem"* to mean *"performance* problem," we realize that we are calling for a far-from-universal usage. Physicians, for example, often use the word *"problem"* to mean *"cause"*—as when they tell a patient, "Unfortunately, your problem is that you have cancer." Many health-sector reformers also do not formulate their analysis in the way we recommend. When asked, "What is the problem in your country?" they answer in terms of some feature of the system: "We don't have enough primary care," or even in terms of some proposed reform: "We need to introduce social insurance." In contrast, we argue that such statements are actually about potential *causes* of, or potential *remedies* for, performance problems. They are not descriptions of a performance problem itself. We can only know if a nation's physician workforce needs changing or its health-care financing needs to be reorganized if these features of the system are leading to unacceptable results.

This leads to our next question—namely, how can a country's performance be judged in relation to the various goals we have identified? In particular, what parameters or aspects of the distribution of health status, satisfaction, or risk protection should reformers be interested in? Again we propose to make such decisions based on the goal of guiding health-sector reform. In that context, a country's overall average performance on one or two simple summary statistics (e.g., life expectancy) is chiefly useful in the early stages of a health-sector reform effort. For example, a nation's poor performance compared to its neighbors', or to its own past performance, can help mobilize public support for reform.

For these purposes, there is little reason to distinguish among various alternative statistical measures (mean, median, and mode). The differences among them involve specific technical issues that are largely irrelevant to the tasks of focusing political attention or marshalling public support. The same is even truer of measures of variation in outcome within the population. While the "average" has some intuitive meaning to many, few have an intuitive grasp of measures of variation like the standard deviation, the inter-quartile range, or the Gini coefficient (Wagstaff and Van Doorslaer 1993). Hence we do not spend much time discussing such statistical alternatives.

It is also the case that the *equity* of outcomes is often of major interest to reformers (and to international donors). We thus suggest that reformers think in terms of a three-by-two matrix: three performance goals and two ethical tests to apply to each. The first ethical test is a comparison to average performance, and the second is an assessment of the equity of the distribution of performance measures. From a reformer's point of view, the distribution of outcomes—across regional, income or ethnic groups—will generally be the most relevant consideration, rather than some statistical measurement. To guide efforts to improve equity, those who are doing badly (such as those in relatively poor health) need to be identified.

Different nations not only *value* equity differently, they *define* it differently. In some countries any difference in service between rich and poor is seen as a problem (e.g., Denmark: Andersen 1984). Other countries focus on improving the situation of the worst-off, while allowing the top to get more (e.g., Australia: White 1995). Countries also might be more concerned with equity when it comes to some performance goals than others. For example, a nation might be more eager to produce equity in health outcomes than in citizen satisfaction.

To choose a particular set of performance goals is to choose a particular focus for public debate about health-sector reform. How should such decisions be made? Our first proposed criterion is political relevance. As we have worked with governments around the world, certain issues have surfaced again and again. Since, as we discussed in Chapter 4, we believe in both the importance and the legitimacy of politics in the reform process, in our view any performance goals should reflect and embody these major political and social concerns. For such concerns have driven (and are driving) health-sector reform around the world. Reformers should be able to recognize and express both their own and others' major concerns within and through the framework we offer.

Second, performance goals should reflect the main alternative philosophical perspectives on the health system as described in Chapter 3. Unless utilitarians, liberals, and communitarians find their views represented, the framework will not be useful to them. Taken together, the set of measures should capture the critical ethical issues at stake in the reform process. Disagreements on those issues should be expressible in terms of different views about the definition of the goals and about the priority of the various ethical tests to be applied.

Our third basis for choosing goals is causal dependence. We want performance measures that are significantly affected by health-policy choices. For example, while the health sector does influence the overall level of citizens' happiness, such well-being also depends on a wide variety of factors outside health care. On the other hand, satisfaction with the health sector itself largely depends on what happens inside the sector. Hence the second, narrower aspect of satisfaction meets the test of causal dependence while overall levels of happiness do not.

As we will see, putting performance measures into usable form requires many additional decisions about definition, measurement, etc. These decisions, too, will necessarily reflect some particular values and priorities. An honest discussion of these details is thus likely to reveal and provoke further ethical debate—and not everyone will be equally pleased with the ultimate formulation.

Health-Sector Performance Goals

Health Status

The health status of the population is our first performance goal. As the subject of much public debate as well as policymaking, it surely meets the test of political relevance. It also meets the test of philosophical relevance. It embodies the central concern of objective utilitarians—for whom health status is a key component of well-being. It is also a critical aspect of opportunity for many egalitarian liberals. In addition, the health status of the population also meets the test of causal dependence. While other factors (e.g., income and education) affect health status, the operation of the health sector does have a significant impact on health itself.

As noted in Table 5.1, constructing a health status index requires many decisions (Arnesen and Nord 1999, Anand and Hanson 1997). Different nations are likely to make these decisions differently. For example, not all countries will count years of life lost at different ages in the same way, nor place the same relative value on current versus future benefits (i.e., use the same discount rate). We believe, however, that all reformers need to begin by focusing on the health status of the population regardless of how they choose to measure that in detail.

In deciding which health problems should be given priority, a country may want to pay special attention to the diseases that are causing the greatest harm. If a country is losing many of its citizens to alcoholism, or to a rise in tuberculosis, or to neonatal tetanus, then controlling those conditions might well be a focus of reform efforts. Countries where sophisticated measures of disease burden like QALYs or DALYs are not available can begin by targeting conditions whose preva-

TABLE 5.1. Decisions Required to Construct a Health-Status Index

- How important are different kinds of disability and disease? For example, in measuring disability, does only functional impairment matter, or are "silent" physiological conditions also relevant?

- What is the relative value of years of life lost at different ages?

- Do the economically productive or socially valuable matter more than the unemployed or retired?

- What impact, if any, should a person's non-health status have on the value of their life? Are some illnesses less serious when they happen to the wealthy, because the wealthy can buy compensating services?

- Should the public attitudes toward different diseases or causes of death matter? For example, should the fact that the U.S. public is especially eager to avoid cancer deaths affect our valuations of the gains from death prevention?

- How does one combine death and disability? Are the non-disabled's lives more valuable than those of the disabled?

- Are future gains to be "discounted" (i.e., valued less than present gains), and if so, at what rate?

- How is uncertainty addressed? Does one just make the best guess of average effects— and ignore differences in the degree of confidence that these will occur—or should one not be so risk-neutral?

lence is higher than in other comparable countries or compared to their own past performance. (The question of whether a country can do anything about such problems is also relevant to its priorities, as we discuss below.)

Reformers who are concerned about the equity of the distribution of health status need information about the variation of health outcomes across the population. For example, are certain regions, ethnic groups or socio-economic strata doing worse on life expectancy or maternal mortality than others (e.g., tribal peoples in India or the island provinces in Malaysia)? In effect, this process uses the country's own average performance as a *benchmark* for identifying performance problems that need attention. (We will elaborate on the various forms of benchmarking when we discuss priority setting in general.)

Once disparities have been identified, nations then have to decide how important it is to correct them. How important is it to improve the lot of those with the worst health status, compared to improving the experience of citizens more toward the middle of the distribution? For example, in China the rural poor have noticeably worse health (Ministry of Health, PRC 1999). But they are often seen as less important politically and economically than urban workers. How should such attitudes affect health-sector policymaking? Similarly, what importance should countries give to helping their disadvantaged ethnic minorities like the Roma in Central Europe (Ringold 2000, Puportka and Zadori 1998) or the tribal peoples in India (Peters et al. 2002), who often have life expectancies five years (or more) below the national average and infant and maternal mortality rates that are twice the national average? Answers to such questions inevitably will be shaped by each nation's values and political process.

As egalitarian liberals we think there are strong ethical arguments for paying special attention to the health of those whose health status is particularly poor. And sometimes extending basic services to the underserved is an efficient way to improve overall (average) health status. Primary care can be very cost-effective. Indeed, some countries with noticeably unequal levels of service across geographic areas (e.g., Turkey) have lower average health status than similar countries (e.g., Chile) with more equal health spending (WHO 1996). This is because of what economists call "diminishing returns." At the margin, the gains from spending more on those who have the most are often less than the gains that could be realized by spending more on those who have the least.

On the other hand, these arguments will not always be true, or if true will not always be compelling. Groups with the poorest health status can be especially difficult to serve. They may live in remote areas or struggle with a variety of social and economic handicaps. In Nepal, for example, there are villages that are several days' walk from the nearest health post. Moreover, not every country's leadership shares our particular values. And various political considerations—from pleasing national elites to placating politically powerful urban workers—can produce pressures to spend even more on care for those who are already well served.

But our views about health equity are not what matters. Reformers need to clarify *their commitments* on these issues, in order to know what problems to focus on and what reforms to advocate. Is it acceptable for the rich to buy better care for themselves, as long as the poor have access to some minimum? Does "fairness" require the state to pay for the poor to have access to the same expensive, life-saving technology that the rich do, even if that technology is not a cost-effective way to produce health status gains? And just how important is it to help the worst off, even if doing so is expensive? In poor countries, where resources by definition are very limited, these can be especially difficult questions. Nevertheless, reformers must seek answers to them to decide how to react to the distribution of health status in their country.

Citizen Satisfaction

Our second performance goal is the degree to which citizens are satisfied with the services provided by the health sector. Philosophically, such a goal is in keeping with the subjective utilitarian view favored by economists. Politically, the system's inability to provide what citizens want is often a significant driver of reform. Moreover, this goal allows us to capture various features of the health system, apart from its impact on health status. For example, how accessible and service-oriented is the care process? By using satisfaction as a performance goal we take account of how citizens themselves evaluate and respond to their care.

Here our approach again departs from the recent WHO formulation, which considers only "legitimate" satisfactions (Murray and Frenk 1999). Our reasons for rejecting that approach are both philosophical and practical. Philosophically, satisfaction is a subjective utilitarian concern. Within that framework, there is no basis for assessing someone else's satisfactions according to our view of their "legitimacy." Furthermore, citizens' satisfaction with the health-care system is likely to depend interactively on various features of that system. For example, many are more willing to tolerate poor service when the care they receive is clinically excellent. In such cases we cannot divide up "satisfaction" and then attribute parts of that total to various bits and pieces of the consumer's experience.

Countries may face tradeoffs between increasing satisfaction, as we have defined it, and achieving other goals. For example, patients might get satisfaction from inappropriate care—like unneeded injections. Responding to such desires can lead a nation to have both lower health status and higher costs than it otherwise would. And those with poor health habits might argue that no effort should be made to change their behavior since those habits increase their own satisfaction. The decision to suppress or avoid such conflicts (by removing what some reformer believes are "illegitimate" satisfactions before making tradeoff decisions) seems to us an awkward and obscurantist approach. Instead, if reformers in a particular country decide for various reasons *not* to respond to certain citizen desires, political accountability requires them to say so explicitly and argue openly for their choices.

Measuring satisfaction—however defined—is not easy. The economist's solution is to try to determine individuals' *willingness to pay* for various kinds of benefits (Weinstein et al. 1996). For example, to put a value on human life, individuals have been asked hypothetical questions about their willingness to take specified risks in return for various payments (so-called contingent valuation studies: Hammitt 2000). These studies have revealed systematic inconsistencies between the behavior that decision theory says is rational and typical patterns of choice. For example, sick people may rate their quality of life as higher than when they were well (Rosser et al. 1992).

An alternative approach to determining satisfaction is to use some sort of customer survey—asking people what they do and do not like about their health care (Cleary 1999). Such surveys do not yield monetary values that are directly comparable to cost estimates. But they can provide valuable guidance to reformers, particularly if they elicit information about specific services or features of the system. Such studies do face certain technical problems (like the tendency of respondents, especially low-status respondents, to answer "yes" to questions). But extensive work has been done in both Europe and the United States to develop and validate reliable survey instruments (Coutler and Cleary 2001).

Judging a nation's performance with regard to satisfaction also involves equity considerations. Are gains in satisfaction to the happy and the unhappy equally important? Here again there are likely to be differences among the adherents to different philosophies. Subjective utilitarians, whose thinking is rooted in economics, will generally argue that total satisfaction—and not its distribution—matters. For egalitarian liberals, a situation in which some are much more satisfied with how they are treated than others would violate notions of equal respect. They would be particularly interested in improving the lot of the groups in the population that are especially unsatisfied.

In summary, we believe that improving citizen satisfaction with the health system should be an important performance goal, despite the need to resolve various methodological and philosophical issues to make these judgments. Citizen satisfaction is heavily influenced by the system, widely discussed, philosophically grounded, and politically relevant. The relevant concern, we have argued, should be *all* reactions of citizens, regardless of whether experts like these reactions or not. Of course, when this goal conflicts with other goals, or when citizens' reactions are ethically problematic, those issues will have to be addressed directly by health reformers who are trying to make priority judgments or evaluate national performance.

Financial Risk Protection

Financial risk protection is a major goal of much health-sector policy-making and frequently a focus of the politics of health reform. It is also greatly influenced by how the sector is financed. In addition, preventing financial impoverishment—and its associated loss of opportunity—is philosophically important to egalitarian liberals. For them, ensuring everyone a minimum level of economic opportunity is as important as preventing early disability or death. In short, there are compelling reasons for including financial risk protection as a critical performance goal.

Providing financial risk protection, however, does not allow the population to avoid all the costs of health care. In fact, that cannot be done. Foreign aid aside, all health-care costs in a country are ultimately paid for by its citizens—directly or indirectly. It is simply not possible to protect those in the middle of a country's income distribution against the costs of routine medical care. If they don't pay those costs directly, they will do so indirectly via various taxes. What is relevant for achieving risk protection is helping people avoid the large and unpredictable costs of a serious illness—that is, to provide a risk-spreading or insurance function, where revenues from citizens are pooled and used to pay for care for those who do get seriously ill.

Measuring financial risk is complicated by the fact that the significance of a given risk depends on both the size of the risk and the economic status (income and assets) of the person incurring the risk. The closer someone is to the poverty level, the smaller the expense that will put them below that line. Hence the more they need financial risk protection.

An additional complication is that financial risk can also affect health status. The seriously ill may not receive adequate care if the financial burden on them contributes to a decision not to seek care. Their injury from a lack of risk protection, therefore, may show up as diminished health status and not as a financial loss.

How can the extent of financial risk protection be described? The simplest data—on the extent of insurance coverage, for instance—are only partially informative, since some nations (e.g., India, Egypt, and many in Eastern Europe) only provide limited health insurance. Instead, they rely more on free (or nearly free) health care in government facilities. Such systems provide some risk protection, depending on the accessibility and quality of the services and the costs that patients have to bear (including medicines, supplies, and any under-the-table payments). When consumers don't fully trust the public sector, however, they may feel compelled to purchase private care when illness occurs, with potentially serious implications for their financial situation (Berman 1998; Nandakumar et al. 2000).

Insurance coverage, moreover, is not a "yes-or-no" variable. Those with only limited insurance may still face significant financial risks when serious illness occurs. (For utilitarians, it is also possible for some citizens to have "too much" insurance in ways that can encourage the cost-ineffective use of care: Gilied 2001.)

We propose to judge the extent of risk protection by the probability (before the fact) or the frequency (after the fact) that individuals will be impoverished by illness or prevented from obtaining adequate treatment by their lack of income. A financing system does well on this criterion when such events are unlikely at the individual level and hence rare in the population. This measure combines both the size of the risk and the individual's economic condition. From an equity perspective, variations in this probability across population groups are critically relevant for deciding on priorities for expanding risk protection. Indeed, it is exactly such risks that have led many middle-income countries in recent years (from Colombia to Taiwan: Colombia Health Sector Reform Project 1996; Lu and Hsiao 2003) to institute or expand social insurance systems.

The measure we have proposed does not take account of the public's satisfaction with the available level of risk protection. Instead, those reactions will be captured through consideration of citizens' overall satisfaction with the health system. Similarly, the effects of a lack of risk protection on health status are reflected in the distribution of health status.

Determining levels of financial risk defined in this way requires household survey data on health care utilization and expenditures. Such studies can be expensive and difficult, especially in poor countries. But a reformer interested in making a careful assessment of national performance on this goal must be prepared to support such research.

Health-Sector Performance in Relationship to the Larger Social and Economic System

In order to complete our analysis of health-sector performance, we have to take account of the fact that health policy both influences and is influenced by the larger social and economic system. Governments do many things in the domestic policy arena apart from health; let's call these activities the "social and economic policy system." The relationships between that system and the health sector are rather complicated. All the variables in each system potentially affect all the variables in the other. In particular, policy decisions act both directly to influence health and non-health performance goals, and indirectly through their impact on various characteristics of the system like efficiency or access. In addition, all these variables are themselves influenced by a variety of more general factors, which include politics, culture, history, and institutions.

These interactions flow in both directions. For example, tobacco taxes imposed to lower smoking could adversely affect economic growth in tobacco-growing regions. Conversely, general social and economic policy developments (for example, a government's commitment to regionalization) can lead to changes in the health sector. Simply put, health-sector policy cannot be evaluated in isolation.

To take account of these connections between the health sector and the rest of the society, two major factors need to inform health-sector policymaking. One is the cost of the system, since that affects the burden the health sector imposes on society and how much money the society has to pursue other goals. The other factor involves the relationship of reform to community norms and cultural practices in the society and the ways these are expressed through the political process.

The Role of Cost in Problem Definition

In Chapter 1 we suggested that the worldwide context for health-sector reform frequently involves a clash within a country between rising costs and rising expectations on one hand, and a limited capacity to pay on the other. Indeed, it is often not the *level* of cost, but sudden *changes* in cost—or even changes in the rate of increase of cost—that attracts political attention. The result of such attention, however, is some form of perceived *cost–performance dilemma*.

International data show that the same level of health spending yields strikingly different results in different countries. Some nations get good results with much lower levels of spending than others. Therefore, spending more money (while it can be helpful) may not be either necessary or sufficient to improve health-sector performance. For example, the existing management system and organizational structure in a country might be such that better performance could be gotten out of existing resources. It might even be the case that added funds would be largely

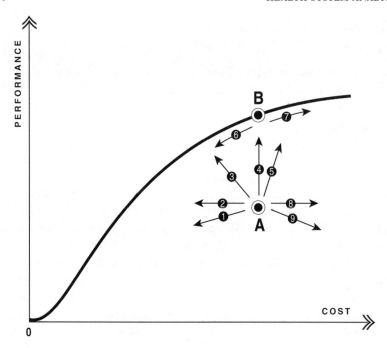

FIGURE 5.1. Cost–performance dilemmas.

wasted, so that the capacity to absorb additional revenue first has to be increased, if more money is to produce better outcomes.

Cost is one major connection between the health sector and the larger social and economic system. In the short run, the amount available for health may be a residual—determined by the country's economy and by other government programs and expenditures. The availability of public funds may be a constraint reformers have to respond to. From a longer-run point of view, however, financing arrangements are not fixed. Reformers can develop schemes for mobilizing new resources either in general (e.g., new social insurance schemes) or for targeted purposes (like user fees in rural hospitals). But again, any money spent on health is money that is not available for other purposes. Such tradeoffs are at the heart of any nation's cost–performance dilemma.

Cost–performance dilemmas can take various forms. Most health systems are not fully efficient. Hence, they are in the situation represented by point A in Figure 5.1, where more performance is possible from current spending. Such nations then face five choices about how to change the relationship between cost and performance, as illustrated by the arrows in the diagram:

1. Accept somewhat reduced performance in order to significantly reduce cost
2. Save as much as possible without reducing outcomes
3. Improved efficiency to both lower cost and raise performance

4. Maximize performance for the current budget
5. Improve performance to such an extent that more money is required.

Consider some specific examples. Countries like Armenia or Tajikistan, in the aftermath of war or civil disorder, may find it necessary to focus on cost reduction, as shown by 1 or 2 in Figure 5.1 (Feachem et al. 1999). On the other hand, countries like Brazil or Russia, which are growing, may be primarily concerned with improving performance—even if cost rises somewhat, as shown by 4 or 5 (Wines and Zuger 2000).

In addition, Figure 5.1 illustrates the choices open to a nation that is fully efficient (i.e., at point B)—a case we believe is uncommon. In that situation, cost and performance have to go up and down together (changes 6 and 7 in the diagram).

In the real world, moreover, changes like 8 sometimes occur. Then the cost increases without any improved performance—for example, when there are political pressures to increase patronage employment. Even moves like 9—when costs go up and performance goes down—are known to occur. Anecdotal evidence suggests that new regulatory controls in recent years have done just that in the U.S. Medicare system.

Different players in the health reform debate often differ about the nature of the cost-performance dilemma facing their country. Ministries of finance often argue that the nation is at point A and a change like 3—more performance *and* lower cost— is required. The ministry of health in contrast tends to argue that the system is at point B and that move 6—more spending for more health—is the only appropriate response. Admitting that the country is at A can be difficult for the health ministry precisely because it reflects on how poorly it is carrying out its responsibilities.

Different aspects of cost tend to become the focus of attention in different contexts. Governments often look only at their own budget costs. On the other hand, even in poor countries, a substantial part of health expenditures comes directly from patients. Hence looking solely at government spending is not sufficient if we are interested in the total burden that the health sector places on the society. Indeed, a comprehensive assessment would include non-money costs, like the time and effort expended by patients and family members, for that is part of the overall economic burden (the *opportunity cost*) of the health sector. In fact, even detailed studies of National Health Accounts do not capture such non-money costs (Sauerborn et al. 1995, Popkin and Doan 1990).

How can a country know whether the cost of its health sector is appropriate? One approach is to compare the gain from spending more *outside* the health sector with the gain from spending more *inside*. Subjective utilitarians would say that the measuring rod for comparing such gains should be changes in consumer satisfaction. In contrast, objective utilitarians have to formulate an index to measure gains from both health and non–health-sector activities. Then, they must ask whether the increases in health, which would come from spending more on health, were worth more or less than the loss that would result from spending less on some other goal (e.g., environmental protection or education).

Whichever method is used, the broader the scope of the analysis, the more difficult it becomes to compare gains and losses. It is difficult enough to decide how to trade physical pain and suffering against the cognitive distortions of mental illness in order to evaluate shifting budget resources from trauma care to mental health. But it is even more difficult to decide how to trade either of these against the gains from expanded primary education, or from increased protection for endangered species.

In practice, societies answer such questions incrementally, by changing spending levels and financing arrangements step by step in search of a reasonable balance. Such decisions are especially difficult when a country is unable to finance a health-care system that will achieve its health-status goals. Unfortunately, this is the situation today in many low- and middle-income countries. Here again, we believe that responsible reformers need to take the lead in telling citizens the truth about the choices they face and in shaping effective social responses. Not all problems can be solved in a world where resources and knowledge are always limited.

Analyzing the Distribution of Costs

From the point of view of setting health sector reform priorities, not only the level of costs, but also their distribution is of major significance. Such distributive issues are often a focus of intense political concern. Such issues are often misunderstood, however, and in fact they are far more obscure than is commonly supposed. Still, this is yet another area in which each nation has to make its own ethical judgments—in this case, about how "pro-poor" it wants its health-care financing system to be.

The first difficulty in accounting for the financing burden of the health sector is that the person who pays a tax may not ultimately bear the burden of it. For example, an employer's social insurance contribution is likely to result in some combination of lower wages to employees, lower profits to owners and higher prices to customers. Determining how the burden of a particular tax is "shifted" will generally require sophisticated statistical research (Gruber 1997, Gruber 1994). On the other hand, the politics of health-sector finance often ignore these complexities as interest groups focus on imposing the responsibility for direct payment on each other.

There are additional complications. Increases in government health spending are sometimes financed by cuts in other government programs. The new activities in effect are paid for by those who lose benefits from curtailed programs. Furthermore, in many countries some or all health expenditures come from general government funds, which rely on many different sources of revenue. But then how can we know which programs are smaller than they would be, or which taxes higher than they would be, because of health expenditures (Rosen 2001)?

In practice it is often easier to answer such questions if we are interested in the *marginal* effect of adjustments in spending—rather than the distribution of the total burden of health spending. It is seldom possible to answer the question "What would all prices, incomes, and tax burdens be like in the economy if the government did away with *all* health spending?" For health system reformers, however, the more tractable marginal question is often more relevant. It is, after all, the incremental effects of any change in the financing system that are likely to provoke an especially strong political response. Moreover, some cost burdens are not that obscure or difficult to analyze—notably the distribution of out-of-pocket costs. And such spending is the proximate cause of financial risk—and of the need for risk protection. On the other hand, technically simplistic, but politically powerful, discussions of the fairness of the entire financing scheme do regularly occur.

In evaluating the distribution of costs, economists tend to focus on what happens to various income groups—a concept they call "vertical equity" (Pechman 1985). For complex historical reasons, the critical reference point for such an analysis is a tax that takes the same *percentage* of income from the poor as the rich. Such a tax is called "proportional." A tax that falls more heavily on the rich (i.e., one that takes a higher proportion of their income) is called "progressive." One that takes a higher percentage of income from the poor is called "regressive."

User fees and insurance premiums are obviously quite regressive. They take the same amount of money from rich and poor, resulting in a much greater burden, in percentage terms, on the poor. (Do note, however, the rich can pay higher taxes than the poor under a regressive system—even if such taxes are a lower proportion of their income.) Social insurance schemes, financed by payroll taxes, are slightly regressive. Earned income (as opposed to investment income) is a greater percentage of all income at lower income levels. Hence a tax on earned income takes a higher percentage of total income from those at lower income. In addition, many nations have an upper limit on the total payroll taxes paid by an individual. This limit significantly increases the system's regressivity. Sales or value-added taxes are also modestly regressive (depending on what, if any, goods are exempt from taxation), since consumption is a higher percentage of income at lower income levels. Only taxes on luxury goods or comprehensive income taxes—where the marginal rates increase—are progressive. On the other hand, even moderately regressive schemes for financing the health sector can be redistributive—if the rich pay more than the cost of the services they receive and the poor less.

To take account of such possibilities, we urge reformers when they are evaluating the distribution of health-care costs to simultaneously take account of the distribution of benefits. For example, in countries with poorly functioning public finance systems, locally collected (and retained) revenues may be the only reliable way to finance increased services in rural areas. When based on user fees, the financing of such schemes is quite regressive. But that is only half the story—improved service being the other half. Egalitarian liberal concerns (that no one be pushed below some minimum level of economic opportunity) can be addressed by exempting the poorest of the poor from such fees.

Economists also analyze financial burden in terms of "horizontal equity." This concept says that people at the same economic level should be treated the same. In the health-reform context, the largest issues in this regard tend to be regional. If a country shifts the financing of health care to local or regional levels, poorer areas need to pay higher taxes to provide the same level of service as richer areas. This is why some schemes for fiscal decentralization (e.g., in Chile) also include an interregional equalization fund. Similarly, since the cost of providing services to scattered rural communities is typically higher, local financing means that rural areas must either pay more or get less. Economists argue such interregional variations violate the principle of horizontal equity. Certain other taxes—on cigarettes or alcohol, for example—can also raise horizontal equity issues. They not only burden selected consumers, but also can have a disproportionate impact on farmers, workers, and businessmen who are part of the taxed industries.

The Cultural Context and the Political Process

The second major connection between health-sector reform and the larger political and social system lies in the values and politics of each specific community. Again, like matters of cost, these forces can be constraints in the short run and modifiable in the longer run. Such interactions are likely to arise in three different contexts: *(1)* in the definition of the performance goals and the relative importance assigned to them—which in turn leads to reform priorities, *(2)* in the reform strategies a nation chooses, and *(3)* in the detailed design of specific policies.

When it comes to defining and prioritizing goals, we have noted above that many apparently technical issues—like how to measure health status—involve value choices. Moreover, as we discussed in Chapter 4, the process of setting reform priorities is always political, involving the tug-of-war of issue entrepreneurs, cultural taboos, and economic and political interest groups.

For those with an economics or mathematics background, the following formulation may help. Performance goals can be viewed as the axes of a diagram defining a "health-sector performance space." But to actually make judgments among alternative outcomes also requires an "objective function" that ranks or compares various outcomes in that space (Edwards and Newman 1986). In practice, that ranking emerges from each country's political system—as influenced by reformers, advocates and political leaders, each acting on their own combination of ethical principles and personal interests. Thus views about equity, about risk, and about the importance of objective health versus subjective satisfaction will and should be played out in the process of setting objectives and assigning reform priorities.

The second way culture and politics enter the reform process is through the broad strategies that countries consider in the policy design process. Is government trusted or not? Are private markets applicable to health care? Can we tax the rich at high levels? Do programs have to be uniform everywhere in the country? Can we trust local governments even—or especially—if these come under the control of ethnic minorities or political opponents?

Broad cultural and political attitudes are likely to be deeply embedded in political discourse and decision-making—in ways that even thoughtful activists may not realize. They reflect broad "strategies" or "standard operating procedures" that have evolved over time in the nation's political system and are not easily modified. Of course, a severe enough crisis can lead to assumptions' being questioned or old rules' being revised. But the energy and effort required to do so may be substantial. Hence, such constraints on what policy is considered will do a great deal to shape the health-sector reform debate. For example, privatizing the formerly public ambulatory-care system was easy to do in Slovakia, but is not even on the agenda in Sri Lanka—reflecting their different histories and cultural attitudes.

The third connection between culture and politics and health-sector reform arises because societies have numerous customs and taboos that directly influence the health sector. The list of potentially relevant cultural norms is far too long to present inclusively, but here are some examples. First, there are beliefs related to issues of life and death, including abortion, resuscitation, and physician-assisted suicide. Second, there are customs related to the use of various substances, from tobacco and alcohol to caffeine and cocaine. Third are norms about sexuality, from prohibitions of homosexual or premarital sex, to views on prostitution and contraception. Many societies also have views about how the body itself (alive or dead) should be treated, which shape the acceptability of practices ranging from transfusion to male circumcision. In Buddhist nations, for example, where the predominant definition of death is "heart death" not "brain death," there is a real shortage of organs for transplantation (Lock 1995).

Broader social dynamics also affect health status—ranging from intra-familial patterns of food distribution (e.g., adult males eat first) to gender-based variations in medical care utilization. Social norms about the role of Western biomedicine also impact the system in many countries. The list goes on and on: the role of traditional birth attendants, whether men and women can be treated by doctors of the opposite sex, the willingness of patients to talk openly to doctors. In evaluating any proposed policy, reformers need to consider the extent to which it would violate such norms, and what that means for its political feasibility and implementability. Hard work can sometimes get controversial policies adopted politically, and creative social marketing efforts (as we will discuss in Chapter 12) can change attitudes. Cultural constraints are therefore somewhat elastic, but they always exist and always need to be considered.

How far reformers go to respect local customs is likely to depend on their ethical perspective. For relative communitarians, local customs and values should be central to any country's health policy. For liberals, individuals should be free to follow traditional customs, if they truly want to. But it is the individual choice, not the community norm, that is worthy of respect. Hence community norms that restrict freedom or opportunity (e.g., the Taliban's opposition to girls' education) can be opposed by egalitarian liberals. For subjective utilitarians, if observing custom increases someone's utility, then that individual should be free to do so. But again, unlike communitarians, and like liberals, for subjective utilitarians custom is a means, not an end in itself. Objective utilitarians are likely to be even more goal-directed—respecting local custom only insofar as doing so increases health status (e.g., by facilitating increased patient compliance).

One set of "customs" we need to call special attention to are current Western views about patient choice and informed consent. These call for patients to make all crucial treatment decisions, and to do so on the basis of complete disclosure by the doctor of the patient's diagnosis and the consequences of different ways of proceeding. Advocates for the universal applicability of such norms argue that treating patients in this way respects their fundamental human rights. Relative communitarians, in contrast, see these norms as a particular cultural practice, and believe they should be followed only in countries where they are widely accepted. In certain East Asian societies, for example, elderly patients are seldom told of a fatal diagnosis, nor would it occur to these patients, their doctors, or their families to have those patients make all the critical decisions about their care.

While nations will have to make their own decisions on this (and all other) ethical issues, one possible compromise is to respect patient choice either where that is the custom in the society, or where a particular patient—contrary to local custom—wants to exercise such choice. Where neither of these conditions is met, and both the society and individual are comfortable with other ways of proceeding, we believe that reformers should not substitute their own judgments or standards for the ones that appeal to the patients and doctors working in a particular national system.

Summary

In this chapter we have presented the case for judging a health sector's performance in terms of three performance goals—health status, citizen satisfaction, and risk protection. Furthermore, we have argued that two kinds of tests or judgments need to be applied to evaluate a nation's achievements in each of these areas—both a country's average performance and how that country does on equity grounds. Insofar as recent international concern with poverty alleviation and meeting basic needs is shared by a country, the equity issue will be of increased importance. We have also argued that in making equity judgments, relatively detailed data on the distribution of outcomes by region, income, and ethnicity are likely to be of critical importance.

We have also explored the connection between the health sector—and judgments about its performance—and the larger social and economic system. We have focused on two such connections: the cost of the health sector, and the influence of social and political processes on health-sector reform. We have contended that any judgment about performance should be reached taking these two kinds of connections into account. As we have stressed repeatedly, costs (and cost increases) often provoke reform. Culture and politics shape problem definition, priority setting, and the kinds of options that a nation can realistically consider.

We noted previously that this focus on ultimate performance does reflect a "paradigm shift" in the way health-sector reform is discussed. Historically, such conversations have not focused on such variables, but instead on structural features of the system or on variables like "efficiency" or "quality" or "access." We believe that such terms are best understood as referring to what we call "intermediate performance measures." Such characteristics of the system help determine the level of performance on system goals, but are not themselves ultimate objectives. Because these "intermediate" variables are both widely discussed and can play a helpful role in the diagnostic process, we will next explore their meaning and role in some detail.

References

Anand, Sudhir; and Kara Hanson. 1997. "Disability-Adjusted Life Years: A Critical Review." *Journal of Health Economics* 16(6): 685–702.

Andersen, B. Rold. 1984. "Rationality and Irrationality of the Nordic Welfare State." *Daedalus* 113(1): 109–39.

Arnesen, Trude; and Erik Nord. 1999. "The Value of DALY Life: Problems with Ethics and the Validity of Disability Adjusted Life Years." *British Medical Journal* 319: 1423–5.

Berman, Peter. 1998. "Rethinking Health Care Systems: Private Health Care Provision in India." *World Development* 26(8): 1463–79.

Cleary, Paul D. 1999. "The Increasing Importance of Patient Surveys." *British Medical Journal* 319: 720–1.

Colombia Health Sector Reform Project. 1996. *Report on Colombia Health Sector Reform and Proposed Master Implementation Plan, Final Report.* Boston, MA: School of Public Health, Harvard University.

Coulter, Angela; and Paul D. Cleary. 2001. "Patients' Experience of Hospital Care in Five Countries." *Health Affairs* 20(3): 244–52.

Edwards, Ward; and J. Robert Newman. 1986. "Multiattribute Evaluation." In: Terry Connolly, Hal R. Arkes, and Kenneth R. Hammond, eds., *Judgment and Decision Making: An Interdisciplinary Reader.* New York: Cambridge University Press.

Feachem, Zwana; Martin Henscher; and Laura Rose, eds. 1999. *Implementing Health Sector Reform in Central Asia: Papers from a Health Policy Seminar Held in Ashgabat, Turkmenistan, in June 1996.* Economic Development Institute. Washington, DC: World Bank.

Gilied, Sherry A. 2001. "Health Insurance and Market Failure." *Journal of Health Politics, Policy, and Law* 26(5): 957–65.

Gruber, Jonathan. 1994. "The Incidence of Mandated Maternity Benefits." *American Economic Review* 84(3): 622–41.

———— 1997. "The Incidence of Payroll Taxation: Evidence from Chile." *Journal of Labor Economics* 15(3): S72–101.

Hammitt, James K. 2000. "Valuing Mortality Risk: Theory and Practice" *Environmental Science and Technology* 34(8): 1396–1400.

Lock, Margaret. 1995. "Contesting the Natural in Japan: Moral Dilemmas and Technologies of Dying." *Culture, Medicine and Psychiatry* 19(1): 1–38.

Lu, Jui-Fen Rachel; and William C. Hsiao. 2003. "Does Universal Health Insurance Make Health Care Unaffordable? Lessons From Taiwan." *Health Affairs* 22(3): 77–88.

Ministry of Health, PRC. 1999. *Reports on the 1998 National Health Services Survey Results.* Beijing, China: Ministry of Health, Center for Health Statistics and Information.

Murray, Christopher J. L.; and Julio Frenk. 1999. *A WHO Framework for Assessing the Performance of Health Systems.* Discussion Paper No. 3, Global Programme on Evidence. Geneva: World Health Organization.

Nandakumar, A. K.; Mukesh Chawla; and Maryam Khan. 2000. "Utilization of Outpatient Care in Egypt and Its Implications for the Role of Government in Health Care Provision." *World Development* 28(1): 187–96.

Pechman, Joseph. 1985. *Who Paid the Taxes, 1966–85?* Washington, DC: Brookings Institution.

Peters, David H.; Abdo S. Yazbeck; Rashmi R. Sharma; G.N.V. Ramana; Lant H. Pritchett; and Adam Wagstaff. 2002. *Better Health Systems for India's Poor: Findings, Analysis, and Options.* Health, Nutrition, and Population Series, Human Development Network. Washington, DC: World Bank.

Popkin, Barry M.; and Rebecca M. Doan. 1990. "Women's Roles, Time Allocation and Health." In: John Caldwell, Sally Findley, Pat Caldwell, Gigi Santow, Wendy Cosford, Jennifer Braid, and Daphne Broers-Freeman, eds., *What We Know About Health Transition: The Cultural, Social, and Behavioural Determinants of Health.* Health Transition Series No. 2 (Vol 2). Health Transition Centre, Australian National University.

Puportka, Lajos; and Zsolt Zadori. 1998. *The Health Status of Romas in Hungary.* Budapest: Roma Press Center. Available from www.worldbank.hu/4roma.html. Accessed June 2002.

Ringold, Dena. 2000. *Roma and the Transition in Central and Eastern Europe: Trends and Challenges.* A World Free of Poverty Series (Vol. 1). Washington, DC: World Bank.

Rosen, Harvey S. 2001. *Public Finance.* 6th Edition. Boston, MA: McGraw-Hill/Irwin, 1984.

Rosser, Rachel; Michaela Cottee; Rosalind Rabin; and Caroline Selai. 1992. "Index of Health-Related Quality of Life." In: Anthony Hopkins, ed., *Measures of the Quality of Life.* London: Royal College of Physicians.

Sauerborn, Ralner; Issouf Ibrango; Adrian Nougtara; Matthias Borchert; M. Hein, Justus Benzler; E. Koob; and H. Jochin Diesfeld. 1995. "The Economic Costs of Illness for Rural Households in Burkina Faso." *Tropical Medical Parisitology* 46(1): 54–60.

Wagstaff, Adam; and Eddy van Doorslaer. 1993. "Equity in Refinance of Health Care: Methods and Findings." In: Eddy van Doorslaer, Adam Wagstaff, and Frans Rutten, eds., *Equity in Finance and Delivery of Health Care: An International Perspective.* New York: Oxford University Press.

Weinstein, Milton C.; Joanna E. Siegel; Marthe Gold; Mark S. Kamlet; and Louise B. Russell. 1996. "Recommendations of the Panel on Cost-Effectiveness in Health and Medicine." *JAMA* 276(15): 1253–8.

White, Joseph. 1995. *Competing Solutions, American Health Care Proposals and International Experience*. Washington, DC: Brookings Institute Press.

WHO. 1996. *Health Care Systems in Transition: Turkey*. Copenhagen: World Health Ogranization. Available from www.who.dk/observatory/Hits. Accessed June 2002.

Wines, Michael; with Abigail Zuger. 2000. "In Russia, the Ill and Infirm Include Health Care Itself." *The New York Times*, 4 December.

6

Assessing Health-System Performance

Experience teaches us that when a health-sector reformer seeks to understand the causes of unsatisfactory outcomes, certain aspects of the system often play an important role. These features of the system are not in themselves either the root causes of performance difficulties or the manifestations of those difficulties at the level of ultimate outcomes. However a reformer will generally be very interested in analyzing features of the system because they are critical links in the chains that connect root causes to ultimate performance goals. We refer to data about these system characteristics as *intermediate performance measures*. In the next chapter, we will discuss in some detail the idea of a "diagnostic journey," a concept we introduced in Chapter 2 (Berwick et al. 1991). Such a journey begins with the identification of a specific performance problem and then moves on to explore the causes of those problems through several successive steps. This process, we believe, will often lead a health-sector reformer to explain performance deficiencies on the basis of certain health system characteristics—like efficiency or quality—and this chapter is devoted to clarifying how those concepts can be defined and measured.

Suppose, for example, a country identifies poor health status in rural areas as a critical priority to be addressed through health-sector reform. In exploring why that situation has developed, researchers might find that rural residents lacked access to services, or that the available services were of poor clinical quality. These discoveries would not be the end of the story, however. A would-be reformer would then have to ask why services were either unavailable or clinically inadequate. Nevertheless, identifying problems in features of the system—in this case, inadequate access and quality—can be a helpful step in diagnosis, since this finding can become a useful focus for further analysis.

As mentioned in the last chapter, these intermediate performance measures have been discussed a good deal in the literature over the years. Poor performance on such dimensions is frequently—and we believe mistakenly—characterized either as "the problem" or "the cause" of other problems in the health sector. Our view is that these conclusions are incorrect. Instead, the variables we are about to discuss are causally intermediate between root causes and ultimate performance goals.

How, then, should one identify intermediate performance measures for special attention in the diagnostic process? Since any list we compile is there to serve as a checklist, we want to identify variables that are important causes relative to our performance goals. Second, we want aspects of the system that are likely to be salient in the political and policy debate. If other observers, critics, and interested parties are likely to focus on a particular measure, health-sector reformers should give that factor special attention in their diagnostic work. Third, the variables we highlight should also be influenced by health-sector reform choices. If they are to play an effective "transmission" role between policy and outcome, they have to be both responsive and influential.

Applying these criteria, we have identified three widely discussed intermediate performance measures that we believe should be singled out for special attention: *efficiency*, *access*, and *quality*. All of these terms have a confusing variety of meanings and uses. We will therefore have to do a good deal of conceptual clarification if we are to offer readers a framework they can use with any precision in the diagnostic process.

After we review each of these terms, we will turn to the question of "strategic problem definition." How can a reformer use information on both the ultimate performance goals and the intermediate performance measures as a basis for setting priorities for health-sector reform?

Efficiency

Perhaps no term in the economics and policy literature has been defined in more different ways than "efficiency." The core idea that ties all these together is that of achieving as much of one's objectives as possible, given finite resources. Since this seems so obviously desirable, "efficiency" has acquired substantial rhetorical value as an apparently uncontroversial objective. This may explain the eagerness of various parties to use the term within their own conceptual frameworks. Here are some selected examples of the many ways the term is used:

• Economists call an economy "efficient" if it produces a particular kind of result that would appeal to subjective utilitarians; that is, no one person can be made

happier unless another person is made less happy. As noted in Chapter 3, such a situation is called "Pareto Optimal" (Reinhardt 2001).
- Industrial engineers call a plant "efficient" if it operates with minimum cost per unit of output (Carr and Howe 1964).
- Business executives describe the use of scarce investment dollars as "efficient" when it produces a maximum rate of return. This language sometimes also shows up in ministries of finance at budget time when comparing spending on different sectors (Bierman and Smidt 1993).

How, then, shall we define "efficiency"? In health-sector reform, two key ideas are relevant: how services are produced and what services are produced. The system as a whole is "efficient" when the right services are produced—given one's goals—and are produced in the right way. This leads us to two specific notions of efficiency.

The first of these is *technical efficiency* (also sometimes called production efficiency). This refers to situations in which a good or a service is produced at minimum cost. An alternative but equivalent formulation is that we get the maximum output for our money. For example, is the cost-per-day in the hospital as low as possible, or are as many patients as possible being treated for the available budget? Included in this notion, therefore, are questions about whether we have the right mix of personnel, equipment, supplies, and facilities. Since "technical efficiency" refers to *how* we produce something, it is primarily the responsibility of health-care system managers.

In health care, there are thousands of different kinds of services. When each is produced at minimum cost (i.e., technically efficient), economists describe the result as being on the "production possibility frontier." This means that the only way to get more of one output is to produce less of another.

A second notion of efficiency is *allocative efficiency*, which refers to whether a nation is producing the right collection of outputs to achieve its overall goals. In other words, is it at the right point on the production possibility frontier? Economists generally use "allocative efficiency" to mean the set of outputs that maximizes customer satisfaction. Health planners are talking about allocative efficiency when they ask whether a particular set of services maximizes health-status gains (a notion they sometimes call "effectiveness"; Crystal and Brewster 1966). Improving allocative efficiency is thus the implicit question that confronts anyone who is trying to change the mix of outputs (e.g., less cosmetic surgery and more primary care) that the health system produces.

Consider the following example: Countries that were part of the former Soviet Union—like Belarus—are being urged by WHO to make significant investments in national measles vaccination as part of WHO's campaign to eliminate the disease. Yet, compared to other uses of funds for immunization (e.g., hepatitis B or flu), it is not obvious that measles control will achieve the maximum health-status gain from the available funds. From a narrow national perspective, the prevalence of the condition is low, the gains from immunization low, and the costs substantial. Deciding whether to spend limited funds on such a program is essentially a matter of allocative efficiency.

Since our overall framework recognizes at least three potentially conflicting performance goals, evaluating allocative efficiency from our perspective is inevitably complex. Someone first has to describe how they propose to judge each goal (including equity aspects), and then they must specify the tradeoffs they are willing to make among them. Only then can reformers know whether they have achieved as much of their goals as possible.

Furthermore, the right output mix may often be a matter of degree. Many medical services exhibit what economists call "diminishing marginal returns." That is, treating the patients who are most appropriate and respond best to a specific kind of cure—even with quite expensive care—can be very cost-effective. As the same treatment is extended to less appropriate cases, however, the cost-effectiveness of care will often diminish, as costs per case increase and case-by-case benefits decline. Hence, the relevant issue is often not "dialysis–yes-or-no" or "cardiac bypass–yes-or-no," but how *much* dialysis or cardiac bypass the system should provide, and to which patients (Weinstein and Stasson 1977).

Since improving technical and allocative efficiency allows a health-care system to do better with existing resources, countries in a cost–performance squeeze often seek to improve efficiency through health-sector reform. Politically, however, it can often be more difficult to improve allocative efficiency than technical efficiency. Lowering the cost of producing outputs to raise technical efficiency is not easy. Workers often resist change, and improving service delivery can require a great deal of effort. Nevertheless, doing so is a relatively straightforward managerial task. In contrast, improving allocative efficiency means altering what is produced, and this is likely to impose very high costs on those involved in the production and consumption of the outputs being reduced. Shifting resources (people and money) from some activities to others—from high-tech services to primary care, for example—is often vigorously resisted.

Given our definitions, what are we to make of the frequent and confusing claim that efficiency and equity are necessarily (or at least often) in conflict? This view is based on using the term "efficiency" very narrowly, to mean maximizing average health status. In that context, serving those in rural areas can be "inefficient," because more DALYs or QALYs could be produced for the same money if it were not spent with an eye to equity. But there is every reason *not* to restrict the definition of "efficiency" so narrowly. In our framework, the "efficiency" of the system (both allocative and technical) is determined by whether or not it reaches society's goals at minimum cost. Thus one could sensibly ask whether a nation's health system is efficient in reaching its equity goals. Does it, for instance, provide health-status gains in rural areas at minimum cost? In our usage, then, there is no reason to set up efficiency and equity in opposition. Properly understood, increased efficiency can actually advance equity—by making it less costly to reach our equity objectives (Reinhardt 2001).

In sum, both kinds of efficiency refer to the relationship of inputs to desired results. Technical efficiency means producing outputs in the "right way," at minimum cost, while allocative efficiency means producing the "right outputs" to maximize the achievement of our goals. Unless a health-care system is both technically and allocatively efficient, it will not achieve as much as it might. This is why efficiency is an appropriate entry on the list of intermediate performance measures. Inefficiency may well be a cause of poor performance. Furthermore, changing the incentives or organization of the system is likely to have an impact on efficiency, at least if it is done properly. We expect that many diagnostic journeys will lead from poor outcomes, back through poor efficiency, to a look at the still deeper sources of that inefficiency as a way of discovering the roots of a nation's failure to achieve its performance goals.

Access

In discussions of health-sector reform, *access* is often a major concern. A lack of access is often introduced as a cause of poor health status in rural areas or of low levels of satisfaction among the poor. Yet to fully understand this concept's role as an intermediate performance measure, we again have to disentangle the various ways the term is used.

First, "access" sometimes simply refers to whether services are offered in a specific area. Here, the question is *physical availability*, which can be measured by the distribution of available inputs (beds, doctors, or nurses) compared to the population. A second notion, one that more closely reflects the intuitive meaning of the term, is *effective availability*; that is, how easy is it for citizens to get care? Differences between physical availability and effective availability can arise because various barriers (e.g., cost, travel time, poor service) may keep people from using facilities that are physically available.

It is not easy, however, to collect enough data on prices, service levels, waiting times, and cultural acceptability in order to evaluate effective availability directly. As a result, the term "access" is often employed to refer to *utilization*. Per capita measures of hospital admissions or outpatient visits are computed for various population groups, and those with low use are said to lack access. In fact, utilization is only partially a reflection of effective availability, as patients may choose not to use services, even if they are available. But if we ignore the possibility that low use might reflect patient choice, and instead argue that low use *always* means that there are barriers to care, effective availability vanishes as an independent concept, since it is no longer measurable separately from utilization.

At first glance, "access," defined as "effective availability," is an obvious intermediate performance measure: it influences both health status and consumer satisfaction. Furthermore, effective availability is clearly influenced by what services are offered at what locations and at what prices, and the financing, payment and organization of the system will affect what is offered and on what terms. This variable therefore meets the test of being both a consequence of policy and a cause of performance.

Some, though, argue for thinking of effective availability as a performance goal—as an end, not a means. Some egalitarians (like Amartya Sen) suggest that government is obligated to make services available and then let citizens use these or not as they choose (Sen 1999). In this view, the effective availability of health care should be the performance goal, not health itself. Similarly, some communitarians focus on the distribution of health services as a matter of fairness to various local communities. And changes in the physical availability of health services (i.e., do we open or close a local hospital) are in fact often a focus of intense political controversy. Indeed, in developed countries, highly contested changes in physical availability will often have little observable impact on health status, because service levels are likely to remain high in any case (Kolata 2002).

On balance, we believe that access fits better as an intermediate performance measure, than as an ultimate performance goal. Effective availability does influence health and satisfaction. In addition, controversies over physical availability can be evaluated in terms of customer satisfaction, which is a performance goal in our framework. (For example, having services available might generate what economists call "option demand"—the value to citizens of having something available, even if it is not used; Pazner 1974.)

We recognize that there are cases where leaders or interest groups argue for expanding physical availability even absent health or satisfaction gains. Sometimes such demands reflect community norms, which (as discussed at the end of the last chapter) can act as constraints on the process of health-sector reform. In other cases, the desire to preserve or expand health services may be a matter of producing patronage or status gains. While such concerns may represent an important political reality, they do not have to be incorporated into our performance goals.

Viewing access (i.e., effective availability) as a tool for improving health status and satisfaction has considerable implications. It means, for example, that we should view with skepticism arguments that every city ought to have certain services—because such a situation is "fair"—if such facilities are not part of a cost-effective plan to produce the desired distribution of satisfaction and health status. Furthermore, if services are valuable only if they produce outcomes, then the reverse is also true. The lack of services is most significant when outcomes are unsatisfactory. We realize that actual debates over health reform are rarely conducted precisely in this way. But, particularly in countries with limited resources, seeing access as a means to reach a country's goals in the desired distribution of health and satisfaction places a useful argumentative burden on those who would contend otherwise.

We believe that this way of thinking promotes greater analytical rigor in conversations about priorities for health-sector reform.

Quality

Quality is our third proposed intermediate performance measure. It is valuable, not for itself, but for its role in achieving a nation's performance goals. Poor quality, like poor access, is often invoked as an explanation for performance failures. Like efficiency, "quality" appears to be something everyone should be in favor of. Since advocates are always trying to appropriate the concept, the term is used in many different ways. Thus, "quality" is sometimes defined from the patient's point of view and sometimes from the perspective of the doctor. It is sometimes applied to the treatment of a particular case, or to the care provided by a particular hospital, or to a national system as a whole. Hence, as before, our first task is conceptual clarification.

The simplest way to think about "quality" is at a disaggregated level; that is, as a characteristic of the treatment of a particular patient in a given encounter. More inclusive judgments (of hospitals or national systems) reflect aggregations (averages) of such encounter-level experiences. But even at the encounter level, the term "quality" refers to several different phenomena (see Table 6.1). In what follows, we try to identify various measurable quality aspects by abstracting from *who* is doing the judging. But we want to stress that different individuals (e.g., different doctors, patients, politicians) may place different levels of importance on different quality dimensions.

Our experience reveals three major uses of the term "quality"—two of which have sub-components. First, as the table indicates, "quality" can be used to mean simply the *quantity* of care provided to a patient, as in: "My aunt got the highest-quality care. They did everything for her." Americans who praise their system for its high "quality" often are using the term in this way.

The second basic meaning of "quality," which health professionals typically use, is *clinical quality*. This involves both the skill of caregivers (e.g., the surgeon's technique) and correct diagnosis and treatment decisions. It also depends on whether

TABLE 6.1. Meanings for the Term *Quality* in Health Care

QUANTITY	CLINICAL QUALITY	SERVICE QUALITY
	Human Inputs: Skill, decision-making	Hotel Services: Food, cleanliness, amenities
	Non-human Inputs: Equipment and supplies	Convenience: Travel and waiting times, appointment delays
	Production System	Interpersonal Relations: Care, politeness, respect

the right inputs (e.g., drugs, equipment) are available to carry out appropriate care. Clinical quality also depends on the system of production that combines the human and non-human inputs into actual delivered services (Berwick et al. 1991).

The third broad definition, which is most often invoked by patients, who find it difficult to judge clinical quality, involves *service quality* (Cunningham 1991). The subcategories here are themselves multidimensional. The first we call hotel services because these include the level of amenity and quality in areas where hotels also act: food, cleanliness, physical design, furnishings, etc. Convenience includes travel time, waiting time, opening hours, and the time necessary to get an appointment. The interpersonal dimension involves whether providers are polite and emotionally supportive, and whether patients are given appropriate information and treated with respect. There are complex issues about the role of patients in the care process—issues that we discussed at the end of the last chapter and to which we will return shortly.

Measuring quality generally requires detailed data. Service quality in particular can be measured in a variety of ways. For instance, administrative systems may be able to generate data on parameters like waiting times and delays in getting an appointment. Special-purpose quality monitoring systems can also be created. For example, in one state in India, hospitals are now subject to periodic (unannounced) quality inspections. An outside contractor undertakes these inspections and forwards the results to a central office at the state level. Patient reports can also be useful in identifying service quality lapses, including deficiencies in the area of interpersonal relationships.

Clinical quality assessment is an activity that has generated an enormous literature in recent years (Brennan and Berwick 1996, Palmer et al. 1995). Comparing clinical care (as recorded in patient records, for example) with expert opinion is one way to determine whether appropriate treatment has been given, as long as those records are themselves accurate. But it is expensive and time-consuming to make such an assessment. Quality can also be measured indirectly by outcome data like infection rates, operative mortality, and so on. Understanding how production systems can produce variations in clinical and service quality—which is the focus of the whole Total Quality Management approach—requires even more detailed studies.

The difficulty of collecting and interpreting sophisticated quality data helps explain why many countries rely heavily on regulating *inputs* (e.g., educational requirements) rather than monitoring and evaluating processes or outcomes in the quality arena (we discuss this point further in the regulation chapter). Indeed, looking at inputs (does the health center have needed drugs and equipment, is a doctor available?) is often the only—albeit highly imperfect—way for patients to assess clinical quality.

Not just the average, but also the distribution of quality (that is, who is subject to poor quality) is often important to the connection between quality and system performance. For example, suppose a country is concerned with patients' bypassing local health posts to seek treatment at regional or national centers. Deciding what to do about such a situation requires an analysis of both clinical and service quality—as well as the quantity of services available—at the local level. If quality at the periphery is poor, then it will be more difficult to prevent bypassing. Furthermore, allowing such poor quality to persist is also likely to raise equity issues, since it will often particularly disadvantage the poor, who cannot afford the time or expense of traveling farther afield for care. Consider, for example, the situation in Sri Lanka, where overuse of hospitals in the largest cities is viewed as a major problem by the ministry of health. The problem is compounded by the fact that under Sri Lankan law, citizens have a right to insist on admission to a hospital. It is also true that doctors are assigned to health posts based on their performance, and that the best-performing physicians generally avoid the most rural areas. Hence dealing with this situation will almost certainly require efforts to improve clinical quality in the periphery.

Deciding whether the quality produced by a health-care system is appropriate involves complex judgments. Just as a car has various quality dimensions (such as fuel economy, acceleration, passenger capacity), so too does any health-care service. Having more of one quality (luggage capacity or patient choice) might lead to less of another quality (road handling or correct clinical decision-making). Increased quality, in cars or in care, also might not be worth the cost, depending on the values of the person making the judgment. Indeed, there are actually three judgments that must be made (Rosen 1974).

The first question a reformer has to ask about health-care quality involves a special kind of technical efficiency. Is each service being produced in a way that results in the highest possible quality given the costs being incurred? For a given cost, a service that produces less than the maximum attainable quality is technically inefficient in the production of quality.

To see this, consider Diagram 1 of Figure 6.1, which depicts the "quality possibility frontier" for a particular health-care service. To make drawing this diagram possible, we have assumed that "clinical" and "service" quality are each a single magnitude, although the "frontier" can be thought of in a space of many dimensions. For a specified level of spending per unit of service, any medical care system can only produce a limited level of clinical or service quality. We have drawn the diagram to imply that if either service or clinical quality is too low, the other aspect of quality suffers; but that is not necessary to the argument. The key is that to be technically efficient in the production of quality, a service has to be organized so that its output is *on* the frontier (X, Y, or Z)—not at some point like Q.

For managers to know whether we are on or at least near the frontier will require some form of benchmarking. For example, we could compare any given health-care facility with those in other countries (or in different regions of our own country) to find those that had similar cost levels. Then we could compare relative waiting times, or the cleanliness of facilities, or patient reports about their care in order to

Diagram 1

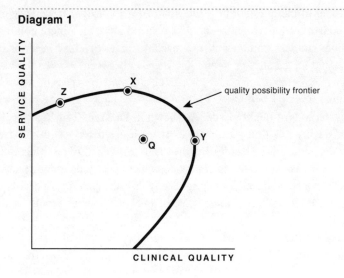

Diagram 2

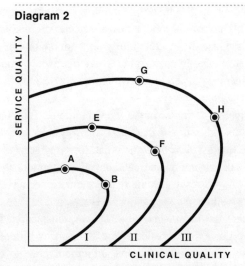

FIGURE 6.1. Quality possibility frontiers for a particular health-care service (Diagram 1), and at three different budget levels: I, II, III (Diagram 2).

evaluate service quality. On the clinical side, we could look at input availability (- were there drugs, was the X-ray machine working?) or output indicators (wound infections, intra-operative death rate). For reformers, the question is, Are we getting all the quality we can, given the budget? This formulation is obviously important for deciding on a reform program. It makes a big difference whether poor quality performance is the result of poor management or because of a low budget, or both.

There is a second quality question. Even if a service is operating on the quality possibility frontier, are the producers offering an appropriate mix of qualities?

This is similar to the question of what kind of car to design. If we have a construction budget for a new clinic, should we spend more on a more comfortable waiting room and less on a new X-ray machine, or vice versa? In terms of the frontier, should we be at X or Y, or somewhere in between? (Given the way we have drawn the frontier, there is no reason to be at Z since it is possible to do better on both dimensions.)

There is yet a third quality issue. As shown in Diagram 2 of Figure 6.1, any number of quality possibility frontiers exist for a given service, each based on a different *budget* level (I, II, and III in the diagram). The third task then is evaluating the *level* of spending for each service, which in turn determines just what quality levels can be produced for that service. This is the *quantity* aspect of quality that we identified initially. The issue is, What level of resources should we devote to each service?

How would different reformers with different philosophical views judge the performance of the health-care system with regard to quality? Objective utilitarians, interested in health maximization, would want to produce the maximum clinical quality for any given budget (i.e., to be on the quality possibility frontier at a point like X in Diagram 1). They would look at how services were managed to see if there was any way to increase the health-status gain from operations. They would then evaluate budget levels based on marginal cost-effectiveness analysis, to see if money was being spent on different services in a way designed to produce the biggest health-status gain.

Notice, however, that the way we have drawn the frontiers implies that objective utilitarians would make a mistake in assuming that they can always increase clinical quality by decreasing service quality. Beyond some point, lowering service levels discourages utilization, lowers patient compliance, and impedes communication, all of which can lead to poorer clinical results. Some real systems (especially public clinics in poor countries) may well be in this paradoxical situation.

Subjective utilitarians, interested in maximizing customer satisfaction, face a slightly different evaluation process. Since patients care about many different aspects of both clinical and service quality, subjective utilitarians have to decide whether the quality mix and spending level for each service represents an optimal response to the varied individual preferences of its customers. The obvious difficulty of such a task helps explain why so many subjective utilitarians favor using markets in health care (and everywhere else). Markets allow everyone to choose (and pay for) the set of services and the mix and level of qualities that they prefer. Of course this assumes that customers (i.e., patients) can judge quality levels, which is doubtful when it comes to clinical quality. Hence, even some subjective utilitarians would regulate markets for quality purposes—as we will discuss in Chapter 11.

For practical reformers, getting more of both service and clinical quality, through better management, is likely to be the first reform priority. This is especially true where budgets are constrained. But when health status and satisfaction outcomes are low and the health services are already well managed, the question of whether or not to increase spending—and hence quality—is likely to be relevant. (This implies wanting a move like 5 or 7 in Figure 5.1.) Similarly, if a well-managed system is producing good health but poor satisfaction (or visa versa), the question of changing the quality mix is also one a reformer may need to address.

In summary, quality is an important intermediate performance measure, affecting both health status and customer satisfaction. We have identified three important but distinct quality issues. First, is quality (on various dimensions) as high as possible given the budget? Second, does the system produce the right mix of qualities given the budget level for each service? Third is the question of quantity. Are budget levels set to produce appropriate levels of quality for each service? In a sense, reallocating budgets across services to improve quality levels is a task very much like changing the mix of outputs to improve allocative efficiency.

The quality characteristics of the system are influenced by numerous policy decisions. The day-to-day responsibility for getting to the quality possibility frontier, as well as for determining the mix of qualities, rests with the managers of health-care services. Many features of the system's organization—including how managers are chosen and rewarded—will influence how they do this job. The financing and payment systems and regulatory regimes will determine the incentives for managers. Hence, these, too, influence the quality performance of the system. Nonetheless, one point is clear. Judging system quality is not simply a matter of "more is better." Resources are always limited, both for the country and for the health sector. Even for a system that is efficient in producing quality, the question remains how much quality—and along what dimensions—will maximize society's ability to achieve its overall goals.

Developing a Strategic Performance Problem Focus

In the last two chapters we have sought to present a framework for defining problems that reformers can use and adapt to their particular circumstances. That framework involves three performance goals, three intermediate performance measures and two ethical tests (average and distribution). It also explicitly considers the roles that cost and culture should play in the analysis, since they represent important connections between the health sector and the larger social and economic system. The complexity of this analytical structure reflects the reality that defining problems and evaluating alternative solutions in health-sector reform is a difficult and complex task. Ignoring that complexity achieves a false simplicity, one that trades rhetoric for relevance, slogans for sophistication.

Having said all that, we would like to offer some advice to would-be reformers about what performance problems to focus on, advice that draws together the various threads of this and the previous chapter. The essence of our advice is this— Think strategically! Choosing a problem definition is the first step in the long process of health-sector reform, and it should be done with an eye on the larger implications of that decision.

As discussed in Chapter 1, the process of reform is often provoked by events outside a reformer's control. The economy goes down, expectations and/or health costs go up, political change occurs, and so forth. What we are urging is that reformers make an effort to take some initiative and influence the problem definition that comes to dominate both political debate and the policy development process.

To clarify their priorities, reformers can ask themselves three questions as a way of synthesizing the ethical, political, and substantive considerations at play in selecting a focus for health-sector reform.

- What improvements in health-sector performance are most important ethically?
- What areas of poor performance can one reasonably hope to do something about?
- What will be the political consequences of taking on this issue?

Paying special attention to the first question involves giving priority to values. The second question requires consideration of whether there are any promising policies or programs available for dealing with ethically important issues, and whether such measures are likely to be politically and practically feasible in one's own country. For only then can a reformer decide if focusing on a particular problem will produce useful results. The cost of such initiatives, compared to the available funds, is a key part of such an analysis. The third question suggests considering political consequences. In a sense politics and feasibility can be viewed as "screens" or "constraints" on a value-based approach. Thus, our advice can be summarized as follows: *Start with what you want to accomplish and then see if there is a technically feasible and politically acceptable way to make that happen.*

The control knobs, after all, are *not* the only forces that determine the performance of the health sector. Instead, non-manipulable factors may be at the heart of a particular performance problem. It will also not always be easy to know whether a politically feasible and effective policy option exists, without doing extensive research into a particular problem area. Our advice is that you consider questions of feasibility as best you can *before* you go too far down the road to reform.

We are well aware that the answers to these questions may *not* all point in the same direction. Leaders sometimes focus on problems where it is unlikely they will be able to accomplish much because such a focus satisfies political concerns. The American "War on Drugs" comes to mind in that regard. We are not saying such symbolic actions are always wrong or inappropriate. Rather, our point is that reformers need to be aware of what is really at stake before choosing a goal whose success appears unlikely.

These questions also remind us that the process of strategic problem definition has to be "agent relative." That is, the political consequences of a given decision are likely to be different for different actors. The minister of finance may well have a different view from the minister of health about the most important goals of health-sector reform, and the two may not be held equally responsible if, for example, the new social insurance fund becomes insolvent. Similarly, focusing on the health status of the rural poor is more likely to be politically advantageous to parties trying to attract the support of small farmers, and less helpful to parties built around a trade-union constituency. In fact, there is no way to pick a problem definition from an abstract point of view—from what philosophers call the "view from nowhere." Instead, choosing a particular problem definition has to be seen as a response to a particular individual's or group's circumstances.

When reformers decide on a problem definition, they often have a question of *scope* to consider. Some might choose to focus quite narrowly on one or two specific performance parameters (like high infant and maternal mortality rates in poor rural areas). Such a problem definition is likely to lead to a relatively targeted set of reforms; the development of new reimbursement mechanisms or selective investment in certain facilities or training programs, for instance. On the other hand, broader problem definitions are likely to lead to a broader and more complicated reform agenda. Concern about widespread simultaneous failures of risk protection, popular dissatisfaction with the health-care system, and high costs could lead reformers to a much more ambitious reform program. The country might decide to create a new social insurance fund, new payment schemes for doctors and hospitals, and new forms of hospital organization—all at once. In making decisions about the scope of problems to tackle, reformers are well advised to think carefully about the administrative and political feasibility of a more or less ambitious agenda.

As a practical matter, one way for reformers to proceed is through "benchmarking," that is, comparing national performance with various standards to see where performance is both inadequate and potentially improvable. This process can take many forms.

- *Ethical benchmarking*: comparing performance to widely accepted norms
- *Internal benchmarking*: comparing performance across groups or regions in the country
- *Historical benchmarking*: comparing performance to a nation's own prior performance
- *External benchmarking*: comparing performance with that of other, similarly situated countries

The first two kinds of comparisons address the issue of ethical importance. If a country's performance is unsatisfactory in light of accepted norms (e.g., the Millennium Development Goals), this suggests an issue that should be addressed. Large internal variations also raise ethical concerns, especially for countries where equity is a priority. The last three forms of comparison (internal, historical, and external benchmarking) can help address the issue of feasibility. If we once did better, or if other countries like us do better, or if we do better in some places—all these suggest that improvement is possible.

We need to note that policy needs to be judged, not just on its effectiveness, but on its cost-effectiveness. As we argued in an earlier chapter, cost is always a part of the problem definition, either implicitly or explicitly. Unfortunately, in a world of limited resources, some very important problems may not be solvable for cost reasons—as the problem of AIDS in southern Africa tragically reminds us. (Of course, cost is far from the *only* obstacle in that situation.)

In the process of choosing priorities, adherents of different ethical theories will tend to emphasize different concerns. Objective utilitarians will focus on the cost-effective improvement of overall health status, while subjective utilitarians' main concern will be customer satisfaction. Egalitarian liberals, who want to get everyone up to some minimum level of opportunity, will tend to focus on the health and economic status of the worst-off in a society. Thus, in addition to health, financial risk protection for the poor will also matter greatly to them. Objective utilitarians will see certain community norms as obstacles to rational resource allocation—even as relative communitarians defend them. Not everyone will agree on the relative importance of clinical versus service quality; nor will they all put the same priority on giving patients a choice within the care process. But that is exactly why deciding on which performance problems to make priorities is a *choice*—one that has to be made both thoughtfully and prudently.

In summary, then, problem definition—picking performance areas for priority attention—is a critical strategic decision for health reformers. It affects how attention is focused, what interventions are tried, and ultimately how the reformers themselves will be judged. It is a choice to allocate scarce political and social resources in one way and not in another. Such choices will have repercussions on many levels—from the individuals and organizations involved up through to the society as a whole—and they need to be made in a transparent and forward-looking way. How else can a reformer establish the best possible base for the difficult work of actually getting reform to happen?—which is, after all, the point of the entire process.

References

Berwick, Donald M.; A. Blanton Godfrey; and Jane Roessner. 1991. *Curing Health Care: New Strategies for Quality Improvement.* San Francisco, CA: Jossey-Bass.
Bierman, Harold; and Seymour Smidt. 1993. *The Capital Budgeting Decision: Economic Analysis of Investment Projects.* 8th Edition. New York: Macmillan.
Brennan, Troyen A.; and Donald M. Berwick. 1996. *New Rules: Regulation, Markets, and the Quality of American Health Care.* San Francisco, CA: Jossey-Bass Publishers.
Carr, Charles R.; and Charles W. Howe. 1964. *Quantitative Decision Procedures in Management and Economics, Deterministic Theory and Applications.* New York: McGraw-Hill.
Crystal, R. A.; and A. W. Brewster. 1966. "Cost Benefit and Cost Effectiveness Analyses in the Health Field: An Introduction." *Inquiry* 3(4): 3–13.
Cunningham, Lynne. 1991. *The Quality Connection in Health Care: Integrating Patient Satisfaction and Risk Management.* San Francisco, CA: Jossey-Bass.

Kolata, Gina. 2002. "Research Suggests More Health Care May Not Be Better." *The New York Times* 21 July.

Palmer R. H.; A. G. Lawthers; J. DeLozier; N. J. Banks; L. Peterson; and B. Duggar. 1995. *Understanding and Choosing Clinical Performance Measures for Quality Improvement: Development of a Typology.* Washington, DC: Agency for Health Care Policy Research.

Pazner, Elisha A. 1974. "Optimal Pricing and Income Distribution." In: Richard E. Caves and Marc J. Roberts, eds., *Regulating the Product: Quality and Variety.* Cambridge, MA: Ballinger.

Reinhardt, Uwe E. 2001. "Can Efficiency in Health Care Be Left to the Market?" *Journal of Health Politics, Policy and Law* 26(5): 967–92.

Rosen, Sherwin. 1974. "Hedonic Prices and Implicit Markets: Product Differentiation in Pure Competition." *Journal of Political Economy* 82(Jan/Feb): 34–55.

Sen, Amartya. 1999. *Development as Freedom.* New York: Knopf.

Weinstein, Milton C.; and William B. Stasson. 1977. "Foundations of Cost-Effectiveness Analysis for Health and Medical Practices." *New England Journal of Medicine* 296: 716–21.

7

From Diagnosis to Health-Sector Reform

Once health-sector reformers have decided which performance problems to focus on—that is, once they have decided on their strategic priorities—they have to go on to the next stages of the policy cycle. This means, first of all, figuring out the causes of the poor performance they are concerned with. This is the process we call "diagnosis." Then they have to decide what to do about the situation—the process we call "policy development." In this chapter we will discuss those activities and offer advice about how to carry them out, so as to produce more effective health-sector reform.

With respect to diagnosis, the fundamental strategy is "Work backwards." Keep asking "why" until you have discovered the causes of the poor performance you want to improve. The goal of this process, called a *diagnostic journey*, is to construct a "diagnostic tree"—an analytical device we describe in detail below—that links aspects of poor performance to the causal factors that might be changed or modified by policy interventions. The subsequent task, *policy development*, involves crafting a set of policies and programs that will alter the causes (or their impact) and thus improve health-sector performance.

In carrying out these tasks, we urge readers to pay attention to some simple guidelines. The first of these is "Process matters." How various health-reform tasks are carried out can have a major effect on what actually happens. For example, whether or not critical actors and interest groups feel they have been consulted will influence their attitudes toward any reform plan. And that in turn can influence both the politics of getting reform measures adopted and how effectively the chosen policy is implemented.

Our second guideline is "Imitate but adapt." Because new ideas are hard to invent, imitating proven approaches has much to recommend it. On the other hand, because local conditions vary, successful imitation involves adapting and adjusting ideas from elsewhere to local circumstances.

Our third guideline is "Use evidence." In recent years, there has been a large movement in medicine away from clinical practice based on received wisdom to "evidence-based medicine," in which decisions follow from careful study of the relevant scientific literature. Advocates of this approach argue that doctors often develop patterns of practice that are not scientifically justified. For example, some physicians routinely remove tonsils or perform hysterectomies when there is no real reason to do so. The same can be said of some health-sector reformers, who routinely urge their favorite remedy—such as "privatization" or "decentralization"—without first determining the performance problems in a particular country and without a careful analysis of whether their favorite intervention will improve that performance. To counter such uncritical enthusiasm, we urge evidence-based reform, whereby policies are based on careful analysis of problems, causes, and likely effects.

Consider the following example. Suppose a newly independent Eastern European country identifies declining male life-expectancy (due to cardiac problems and rising suicide rates) as a priority performance problem. Suppose, too, that some reformers urge that country to develop competitive private health insurance in order to help improve the performance of the health-care system. Such a move would not make sense unless advocates could explain how and why these new financing arrangements would have a positive impact on male life-expectancy (in fact we doubt such a link exists).

In carrying out diagnosis and policy development, we urge reformers to utilize the framework we outlined in Chapter 2; namely, the five "control knobs." Each control knob focuses on certain features of the system and the strategies that governments can use in each arena to improve health-sector performance. For example, governments can change what taxes are used to finance health care, or how physicians are paid, or how they organize and manage hospitals. In Part II of this book, we review each of these sets of policy options in some detail and discuss the likely consequences of different approaches.

The control knob framework can also be a helpful organizing device at the diagnostic stage. For at that stage the task is *not* just to identify causes but to identify causes that can be *changed* by government action. The control knobs thus provide a menu or shopping list—a set of possible endpoints to the diagnostic journey that can in turn be the basis for government action.

Let us put this point another way. Identifying potentially effective changes in one or more control knobs is the end of the diagnostic task and the beginning of the policy development task. Analysts first work *backward* to causes. Next, they have to look for policies to change those causes, and then work *forward* from causes to forecasts of improved health-sector performance as a result of various policy changes.

In this chapter we begin by working through an extended example of a diagnostic tree and discuss how to link diagnosis to the control knobs. Before offering a "one-problem" analysis, however, we discuss the circumstances under which reformers are likely to conclude that a more ambitious, multifaceted effort—that is, major health-sector reform—is really needed.

In the second half of the chapter, we shift our focus to policy development. We first discuss some process concerns and then explore some screening criteria by which to judge alternative proposals. Finally, we discuss how to find and use evidence in both phases of the process, and conclude with a few final cautions and observations.

The Genesis of Major Health-Sector Reform Efforts

So far we have been discussing the process of health-system diagnosis and policy development as if it focused on one specific performance problem at a time. Such an approach is likely to provoke piecemeal, programmatic initiatives; a new maternal health program, for example, or an expanded effort at childhood immunization. But as we have noted before, countries often confront a number of interlinked performance problems. The diagnosis for each specific problem may well reveal that certain common features of the health-care system are important causal factors. To deal effectively with these multiple problems, multiple interventions may be required. This kind of analysis, then, is one path that can lead a country to major health-sector reform efforts.

In this connection, we have to return again to the key role of cost, as described in Chapter 5. A nation unhappy with its health sector's performance—and yet facing cost constraints—will often be forced into a complex and multipart analysis as it seeks to explicate the causes of its difficulties. Many different causes are likely to emerge, including technical inefficiency (due to poor incentives produced by the payment system and poor management due to faulty organization), allocative inefficiency (due to poor resource allocation from the financing system), poor quality, and limited access. And program-by-program fixes will not be possible, precisely because there is not enough money to pay for a whole series of uncoordinated new initiatives. Again, a multipart reform, in which major changes are made to several control knobs in an effort to fundamentally alter the system, is likely to be the answer (Colombia Health Sector Reform Project 1996).

There is also a matter of coherence here. Multiple programmatic efforts run the risk of being uncoordinated and even inconsistent. Someone may urge decentralization of primary care to the provincial level, even as someone else urges carrying out a centralized national vaccination program. Dealing with such conflicts in an integrated way may require a coordinated look at, and a plan for, the revision of the system as a whole.

There is also the issue of the limited political and technical resources typically available to reformers. Tackling a large number of performance problems in isolation from each other can place far too great a demand on those resources. Focusing instead on certain common and more fundamental problems can potentially be a cost-effective use of limited reform energies—assuming, of course, that such changes are possible.

Finally, an integrated and extensive reform effort may have political value, in that it often appears more dramatic and attention-getting than a series of narrow programmatic initiatives. By promising more to the population, broad reform can seem like an effective political strategy—especially when the population is dissatisfied with the current system (Edelman 1984).

Consider the following example. Suppose a country is concerned about both an apparent excess of maternal deaths and the low overall life-expectancy among the rural poor. The diagnosis seeking the causes of these problems is likely to produce similar results. Poor service quality and lack of utilization will appear again and again. Since the same budget-based public system provides care in all these arenas, an appropriate response to such a situation could be a multipronged attack, using several control knobs to improve service and increase utilization in the rural areas. This could lead to a complex program of health-system reform, designed to improve performance without raising costs. For example, substantial authority could be delegated to local communities, who would also be allowed to set up local insurance schemes (community financing) to generate some added funds. These communities could also be allowed to contract with NGOs or private practitioners on either a capitated or incentive basis to operate local health centers—to get better results from the available resources.

Such a scheme, involving a number of significant changes, would involve substantial risks and demands, but it would also be dramatic enough to have the possibility of rallying significant political support. It also offers the hope that one set of reforms would deal with many issues at once, in an integrated and consistent fashion.

Here is another example. Suppose a nation is concerned about differences in health status and risk protection between those who work in the formal sector (government and large employers) and those who are self-employed or who work in the informal sector. The diagnostic journey for each of these problems is likely to reveal that only those in the formal sector are covered by social insurance, while other segments of the workforce largely utilize public hospitals or private doctors and pay for care out-of-pocket. Such a nation might well decide to establish a new unified social insurance system. This would both increase access to care among workers in the informal sector and give them the risk protection they now lack. It might also join this with efforts to institute selective contracting by the new insurance fund, together with reform of the hospitals themselves to give them more autonomy and their managers more authority. Such a multifaceted reform should be based on a series of specific diagnostic journeys. But the need for an interlinked portfolio of changes arises because of the complex intersecting set of causes that must be dealt with. And, as always, calculations of *political feasibility* and *administrative implementability*, as we discuss later in this chapter, should influence a reformer's decision to proceed in this way.

It is possible that this kind of analysis is implicit in the arguments of those reformers who advocate substantial policy changes without linking their proposals to any particular expected performance gains. In our experience, however, that is not typically the case. The failure to offer any systematic diagnostic analysis is more likely to reflect badly designed or poorly thought-through reform ideas. In fact, a complex reform program, designed to improve performance on multiple dimensions, requires more, not less, thought than simpler and more modest reform alternatives. The potentially complementary and conflicting consequences of such complex programs are in particular need of explicit analysis.

Developing a Health-System Diagnostic Tree

Before presenting a specific example of how to do a diagnosis, we need to calibrate our expectations about what such a process is likely to find. Given the complexity of the health sector, it will seldom be the case that A is caused by B and only B, and that B is caused by C and only C. Instead:

- There are likely to be several stages or series of causes
- Each effect may well be produced by more than one cause
- Each cause is likely to have multiple effects
- Causes and effects may interact and reinforce each other in various ways
- Not every cause will be manipulable by public policy
- Change may well require acting on more than one cause at a time—that is, changing more than one control knob.

With these cautions in mind, let's look at a specific example of a diagnostic journey. To do this, we will use an analytical tool we call a *health-system diagnostic tree,* which is similar to, but different from, two other kinds of tree diagrams the reader may be familiar with. One kind is a decision tree, which is used for analyzing decisions under uncertain circumstances. At each branching point in a decision tree, one of a set of mutually exclusive *events* occurs (either by chance or by the choice of the decision-maker; Behn and Vaupel 1982). In a health-system diagnostic tree, however, an analyst represents various possible *causes* for a particular situation at each branching point, and it may well be the case that several of the causes are in fact operating at the same time. Unlike the decision tree, there is no presumption that paths are mutually exclusive.

The health-sector diagnostic tree is also different from the kind of tree diagram implicit in the diagnostic process in clinical medicine. While these trees also involve causality, normally at each branch, only one out of a set of alternative causes will be selected. The patient has *either* this disease *or* that one (Tierney et al. 2001). In health-sector diagnosis, more than one cause (more than one "disease") is generally operating at the same time.

Consider the following example. Suppose the government of a country decides that, compared to other similar countries, it has a noticeably higher rate of maternal mortality, especially among the rural poor. Suppose further that on both political and philosophical grounds the government decides to make improving this rate a priority. We will work through this example to see how the diagnostic process operates.

The first step is to consider *broad categories* of causes. Figure 7.1 lists three possible causes that often contribute to such health problems in developing countries: high-risk behavior, inadequate health care, and poor socioeconomic conditions.

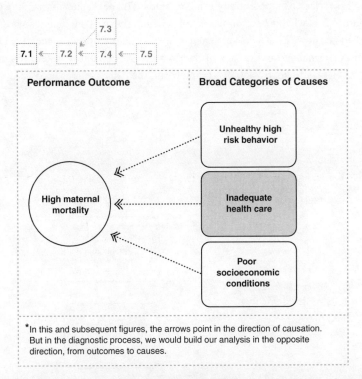

*In this and subsequent figures, the arrows point in the direction of causation. But in the diagnostic process, we would build our analysis in the opposite direction, from outcomes to causes.

FIGURE 7.1. Starting to work back* along the causal chain.

As part of health-sector reform, a country will not be able to address causes outside the health-care system. Nevertheless, these should be still considered in the analysis to keep realistic expectations of the role that health-sector reform can play in solving the problem (WHO 1986).

One way to determine which links are significant is to look at one's own situation compared to similar countries that do better. A possible causal factor that operates similarly in both nations is not likely to account for differences in their performance. For example, if known behavioral risk factors (e.g., hard physical labor, smoking) are similar in our nation to those in countries that do better, then these causes are not likely to account for our high maternal mortality. A second line of analysis is to take advantage of any variations in outcome within a country; for example, by region or socioeconomic group. We can then look to see whether there are any variations in potential causes that are parallel to variations in outcomes. Such an association does not prove that there is a causal connection, but it should make one suspicious enough to explore the matter further (Rossi and Freeman 1998).

Suppose other countries with similar socioeconomic conditions and behavior patterns do achieve better levels of maternal mortality. This implies a need to focus on health services as a potentially critical factor. The next question, as illustrated by Figure 7.2, is what aspects of the nation's health services are "inadequate." This second stage shows how a causal analysis reaches back through successive causes of poor performance (and causes of these causes). The health-system diagnostic tree is just a way to keep track of, and map out, the causal chains involved.

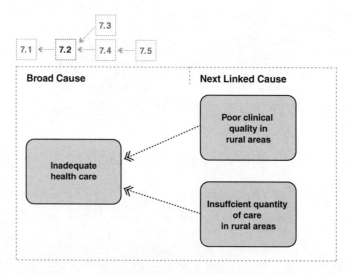

FIGURE 7.2. The next step back along the chain.

The first step in sorting out the relative contribution of the two causes described in Figure 7.2 is to look at utilization. What care do citizens receive? If, for example, antenatal care visits per capita and the rate of hospital deliveries are similar to those of better performing nations, quantity of care is not likely to be the problem. Lower utilization rates, on the other hand, do suggest a quantity issue. Similarly, the death rate among patients who are admitted to a hospital (again, versus international benchmarks) could provide information on clinical quality. Since maternal death rates among the rural poor are of special concern, it would be important to compare the quality and quantity of care for that population vis-a-vis the rest of the country. In addition, as we noted initially, at each juncture in the tree, the options are *not* mutually exclusive. There could well be both quantity and quality problems to varying degrees in different regions of the country.

As analysts move back through the causal tree, they should seek to identify factors that can be altered through new policy initiatives. For example, suppose data suggest that poor clinical quality of care—especially in rural areas—contributes to maternal deaths. This implies a deeper look at possible causes of that poor clinical quality is in order, as illustrated in Figure 7.3. The first two branches of that diagram are straightforward. First, is there a problem with the providers? As discussed in Chapter 6, evaluating skill and decision-making will generally involve looking at clinical records, and investigating the care given in a sample of maternal death cases would be one way to proceed (Lockyer and Harrison 1994). If this study does reveal clinical quality issues, this should provoke still further inquiry. First, were the right decisions made about how to care for patients? Alternatively, was it the case that while providers tried to act correctly, they could not because they lacked critical inputs, such as personnel, facilities, equipment, drugs, or other supplies (Berwick et al. 1991)?

Another possibility is that we could discover problems in clinical systems—poor communication, lost records, and so forth. The third branch of Figure 7.3 reflects this last possibility. As we mentioned in discussing clinical quality, it is often the way the care system is organized that accounts for poor results. As we will see in Chapter 10 (Organization), much of the thrust of the total-quality-management movement has been aimed at making changes to such systems (Deming 1982, Juran and Gryna 1980).

Each of these causes gives rise to still further questions. Suppose wrong decisions are made. Is it because people don't know better (training), or because they are not trying hard enough (motivation)? If inputs are limited, is it a matter of overall budget resources or how purchasing and staffing are carried out? If clinical systems and processes are faulty, is it poor management within institutions, or the way care is organized across the system, or both? As we move backwards up the causal chain, we should be mindful of the imperative to base our work on evidence, not speculation.

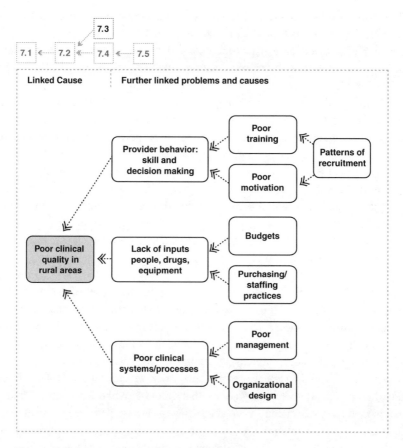

FIGURE 7.3. More steps back along the chain.

Going back still farther begins to reveal factors that are subsumed under the control knobs. If workers are not motivated or clinical systems are not well constructed—because of poor management—why is that? Is it because there are no incentives for the organization to produce quality, or are there no incentives for managers to do better? Or is it that managers lack the skill and the authority to do better (Roberts 1975)? Here we see the expression of the principles noted initially—that causes can have more than one effect, and effects can have more than one cause. Obviously, each of these endpoints could, in turn, provoke further analysis. Why, for instance, isn't training better, or why are doctors not more motivated?

Alternatively, suppose the assessment depicted in Figure 7.2 revealed that an insufficient quantity of services being used in rural areas is a critical cause of poor performance. The further study then required is shown in Figure 7.4.

Why might the quantity of care be insufficient? The explanation could lie on either the supply or the demand side. On the supply side, the most direct

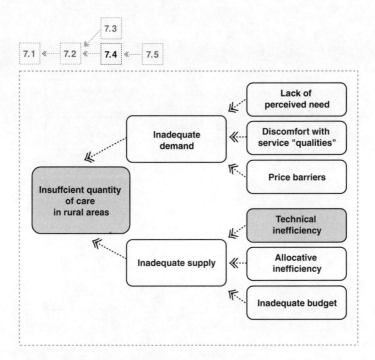

FIGURE 7.4. Possible causes of low service use.

explanation might involve simple physical availability. Are there clinics and hospitals with staff, supplies, and the capacity to deliver more services? If that is the case, then either patients are not using the services that are there, or there are barriers preventing "physical availability" from becoming "effective availability" (as we defined those concepts when discussing "access" in Chapter 6). If services are not physically available, asking "why" leads to various possibilities—perhaps the budget for these activities is too low. Alternatively, if spending levels are comparable to other regions or other countries with higher utilization, then the lack of services could be due to either technical inefficiency (i.e., high unit cost leading to lower volume) or allocative inefficiency (i.e., the wrong mix of services is being produced from the perspective of cost-effective performance). And if any (or all) of these turn out to be the case, we are coming closer to the point of identifying causes that might be changed by acting on the various control knobs.

On the other hand, if services are physically available but unused, the issue is on the demand side. First, there might be a lack of perceived need—that is, the local culture may strongly favor noninstitutionalized or traditional delivery. Alternatively, service "qualities" may make the service unattractive (Mehrotra and Jarrett 2002); so, too, might the presence of user fees, either explicitly to the institution, or in the form of informal payments to providers, or the requirement that patients

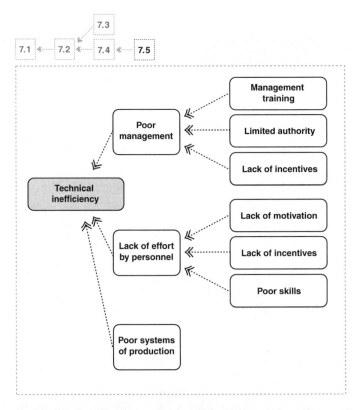

FIGURE 7.5. Possible causes of technical inefficiency.

pay for drugs and supplies. This example shows how supply and demand are not fully separable, because low demand may be due to the nature of the supply.

To see this, let us trace out one further set of causal connections, as in Figure 7.5. Suppose the system is technically inefficient (high cost). Why might that be the case? Is it poor management, lack of effort from workers, or failures in the system of production? Suppose, for example, studies reveal that while clinics theoretically have adequate staff, doctors actually only work a few hours a day and spend the afternoons in private practice (Berman and Sakai 1993). Hence, reported case-loads per doctor are low and average costs are high. To account for this, the diagnostic journey has to go even deeper and look at staff incentives, organizational culture, systems of accountability (or their absence), how managers are selected and rewarded, and other matters of this sort. This analysis can lead to the end of the journey; namely, identifying features of the situation that are potentially changeable. Remember, however, that multiple, interacting causes may well be at work, and multiple interacting policies may be required to produce better results.

Notice that as we have done this analysis, quite a number of the intermediate performance measures identified in Chapter 6 have made an appearance: various aspects of efficiency, access, and quality have played a role in all the potential causal chains. Notice, too, however, that categories like "technical efficiency" and "clinical quality" do not appear at the ends of the diagnostic tree branches. Rather, they appear in the middle of the journey, and their appearance itself requires further explanation.

As noted, the pathways in these diagrams are not mutually exclusive. Going back to Figure 7.2, we could have both a quantity and a quality problem—the same causes could be producing both. For instance, hospitals might be paid in a way that does not generate any incentives for performance. This, in turn, can produce both poor-quality clinical care and technical inefficiency that limits the quantity of care. Moreover, if we view the full tree in all its branches, we would see that many of the factors that contribute to poor quality are also potential causes of technical inefficiency. This is because poorly performing organizations are typically inefficient in the production of everything: quantitatively as well as qualitatively. Moreover, one deficiency could be the result of several interacting causes.

As we work back along the causal chain, we identify more and more specific causes that in turn begin to allow us to identify specific remedies. This process of diagnosis leads us back to the health system control knobs.

Linking Diagnosis to the Control Knobs

We have argued all along that the "control knobs" provide a framework for considering possible interventions to improve health-sector performance once we have embarked on a diagnostic journey. In effect, they provide a list of options. As a way of illustrating their use, we now explore the high-maternal-mortality example one step farther.

- *Financing*: If we do have a quantity-of-service problem, can we tap new or additional sources of funding to expand the budget for this service? Alternatively, can we alter how we spend existing funds to increase allocative efficiency?
- *Payment*: If we discover we have a problem of motivation, whether at the level of the organization or of the individual provider, can we change how we pay, or the rates we pay, to improve both the quantity and quality of services?
- *Organization*: If we are not organized to facilitate economies of scale and coordination, if patients experience cultural barriers or have preferences for certain types of providers, what changes could we make in who offers various maternal health services to overcome these problems? If the issue is technical efficiency and/or clinical or service quality, can we change how providers are organized in ways that would increase their performance?

- *Regulation*: Are there regulatory devices we can deploy to increase the quality and quantity of services or to increase their utilization?
- *Behavior*: If there are important causes on the demand side, could we seek to influence mothers to increase their use of the services that are available?

Notice that to get significant improvements in maternal mortality, we will probably have to take several actions simultaneously. For example, suppose we reorganize to give managers increased authority to improve efficiency. This is likely to have much less impact if done in isolation than if it is done in conjunction with payment reform (e.g., incentive contracting) of a sort that gives managers a strong reason to improve their performance. Similarly, raising more money (via financing) to push into a system of care that performs poorly may have very little impact without complementary changes in payment and organization.

Similar kinds of interacting effects are likely to operate when it comes to producing changes in behavior on the demand side of this problem. Suppose we are trying to persuade skeptical patients to increase their utilization of our reorganized maternal health services. That reorganization has to deliver changes in clinical quality and service "qualities" that will produce positive experiences for those who utilize the service. Indeed, to truly make a difference, we may need to raise more money (finance) and deliver it via new incentive schemes (payment) to restructured providers (organization), even as we seek to convince patients that the new services are worthy of their patronage (behavior).

The relative importance and relevance, as well as the content, of these interventions will depend on the specifics of a country's situation. For example, if services are largely provided in facilities directly operated by the ministry of health, it will be easier to influence their internal organization than if they are offered by independent practitioners. In the latter case, it is likely that incentive payments and/or regulatory constraints will play a larger role. Similarly, a nation with a public delivery system manned by reasonably well-motivated employees who are hamstrung by restrictive budgetary practices and poor management will need different organizational changes than one in which staff are cynical and uninvolved.

We also need to recognize that not every health-sector reformer will decide on an ambitious program of multiple major changes. They may lack the authority or the resources, or political and administrative feasibility may point toward a more modest effort. If so, we believe that decision should emerge as a result of the kind of analyses we have described.

The Process of Policy Development

Before we say more about the substance of health-sector reform, we need to say more about the process. Experience shows that process can matter as much as substance; indeed, these two are deeply intertwined. In particular, involving interest groups in the process of policy development serves at least four functions.

First, participation by those affected allows policymakers to hear and take into account interest groups' concerns. This can improve both the acceptance and the effectiveness of reform initiatives. As we discussed in Chapter 4, one way to assemble a support coalition is to compromise with key constituencies on features of a reform that matter more to them than they do to the reformers. Allowing constituencies to participate in the policy-development process is one way to learn about those concerns and take them into account (Heymann 1987).

Furthermore, being aware of such concerns can improve a policy's chances of successful implementation. For example, compliance with a proposed new regulatory system might simply not be practical, given hospitals' existing data systems and administrative capacity. Learning about such issues in the policy-development process can be critically important in creating a scheme that will function as intended.

Second, participation can increase the acceptance of a plan, because it increases the psychological and philosophical legitimacy of the process that developed it. Being heard can "co-opt" participants, who then feel that their concerns have been acknowledged even if they don't get everything they want (Cobb and Ross 1997). Exclusion, on the other hand, operates both emotionally and prudentially to generate hostility and suspicion. Furthermore, in democratic societies, allowing interests to be heard is likely to increase the legitimacy of the process (and its product), not only among those who do participate, but for everyone else (Almond and Verba 1963).

Third, participation can serve to educate interest groups about the concerns of, and pressures exerted on reformers by, other constituencies. For example, the doctors are likely to learn what the hospitals, unions, and consumers are demanding. This gives reformers both an excuse and an explanation for why they cannot necessarily respond favorably to any one interest group's demands.

Fourth, participation educates the participants about the details of the proposals that ultimately emerge. If, for example, local governments have been involved in crafting a health-sector-decentralization proposal, they are more likely to know what it means for their own responsibilities. This allows the relevant groups to understand any reform, makes them better able to predict the consequences to them of it, and prepares them for those consequences. This in turn is likely to lower their uncertainty and anxiety, and hence decrease at least some of their resistance to change.

At the same time, it is also true that participation can go too far. There is a great deal of evidence that the skill and ability of interest groups varies widely when it comes to influencing policy development (Kweit and Kweit 1987; Kathlene and Martin 1991). Groups with more resources and expertise tend to have more impact. Thus, the balance of forces in a participatory process may be quite different from the relative importance reform advocates place on the concerns of various interest groups.

As we have suggested several times, when it comes to health-sector reform, this imbalance often lends a conservative bias to the process. Organized groups, especially providers, can overwhelm the inexpert and unorganized. Poor, rural consumers, for example, seldom have the resources to have an effective voice in reform discussions, especially on more technical issues. Furthermore, the new institutions or organizational forms that might be created by reform do not yet exist to advocate their interests.

In addition, participatory processes can easily degenerate into a demand for unanimity. This gives entrenched interests a veto that can cripple any hope for real change. It can also lead to reports or legislative language that are intentionally vague—for the precise purpose of allowing those with diverse perspectives to agree to the compromise. This outcome only defers hard choices to the implementation stage—where, again, well-organized interests can often prevail (as we discuss in Chapter 11 on Regulation; Ackerman 1974, Landy et al. 1990). Indeed, powerful interests sometimes strategically support vague language to defer important issues to a less publicly visible administrative process in which they expect to have more influence.

All of these observations suggest that participation by interest groups raises, not lowers, the need for leadership by reformers. Reformers can do much to shape any participatory process by defining its procedures and its membership: they can formulate questions, set agendas, specify alternatives, and analyze implications. They can, and should, honestly explain the limits of the conversation and specify what options and spheres of action are, and are not, on the table.

Moreover, those in charge of managing a diagnostic or policy-development process need to understand that large groups of people are seldom capable of serious analytical work. At the front end, they can "brainstorm" and generate new ideas, and at the back end they can make selective criticisms of proposals once on the table. But the hard work in the middle, of going from a "brainstorm" to a developed policy option, together with an analysis of its implications, is not the work of a large meeting. Instead, it requires organized and disciplined staff resources. Sophisticated managers know that the background, training, politics, and biases of those doing the staff work can affect the result. This is especially so when data are scarce or inconclusive, as is often the case in health-sector reform (a point we return to shortly). This only reinforces the need to manage a participatory process—and the associated staff work—in a disciplined and sophisticated manner.

To get this work done health-reform advocates often organize a "change team" to manage the processes of policy design and adoption (González-Rosetti and Bossert 2000). These teams are responsible for working with diverse groups—both inside and outside of government—to manage the complexities of promoting policy change. The change team requires, not only technical capacity for policy design, but also the political capacity to mobilize relevant groups and individuals. The location of the change team varies, depending on the institutional setup and the location of the reform advocates. The change team can be an advisory group in the president's or prime minister's office; the team can also be a legislative commission or an adhoc committee to advise the minister of health. As has been found with economic policy reform (Waterbury 1992), the composition, location, incentives, and power of the change team can make a critical difference in the chances for successful health-sector reform.

An analysis of change teams in three Latin American cases of health reform (Chile, Colombia, and Mexico) found several common traits: ideological cohesiveness, high technical skills, work in isolation, and the use of policy networks (González-Rossetti and Bossert 2000, 50). The teams in these countries worked with several ministries and agencies, especially the ministry of finance, the ministry of planning, the office of the president, and sometimes the military. While composed of technical people who could formulate a new policy, they also needed to engage in bureaucratic battles with government agencies, manage the pressures from interest groups, navigate the legislative process of producing a new law, and initiate implementation of the reform. The creation of a change team thus represented a significant political strategy in itself in these cases. But the teams also constructed additional political strategies to address these challenges of the health-reform process—and sometimes required support from the highest political levels to achieve change, as occurred in Colombia and Chile.

Finally, we need to say a word about the process of generating policy alternatives. Much research on human problem-solving and cognition supports the notion that new ideas are extremely difficult to generate (Barzelay and Armajani 1992). People in general have a difficult time thinking "outside the box" of their familiar concepts and paradigms. All of this implies the lesson we announced at the beginning of the chapter: "Imitate but adapt."

Imitation can take various forms. Ideas from health-sector initiatives in other countries are one obvious source. Another possibility is ideas developed in other policy areas that can be adapted to the health context. For example, if decentralization has worked well in education, perhaps it can be applied to health services. If contracting out in the highway department has improved the quality of work, maybe there are lessons to be learned for hospital laundries or food services.

General theoretical arguments can also provide new ideas. Perhaps ideas about competition in economics or tort liability in law can suggest reform initiatives. Here, however, we need to issue some words of warning. Economists in particular easily become overly enthusiastic about using markets to solve every problem—based on theoretical models that don't always apply to the health sector (Reinhardt 2001). For these and other new ideas, it is important to observe the "but adapt" part of our guideline.

To summarize: process has an impact on content, politics, and implementation. Participation is not just a ploy. It is both a learning and a teaching device, and can improve a policy substantially and have a major impact on its acceptability. But it can also get out of hand and make the life of a reformer extremely difficult. Therefore, the process of policy development needs to be managed strategically. As with everything else about health-sector reform, foresight, careful analysis, and self-critical thinking can make substantial contributions to the prospects of success or failure.

Screening Tests for Policy Interventions

Once plausible policies have been identified, reformers need to do a serious feasibility and implementation analysis. That analysis has to take account of the likely politics before and after a program is adopted; of local customs, capacities, and institutions; and of the available financial and human resources. The analysis has to lead to a plausible story about how the policy interventions will act to produce the desired performance changes. This is not always easy to do. Our knowledge of the health sector and of the social and economic systems connected to it is far from exact or complete. We are therefore often unable to fully predict the impact of all possible reforms on all possible outcomes. There are, however, certain characteristics of reform proposals that have general predictive value—characteristics we can look for to test the likely efficacy of a particular proposal.

Implementability

What matters is what actually happens to the system's performance when a reform is implemented. Reformers therefore have to explore whether their country has the institutional and social prerequisites needed to support a proposed innovation. For example, do the government agencies that will have to carry out the new program have the necessary technical skills and managerial sophistication? Can the existing systems of data collection produce the information that will be needed? How reliable are the courts and police when it comes to enforcing proposed regulations? There is also the matter of influence from special interests. What role will various groups—from tribal leaders and political parties to the medical society—have in the implementation process? Will this influence undermine a program's real impact? All these factors will help determine what a particular policy will actually accomplish (Pressman and Wildavsky 1973, Davies and Davies 1975).

Social and cultural conditions and norms will also have an impact on implementation. How deferential to authority is the population? How willing is the government to use coercion to get its way, and how legitimate will such efforts be in the eyes of the population? Is rule compliance itself widely valued, or widely flouted and disrespected? Will people lie or tell the truth when asked to report on their own behavior?

As we stressed in discussing the policy cycle (Chapter 2), wise policy designers carefully consider such issues in the process of policy development. They don't propose payment systems that will tempt the unscrupulous or regulations that require unavailable data for their monitoring. Wise reformers do *not* presume that an idea from Denmark can automatically be replicated in Uganda. They will instead look for schemes that fit the cultural milieu and organizational capacity of their environment.

Political Feasibility

Those doing policy development also need to anticipate the process of political decision-making. In Chapter 4 we discussed the ideas of political analysis and political strategy, and showed how these affect political feasibility. That chapter emphasized that feasibility is not a "yes" or "no" judgment. It depends not only on who starts out in favor of or opposed to a plan, but on who is prepared to expend what resources, and take what risks, to get a plan adopted. It also depends on the political skill of a plan's opponents. Even then, the outcome is almost always uncertain.

Reformers therefore need to ask themselves how hard they and their allies are prepared to fight to get a particular scheme adopted. Their real choice may be between a plan that it is easier to get approved and one that is politically more difficult to adopt, but that promises more impact. Thus a political cost-benefit calculation, based on the particular situation (e.g., political resources, goals, philosophy) of reform advocates, is implicit in any "screening test" for political feasibility. As we noted in Chapter 4, the critical tradeoff may involve personal costs to the reformer versus benefits to the society as a whole.

Political Controllability

A final consideration in policy design is whether new arrangements and institutions will be subject to effective democratic political control. Such control depends on many features of the situation. First, will the results of the policy be publicly knowable? i.e., are the consequences measurable and those results transparent? Second, once we know the results of a policy, are there mechanisms in place to change it in response to information about its performance? Finally, are those who have the power to make such changes *themselves* politically accountable? That is, if citizens are unhappy, do they have channels of political action available to effectively express their dissatisfaction and through which to push for further reform?

The general argument for such controllability is based in part on the likely imperfection of any reform. If we create new institutions and arrangements that are difficult to change, our initial efforts can easily become an obstacle in later rounds of reform (Rawls 1996). Political controllability, we believe, will also generally produce better outcomes in the long run. Consumers, patients, and citizens who have a political voice are more likely to demand, and get, better performance from the health system. Moreover, results aside, as egalitarian liberals, we believe that people ought to be able to shape public policies that have a large impact on them.

This test is also controversial, however, and some people within the health sector want to limit political control over the products of reform. For example, in transitional economies in Eastern Europe, physicians have often favored the establishment of social insurance funds isolated from the general budget process (Feldstein 2001). They do not trust their country's political institutions, pressed by many competing demands, to produce the funding levels for health care that they desire.

We realize that political accountability can produce undesirable consequences in specific cases. For example, transparency can increase the influence of special interest groups, who use information about what is occurring to exert pressure on the legislative process. Such arrangements also can make it more difficult for legislators to support proposals they believe are in the national interest, when those same proposals undermine the parochial interests of their constituents.

Benevolent dictators or powerful technocrats can produce "good" results, if one happens to agree with their particular substantive values. But this is a risky long-run strategy. In addition, the inability to predict the full consequences of one's policy proposals is a strong argument against trying to prevent revisions. Thus, we urge that transparent mechanisms for political accountability be built into institutions as part of health-sector reform.

Finding and Using Evidence for Diagnosis and Therapy

Evidence-based health policy requires . . . evidence! Yet many lower and middle-income countries lack adequate evidence. Ironically, however, even when data and information are available, they are often not well utilized. We therefore need to be concerned both with the availability of information and with its effective use. The recent report of the Global Forum for Health Research noted that, "like other global public goods, global health and global health research suffer from insufficient investment" (2000).

What kind of knowledge can we use to identify the causes and predict the consequences of health-sector reform? Most desirable are well-designed studies that produce reliable statistical results linking policy to performance. Such studies, though, are far less common in health systems work than in clinical medicine.

Health-care systems are complex and varied, and there are few cases to study—i.e., relatively few countries. It is difficult, therefore, to get a large enough sample to deal with the many potentially relevant variables. In addition, because data are difficult to collect, they are often incomplete or unreliable (Williams 2000). Furthermore, it is almost impossible to run controlled trials on even a single health-care system—never mind a large number of systems—the way we can study a large numbers of patients.

Another desirable source of evidence is well-designed studies of demonstration projects that cover both experimental and nonexperimental sites (to serve as control groups) and report comparative performance data. But these, too, are relatively rare. Comparative analyses of similar interventions in different countries are more frequent and can be quite helpful in suggesting possible patterns of causality (Frankel and Doggett 1992). Suppose, for example, we look at a selection of community financing initiatives, some of which went well and others, badly. We might then be able to develop some ideas about the preconditions for the success of such interventions. More difficult to use, but still of value (and perhaps most common, especially for national-level changes) are reports about the effects of a policy change in a single country (Collins et al. 1996). It can be hard to disentangle causes of success or failure in such reports, but they can still be provocative or suggestive.

In addition to studies of various kinds, general theoretical arguments—about the effects of economic incentives or of political symbols—can also be brought to bear on a particular case. For example, if we pay doctors more to do X than Y, they often do more X and less Y. We do, however, have to be cautious, because theoretical arguments may miss important local details, such as whether hospitals will report accurately or whether local markets are competitive. This leads to a third basis for diagnosis and prediction; namely, an analyst's own experience and judgment as informed by detailed local knowledge. This can help someone see why a particular policy or program might not work in a specific country.

It is beyond the scope of this chapter to provide extensive guidance on the many facets of health systems research that could support diagnostic journeys for health reform. But to help get things started, here are some brief suggestions.

In the 1990s, there have been important advances in compiling data on health system performance. For the lower and middle-income countries, this has included the reports of the International Commission on Health Research for Development, the World Bank's 1993 report *Investing in Health*, and most recently WHO's *Health Systems: Improving Performance* (2000). The annual publication of the Organization for Economic Cooperation and Development, *Health Data*, provides an invaluable source of data on OECD member countries. The national reports on Central and Eastern European countries, produced by the WHO and the European Observatory on Health Care Systems (the "Health Care Systems in Transition," or HIT series), are also very helpful. Each of these major reports includes a good amount of information on health system characteristics and outcomes.

Yet the availability and quality of the data in these global references is very uneven. The response of various nations to the World Bank's 1993 report and WHO's 2000 report was quite mixed. Various criticisms revealed that individual country figures were sometimes extrapolated from regional averages. In addition, national health-expenditure information was sometimes based on significant "data-filling." Where good local sources are available but not known to international compilers, they can be a more trusted (and trustworthy) alternative.

Of the three main performance criteria, evidence on health status is by far the most developed. Traditional health-status measures, like infant and under-five mortality and life expectancy, have now been augmented with new composite measures of disease burden like DALYs (WHO 2000). Many countries now collect significant national health status information using standardized survey instruments such as the Demographic and Health Surveys (DHS) and the Living Standards Measurement Surveys (LSMS). These can be supplemented with data from well-done, smaller local studies, which may provide additional details on specific health problems and population groups.

Evidence about financial protection and citizen satisfaction is more limited, especially in low- and middle-income countries. For example, evidence on the distribution of the financial burden of health care may be available from national health accounts studies or household surveys (Makinen et al. 2000). But the concept of risk protection implies concern with the impact of the financial burden of care on household financial status. Here there are few general data available. Such outcomes depend not only on the health system, but on other socioeconomic factors. Measurement of customer satisfaction with health systems has been extensively done in the OECD countries using polling methods, but little evidence on satisfaction is available from the low- and middle-income countries. The effort by WHO (2000) in the report *Health Systems: Improving Performance* is worth noting, but this information is often not detailed enough to be used for diagnostic purposes.

Individual countries may have some evidence on both financial protection and customer satisfaction from national surveys and specific studies. We strongly encourage diagnosticians to assemble and review this information and improve upon it if they can.

When it comes to many intermediate performance characteristics and other factors that help determine health-system performance, the good news is that significant evidence is available. Here are some of the key data sources:

• National health accounts, health-care costing studies, and financial reports of insurers and other payers on financial resources provide data on costs and outputs that can be used to assess efficacy;

- Household surveys and health information system reports shed light on access and utilization;
- Quality studies and health information system reports provide information on the clinical quality of care;
- Government statistics, professional organization statistics, and facility-based studies provide data on the availability of facilities, manpower, equipment, and supplies, as well as on service volumes;
- International pharmaceutical market data and government and private market statistics provide information on pharmaceutical availability and use.

We know from experience that there is a lot of relevant information available for health systems analysis in almost every country. But we also know that this information may not be easily accessible and that it often needs to be used with caution. Much of what is helpful will be unpublished, in studies done by government or international agencies, local or foreign foundations and consulting companies. Hence "data entrepreneurship" may be required in tracking down the relevant information.

Here are some of the ways reformers can make more efficient use of the available evidence:

- *Know the literature*: It is increasingly easy to access up-to-date information through international publications and the Internet. Take the time to identify the relevant literature and become familiar with it. It is unlikely that you are the first person to confront or think about the problem that you are trying to solve.
- *Get advice*: National and international expertise is often available to help you sort through the literature and experiences of other countries. The major international organizations can be helpful, as can international networks like the European Observatory or the Alliance for Health Systems Research. But *caveat emptor* (let the buyer beware). Be skeptical of advice as well, especially advice that comes from those with something to sell, like a costly computerized information system.
- *Do rapid assessments*: Many questions do not require a major research project in order to develop a plausible account. Just because detailed evidence on an important point isn't available doesn't mean there aren't quick and relatively inexpensive methods to get plausible estimates. And those estimates may be sufficient for policy purposes.
- *Support good research*: Despite the last point, there may be real problems with "quick and dirty" studies and assessments. Sound applied research can provide more valid and reliable evidence. The bigger the stakes, the costlier it will be to make mistakes. In our experience, most low- and middle-income countries seriously underinvest in health systems research. But since such research takes time, planning, and resources, a good deal of foresight and forward thinking is required if you are to have the data you need when you actually need it.

Diagnosis and Policy Development: Some Final Observations

To do a good job of national health system diagnosis, the health-system reformer must be well prepared, curious, careful, and willing to learn from experience. The "science" of health-sector reform is still in an early stage of development. Here are some final points we urge you to keep in mind.

- *Work backwards up the causal chain until you can identify potentially manipulable variables*: The job of health-sector diagnosis goes from symptoms to causes, from unsatisfactory performance on critical goals to what is producing these results. This process is not always obvious. Policies can produce unintended consequences, and they can be badly managed. Individuals can claim to be doing one thing and in practice be doing something else. An open and skeptical mind and a high degree of energy and curiosity are often required.
- *Do not jump to quick conclusions*: It is tempting to decide early on what the problem *really* is, based on ideology or preconceptions. Unfortunately, it is not uncommon for a committed true believer to short-circuit the diagnostic process. This can be unfortunate, since identifying the wrong causes can lead to badly designed policies. This will not only divert valuable energy and waste a valuable opportunity, it can also discredit reform generally.
- *Be scientific, not judgmental*: Diagnosis can go astray when evaluative judgments cloud scientific analysis. If institutions or individuals behave in ways we disapprove of, we are quite likely to decide that they are the problem. In fact, not every bad actor is important, and bad behavior may be the result of larger forces. Thus it is important to remain dispassionate in the diagnostic process. There will be plenty of time (and need) for passion, once you are trying to mobilize political support for a particular policy. Meanwhile, clear, self-skeptical analysis is called for.
- *Use numbers*: We do not believe that everything important to health-sector reformers can be reduced to numbers. Still less do we believe that every country will have—or can afford—all of the good-quality data an analyst might like. And ignoring problems that cannot be documented in numbers can be very foolish. Disaster planners know that after earthquakes, the *silent zones* that they don't hear from can be the most badly affected. The same is true for health system performance. We may get no data at all from the poorest and worst-off areas. Yet, for all of that, data can be very helpful. Data can be a check on bias and premature judgment. Data can help support a scientific attitude. Whether they are DALYs or other health status indicators, whether they are National Health Accounts or surveys of citizens' attitudes, data can be a great leveler of prejudices. To use information wisely, reformers have to know where it comes from, and its limitations, omissions, and assumptions. But that only increases the need for making the requisite investment in such understanding.

References

Ackerman, Bruce A. 1974. *The Uncertain Search for Environmental Quality.* New York: Free Press.

Almond, Gabriel A.; and Sidney Verba. 1963. *The Civic Culture: Political Attitudes and Democracy in Five Nations.* Princeton, NJ: Princeton University Press.

Barzelay, Michael; with Babak J. Armajani. 1992. *Breaking Through Bureaucracy: A New Vision for Managing in Government.* Berkeley, CA: University of California Press.

Behn, Robert D.; and James W. Vaupel. 1982. *Quick Analysis for Busy Decision Makers.* New York: Basic Books.

Berman, Peter; and Suomi Sakai. 1993. "The Productivity of Manpower and Supplies in Public Health Services in Java." In: Anne Mills and Kenneth Lee, eds., *Health Economics Research in Developing Countries.* New York: Oxford University Press.

Berwick, Donald M.; A. Blanton Godfrey; and Jane Roessner. 1991. *Curing Health Care: New Strategies for Quality Improvement.* San Francisco, CA: Jossey-Bass.

Cobb, Roger W.; and Marc H. Ross. 1997. "Denying Agenda Access: Strategic Considerations." In: Roger W. Cobb and Marc H. Ross, eds., *Cultural Strategies of Agenda Denial: Avoidance, Attack, and Redefinition.* Laurence, KS: University Press of Kansas, 25–45.

Collins, David H.; Jonathan D. Quick; Stephen N. Musau; and Daniel L. Kraushaar. 1996. *Health Financing Reform in Kenya, The Fall and Rise of Cost Sharing, 1989–1994.* Stubbs Monograph Series No. 1. Boston, MA: Management Sciences for Health.

Colombia Health Sector Reform Project. 1996. *Report on Colombia Health Sector Reform and Proposed Master Implementation Plan, Final Report.* Boston, MA: School of Public Health, Harvard University.

Davies, J. Clarence, III; and Barbara S. Davies. 1975. *The Politics of Pollution.* Indianapolis, IN: Pegasus.

Deming, W. Edwards. 1982. *Quality, Productivity, and Competitive Position.* Cambridge, MA: MIT Center for Advanced Engineering Study.

Edelman, Murray. 1984. *The Symbolic Uses of Politics.* Urbana, IL: University of Illinois Press.

Feldstein, Paul J. 2001. *The Politics of Health Legislation, An Economic Perspective.* Chicago: Health Administration Press.

Frankel, Stephen; with Aileen Doggett, eds. 1992. *The Community Health Worker: Effective Programmes for Developing Countries.* New York: Oxford University Press.

González-Rossetti, Alejandra; and Thoams J. Bossert. 2000. *Enhancing the Political Feasibility of Health Reform: A Comparative Analysis of Chile, Colombia, and Mexico.* Boston, MA: Harvard School of Public Health/Data for Decision Making Project, June.

Heymann, Phillip B. 1987. *The Politics of Public Management.* New Haven, CT: Yale University Press.

Juran, Joseph M.; and Frank M. Gryna, Jr. 1980. *Quality Planning and Analysis.* New York: McGraw-Hill.

Kathlene, Lyn; and John A. Martin. 1991. "Enhancing Citizen Participation: Panel Designs, Perspectives, and Policy Formation." *Journal of Policy Analysis and Management* 10: 46–63.

Kweit, Mary G.; and Robert W. Kweit. 1987. "Citizen Participation: Enduring Issues for the Next Century." *National Civic Review* 76(May/June): 191–98.

Landy, Marc K.; Marc J. Roberts; and Stephen R. Thomas. 1990. *The Environmental Protection Agency: Asking the Wrong Questions.* New York: Oxford University Press.

Lockyer, Jocelyn M.; and R.Van Harrison. 1994. "The Role of Chart Review, Analysis and Continuing Medical Education in Physician Performance Enhancement." In: D. A. Davis and R. D. Fox, eds., *The Physician as Learner—Linking Research to Practice.* Chicago: American Medical Association.

Makinen, Marty; H. Water; Margie Rauch; Naila Almagambetova; Ricardo Bitran; Lucy Gilson; Diane McIntyre; Supasit Pannarunothai; A. Loreno Prieto; Gloria Ubilla; and Sujata Ram. 2000. "Inequalities in Health Care Use and Expenditures: Empirical Data from Eight Developing Countries and Countries in Transition." *Bulletin of the World Health Organization* 78(1): 55–65.

Mehrotra, Santosh; and Stephen Jarrett. 2002. "Improving Basic Health Service Delivery in Low-Income Countries: 'Voice' to the Poor." *Social Science and Medicine* 54(11): 1685–90.

Pressman, Jeffrey L.; and Aaron Wildavsky. 1973. *Implementation: How Great Expectations in Washington Are Dashed in Oakland.* Berkeley, CA: University of California Press.

Rawls, John. 1996. *Political Liberalism.* New York: Columbia University Press.

Reinhardt, Uwe E. 2001. "Can Efficiency in Health Care Be Left to the Market?" *Journal of Health Politics, Policy and Law* 26(5): 967–92.

Roberts, Marc J. 1975. "An Evolutionary and Institutional View of the Behavior of Public and Private Companies." *American Economic Review* 65(2): 415–27.

Rossi, Peter; Howard Freeman; and Mark Lipsey. 1998. *Evaluation: A Systematic Approach.* 6th edition. Thousand Oaks, CA: Sage.

Tierney, Lawrence M.; Stephen J. McPhee; and Maxine A. Papadakis, eds. 2001. *Current Medical Diagnosis and Treatment 2002.* 41st edition. New York: McGraw-Hill.

Waterbury, John. 1992. "The Heart of the Matter? Public Enterprise and the Adjustment Process." In: Stephan Haggard and Robert R. Kaufman, eds., with contributions by Peter Evans. *The Politics of Economic Adjustment: International Constraints, Distributive Conflicts, and the State.* Princeton, NJ: Princeton University Press.

Williams, Alan. 2000. "Science or Marketing at WHO? A Commentary on 'World Health 2000'." *Health Economics* 10(2): 93–100.

World Health Organization. 1986. *Intersectoral Action for Health: The Role of Intersectoral Cooperation in National Strategies for Health for All.* Geneva: World Health Organization.

——— 2000. *World Health Report 2000, Health Systems: Improving Performance.* Geneva: World Health Organization.

II

THE CONTROL KNOBS

8

Financing

The first control knob we explore is financing—the mechanisms by which money is mobilized to fund health-sector activities, and how it is used (i.e., allocation). How the money, once raised, is paid out falls under the heading of the "payment" control knob, which we consider in the next chapter.

Financing has an extremely important impact on the performance of a health system. It determines how much money is available, who bears the financial burden, who controls the funds, how risks are pooled, and whether health-care costs can be controlled. These factors, in turn, help determine who has access to care, who is protected against impoverishment from catastrophic medical expenses, and the health status of the population. There is no magic solution to financing problems. All the money raised through any financing method (except for foreign contributions) comes, directly or indirectly, from citizens. What each nation has to decide is what sources to use, and to what extent. These questions are the subject matter of this chapter.

Our discussion is organized as follows: The next section lays out the key criteria to be used when a nation considers which combination of financing methods may be best suited to it. We will argue that the mixture does and should depend greatly on social values and politics. Then we describe the different methods of financing and discuss their advantages and disadvantages. Next we discuss the question of how to allocate the funds that the financing system generates. We close with some conditional advice about which financing schemes are feasible for countries at different stages of socioeconomic development.

Considerations in Choosing a Financing Strategy

Implicitly or explicitly, every nation has to decide on a financing strategy—on what combination of financing methods to use to fund its health system. Five methods are described in this chapter: general revenue, social insurance, private insurance, direct payments by patients, and community financing. Most countries use a combination of methods. For example, the United Kingdom is widely perceived as a nation that relies on general revenues to finance its health system. In reality, however, only 76% of its health funds come from general revenues; 12% comes from social insurance contributions, 10% from private insurance, and 2% from direct out-of-pocket payments (OECD Health Data 2002). India also is viewed as relying mostly on general revenues to finance health care. In reality, however, only 20% of total health expenditure comes from general revenues, with over 70% from patients out-of-pocket and less than 10% from other sources (Peters et al. 2002).

When nations search for better financing strategies to improve the performance of their health systems, several essential factors have to be considered.

Socioeconomic Development

To state the obvious, the same structure in financing and its organizational arrangement cannot be applied to all nations. What works in the United Kingdom may not work in Kenya. On the other hand, do we have to treat every nation differently? Can we group nations into categories and derive general conclusions for the nations within each group? For several reasons we believe it is possible to do this based on per capita GDP (Hsiao 2000).

A nation's ability to mobilize funds is highly correlated with its per capita income. Income determines households' capacity to pay for health care and their demand for services. Other major factors highly correlated with income include the tax base from which a nation can raise tax revenues; the number of workers employed in the formal sector, which influences how much can be raised through social insurance; and the number of poor households that have to be subsidized.

Different methods also place greater or lesser demands on a nation's infrastructure and its competence in public and private management. These factors, too, are highly correlated with per capita income. Lower-income nations, on average, also differ from higher-income nations in having a much higher percentage of economic activity in the shadow economy (unrecorded legal income and proceeds from illicit activities). Schneider (2002) estimated that the shadow economies of Mexico, Philippines, Egypt, and Thailand are more than fifty percent of their official GDP.

High-income nations such Japan and the United States have shadow economies that are less than ten percent of their official GDP. This is relevant to financing choices because it is impossible to collect taxes or social insurance contributions from the income of the shadow economy. For these reasons, we use per capita GDP as a way to group nations into categories (Hsiao 2000).

Sorting nations by income level helps us analyze the financing methods that are available to them, the amount of money that can be raised through various sources, and thus the potential to pool the financial risks of poor health. Our first category includes all low-income countries. Here tax funds usually finance 40% to 60% of total health expenditures, 10% to 15% is financed by social insurance (most likely covering civil servants), and 40% to 50% comes from patients' direct out-of-pocket payments. Private insurance is negligible or nonexistent, because few households can afford to buy private insurance, and the necessary administrative safeguards are not in place to prevent fraudulent insurance claims.

As a country industrializes and per capita income grows, making it a middle-income country, social insurance usually expands, because the number of workers in the formal sector grows. Private insurance begins to emerge but still plays a small role. The major portion of total national health expenditures is still financed by general revenue or patients' direct payments. These countries are included in our second category. The major difference between the first and second categories is the relative proportion of total health expenditures financed from different sources, and the size of the private-insurance and social-insurance-funded services. Such services generally develop once these other sources of funding are available, and they often offer a noticeably higher quality of services than what is available in directly operated public-sector facilities.

The third category includes all high-income nations, which (except for the United States) have established a system of financing to assure universal access to health care. Table 8.1 presents these three stages of health financing development, with examples of countries in each category, as well as a summary of the financing and organization of health care typical of each stage.

Fiscal Capacity

A key question for a financing strategy is, can it mobilize enough money to meet the desired level of expenditures in the health sector? Fiscal capacity is contextual. The results of any strategy will depend on the economic structure of a society (are there many workers in the formal sector?), and the government's administrative capacity. Moreover, the amount of money that can be raised may well depend not only on its economic base but also on what a country is willing to give up in other arenas (such as in international competitiveness from higher labor costs or lower spending on pensions or education) in order to increase its health-sector spending. Thus, it is useful to think of the match or mismatch between a given

TABLE 8.1. Evolution of Health-Care Financing and Provision Systems at Various Stages of Economic Development

	STAGE I (THREE-TIERED SYSTEM)		STAGE II (COMPARTMENTALIZED FINANCING AND PROVISION)	STAGE III (UNIVERSAL COVERAGE**)
	Poor (less than $1,800)*	Low-Income ($1,800–$4,800)*	($5,000–$12,000)*	(greater than $12,000)*
General Revenue Financed and Donor	Public health, prevention Government-health facilities (clinics, hospitals) (50%–60%)	(40%–50%)	Public Health Service (20%–40%)	National Health Service (U.K., N.Z.) Medisave and Catastrophic Insurance (Singapore)
Social Insurance	For civil servants only	(10%–20%)	Social Insurance (Direct/Indirect Provision) (30%–60%)	National Health Insurance (Canada, Australia) Bismarckian Social Insurance (Germany, Japan)
Private Insurance	Negligible	(5%–10%)	Private Insurance (15%–40%)	Managed Care and Medicare (U.S.)
Self-pay	Private hospitals and clinics Pharmacists Indigenous providers (35%–45%)	(20%–40%)	Self-pay (15%–25%)	Self-pay (15%–25%)
	Mali, Nigeria, Tanzania, Kenya, Yemen, Bangladesh, India	China, Egypt, Peru, Ecuador, Philippines, Indonesia	Turkey, Chile, Mexico, Argentina, Brazil, Lebanon, Venezuela, Thailand, Malaysia	

* GDP per capita, 1997 PPP $
** Except U.S. & Hong Kong
Source: Hsiao 2000.

financing strategy and a nation's health-sector funding goals. When reformers discuss the "sustainability" of a nation's health financing system, they are, in effect, focusing on this question. Let us take a quick look at each financing method from this perspective.

The capacity of a nation to raise money from general revenue depends on the size of various tax bases—the volume of economic activity subject to a particular tax. While this capacity correlates closely with the overall level of economic development, particular factors may also play a role (e.g., the presence of easy-to-tax resources like oil, or a large role for hard-to-tax sectors like small farmers).

For social insurance, fiscal capacity depends on the ability to collect contributions from employers and workers. Smaller firms, however, may not keep appropriate records, and even at a conceptual level, separating a small farmer or business owner's earnings (labor income) from their profits (capital income) is not easy to do. Yet only the labor income is supposed to be subject to tax. Some countries have resorted to a standardized contribution from the self-employed to solve this problem. In Hungary, for example, this is based on the income of someone earning the minimum wage, a rule very favorable to small-businessmen.

In general, the more sophisticated a country's administrative infrastructure, and the more cooperative its citizens, the farther down the business size scale a social insurance system can reach. But in low- to middle-income countries, that is not very far. In such cases, social insurance can generally be effectively implemented only for workers who are employed in larger companies (e.g., more than ten employees) and in the formal sector.

Private insurance can mobilize funds from people who can pay and wish to be insured. Upper-income people may be more willing to buy private insurance, to cover expanded or higher-quality services for themselves, than to pay taxes that benefit others. But funds mobilized through private health insurance cannot easily provide financing for the poor. In such a system, those who do not have private insurance—because they cannot afford it—can end up in desperate straits, without access to health services.

Community financing, especially in poor rural communities, has only a limited capacity to raise funds for health care. Yet resources mobilized in this way can produce modest but important gains in funding for primary health services and some hospital care.

Finally, direct out-of-pocket payment by patients is common in most low- and middle-income countries. Recent National Health Accounts (NHA) studies suggest that there may be substantial willingness and ability to spend on outpatient care, even among relatively poor people in poor countries—especially when we include informal payments to physicians (and nurses) and payments for drugs and supplies that clinics do not provide. The NHA studies show that even in countries with extensive tax-funded public health services, independent private practitioners provide a high proportion of outpatient care, paid for directly by patients.

In higher-income countries, the capacity to use out-of-pocket payments is even greater because household incomes are higher. In such countries, selected services may not be covered by insurance (such as drugs or dentistry). In other situations, patients may have to pay something, officially, even for some publicly provided or insured services (user fees or co-payments). There may also be gaps in what insurance covers in the form of deductibles (at the front end) or limits (at the back end).

Implementability

Raising funds requires spending money to create records, establish accounting and auditing systems, and organize administrative agencies. If there are competitive, private insurance companies, money also will be spent on marketing, sales, and profits. Thus an important question is how much of total spending goes for administrative expenses and profits under various financing arrangements.

Private insurance in particular has very high administrative costs. U.S. insurance companies often spend 25% to 30% of total revenue on expenses other than patient care (sales, administration, and profit). In addition, doctors and hospitals also have substantially higher administrative costs in the United States than they do in other countries. Studies report that advanced American hospitals have two full-time administrative employees for each occupied bed, about ten times as many as do comparable German hospitals (Köeck et al. 1998).

The right regulations (e.g., specifying uniform claim forms to be used by all insurance companies) can somewhat reduce these costs. Nevertheless, the burden remains substantial. Private health insurance markets are very complicated systems. Nations that go the private insurance route, therefore, must be prepared not only to pay these high transaction costs, but also to develop substantial capacity to monitor, analyze, and regulate these markets. Otherwise they are unlikely to achieve various social objectives.

A second key aspect of implementability is a country's administrative capacity. Does the nation have the administrative systems and human resources it needs to operate a financing scheme effectively? These concerns lead countries with weak administrative systems to rely on the taxes that are easiest to collect (e.g., import duties and value-added taxes), even if they are not desirable revenue sources on other grounds. For example, sales taxes are often easier to collect than income taxes, because there are fewer businesses to collect sales taxes from than there are households to collect income taxes from, and businesses tend to have better records than households. Moreover, income from "black" or "gray" sources can be taxed when spent (through consumption taxes), but these sources are not likely to be reported to income tax collectors. Both payroll and sales taxes, however, can be difficult to administer when there are many small sellers in the informal sector, as is the case in many poor countries.

Implementability also depends on the social acceptability of a financing scheme. Will citizens cheat or not? The reach of any system depends greatly on the attitudes of the public toward government in general, and tax-paying in particular. Levels of voluntary compliance vary enormously both inter- and intra-nationally, and using schemes that the population sees as legitimate is much more likely to be success-ful. (Many of these issues of enforceability will arise again in our discussion of regulation in Chapter 11.)

One particular example of this issue is that the social contract implicit in many social insurance schemes can have a major impact on their acceptability and hence on their ability to raise revenue. Citizens often feel that they are more likely to get services in return for their contributions when the funds are segregated, and when non-contributors are not part of the pool. This is partly why Colombia es-tablished two separate social insurance funds for the formal and informal sectors. Whether such arrangements are in a nation's best interest is a complex political judgment that requires a case-by-case analysis beyond the scope of our current discussion.

Political Accountability

In a democracy, decisions about how to spend money and about how much to spend are a basic expression of government power. From the perspective of demo-cratic political theory, these choices must be made in a way that allows citizens appropriate control over the process. Several features of the financing system affect this accountability. Is someone who has authority over the financing process subject to selection by democratic process? If the administrator is an appointed technocrat, does a chain of accountability exist to connect the administrator to someone whose authority is subject to electoral decisions?

The ideal of political accountability, however, is controversial in many nations. Where distrust of the political process is great, some prefer that health financing decisions be made by agencies that are insulated from political processes. This tendency is particularly true of countries whose public budgets are under great pressure. Interest groups in those countries hope that isolating health financing from the general budget process will increase the flow of resources into the health sector and thereby produce more income for providers. This helps explain why new social insurance schemes have been supported by the medical societies in a wide variety of nations (for example, both Poland and Colombia).

Criteria for Judging Financing Methods

In addition to the four considerations just reviewed, several other key criteria have to be considered in evaluating a financing method and its associated organization-al arrangements. In particular, these are equity, risk pooling, and economic effects.

Equity: Since financing directly affects the distribution of the cost of health care, one obvious question is, Who bears the financial burden? Since how the funds are used directly affects the distribution of health care, a second obvious question is, Who receives the benefits? Assessing the distribution of burden and benefit has two different dimensions. Vertical equity refers to the distribution of the burden between the rich and the poor. Horizontal equity has to do with creating fairness among those at the same income level, including people living in different regions.

Risk Pooling: Illnesses, and the health-care costs associated with them, do not fall evenly throughout the population. Cancer strikes some people but not others, and diarrhea hits some children but not others. On the other hand, some groups of people do face higher health risks. Older people have more sickness and disability than the young, and diabetics need much more frequent health care than the average person. The uncertainty of illness calls for a financing strategy where risks can be pooled. But the task is not so easy when there are identifiable high- and low-risk groups. Low-risk groups, such as the young and healthy people, do not want to be pooled with the high-risk groups, because pooling pushes up the cost for low-risk groups. For example, China found that the joint-venture companies that tend to employ younger workers strongly resist being pooled under social insurance with workers in established industries that tend to have older workers.

The ability to pool health risks varies widely among the five methods for mobilizing funds. General revenues pool risks if they are used for health services accessible to all or to subsidize the premiums of high-risk groups. Mandatory social insurance can provide substantial risk pooling, provided coverage is more or less universal. Private group insurance only pools health risks within a selected group, such as for the workers of a particular company or the members of an occupational group. Patients' out-of-pocket payment, of course, offers no risk pooling.

Economic Effects: When a government compels a firm or individual to pay a tax on a selected activity such as wages, the firm and individual may alter their decisions about how much to work and earn. Various options have differential impacts on deterring or encouraging investment, employment opportunities, and labor supply, thereby influencing both the mix and the level of economic activity in the short and long run.

Financing Options

Our typology of financing options is a mixture of the fiscal and organizational aspects of the money-raising process. It reflects both the economic sources used by alternative methods and the organizational arrangements through which financing is carried out. Our options are best thought of as a set of "ideal methods"—each alternative is a highly stylized pure case.

In practice, however, most financing systems are *not* pure. Instead, most nations have chosen a mix-and-match approach, combining methods in complex ways that reflect the trade-offs in objectives that a nation is willing to make, based on its particular political and economic history. For example, general revenue systems in low- and middle-income countries often require patients to pay user fees and do not cover certain kinds of medical expenses, such as drugs. Likewise, most private insurance schemes require patients to make substantial direct payments to providers.

Our categories are intended to provide a framework for characterizing and analyzing actual financing systems. We discuss the five major methods of financing in turn.

General Revenue

In general revenue financing, many kinds of taxes are used to support the full range of government activities. The health system, therefore, has to compete for funds with other government-funded programs and obtains its resources via the regular government budget process.

Government revenues range from income and profit taxes, to value-added and sales taxes, to import duties, to taxes on profits from minerals. Each places burdens on different groups of citizens. The mix of taxes used by a particular country generally depends on its situation. Low-income countries tend to rely more on easy-to-collect sources of revenue, like import and export fees, or canal tolls—if you are Egypt or Panama. Other sources (income and value-added taxes) require more extensive data systems and a higher level of voluntary compliance.

Broad-based taxes automatically generate more resources for health as the economy grows over time. On the other hand, collections also rise and fall in the short-run over the business cycle. Some taxes, such as progressive income taxes and taxes on profits, are more sensitive than others to both short-run business cycles and long-run growth. Growth moves people into higher income tax brackets, increasing both marginal and average collections, while profits also are quite sensitive to the business cycle. In contrast, payroll and sales taxes change slightly less in percentage terms than the gross domestic product (GDP). When there are large swings in national income (as in the Asian economic crisis of 1997 or the recent troubles in Argentina) governments can find themselves hard-pressed to maintain health spending regardless of which mix of taxes they use, especially since the demands on government for other types of spending also rise in a recession.

General tax financing offers a high degree of political accountability in democratic political systems, since the key decisions pass directly through the legislative process. Thus, the level of funding can be controlled, and decision-makers held accountable for their actions. On the other hand, implicit tax support through mechanisms like tax concessions (e.g., allowing expenditures on health care to lower a person's income tax liability) is neither transparent nor controllable. It is difficult to know how much revenue is lost via such schemes, and difficult to control who benefits from them.

A related tax structure issue, raised by general revenue financing, is the question of the distribution of the financing burden by levels of government. As we discuss in more detail below (in Chapter 10 on organization) nations occasionally devolve responsibility for operating health-care systems to local and regional governments. This is sometimes done by fiscally hard-pressed national governments to force the local or regional governments to raise their own taxes to support the delivery system.

For example, some years ago Poland tried to get the largest cities to assume operating responsibility for local hospitals under the so-called Large Cities Law (Roberts and Bossert 1998). A majority of cities turned these institutions back to the national government when they realized the obligations they were incurring. In other countries (e.g., China and India) the bulk of the health budget comes from state or provincial revenues. As we discuss in the next section, such arrangements can raise substantial equity issues when (as is typically the case) there are large interregional variations in fiscal capacity.

Vertical and horizontal equity of alternative taxes

As we discussed in Chapter 6, the tax burden may not fall only on those who pay taxes. Instead, governments may curtail other services when they appropriate more money for health. In this case, the beneficiaries of other services that are now *not* being provided are the ones paying for higher health-sector costs. The same is true when government subsidizes some activities through tax concessions. The payers might be those who pay the other taxes raised to make up for the lost revenue or they might be the potential beneficiaries of other activities that were curtailed because of money lost to tax concessions.

In addition, those who directly pay a tax may not be those who ultimately bear the burden. For example, employers generally shift some of the cost of payroll taxes back to workers in the form of lower salaries. Similarly, property taxes on landlords may be passed on to renters in the form of more expensive rents. Whether such shifting occurs, and to what extent, depends on a variety of features of the relevant markets. There is vast economic literature on such issues (Musgrave and Musgrave 1989; Atkinson and Stiglitz 1980).

Vertical Equity: We have already introduced the distinctions among progressive, proportional, and regressive taxes (see Chapter 5). In most countries, only comprehensive income taxes, including taxes on capital income, can be truly progressive, since only such taxes can take a higher proportion of the income of people at higher income levels. In contrast, payroll taxes are mildly regressive, because the proportion of total income that comes from payrolls falls at higher income levels. Such schemes become even more regressive if there is a limit on any one person's payroll tax contribution (as is sometimes the case). Taxes on consumption—sales and value-added taxes—are also moderately regressive, because the percentage of income that is spent and taxed, as opposed to saved, is lower at higher incomes. This is why some consumption tax schemes exempt, or tax at a lower rate, commodities on which the poor spend a higher percentage of their income, like food. For similar reasons, we often find a higher tax rate on luxury items, where the rich spend more of their income.

To understand the vertical equity of a tax system—how redistributive it is on balance—we have to look not only at burdens but also at the distribution of benefits by income groups. In the final analysis, the vertical equity of net benefits—the benefits minus burden—will be of special interest from an equity perspective. Even regressive taxes, where the rich pay more absolutely, if not relatively (like payroll taxes), can support a redistributive system. If services are widely available, then the poor are likely to pay less than the cost of the services they receive, while the rich pay more.

Horizontal Equity: The horizontal equity of tax-based financing varies with the kind of taxes being levied. Broad-based national taxes do not raise horizontal equity issues, but narrower taxes (e.g., on tobacco or alcohol) may do so. Is it really fair to ask drinkers or smokers to pay more, especially if, as appears to be the case, moderate alcohol consumption improves health?

In recent years, many countries have shifted both control and fiscal responsibility for health care to the subnational level. Such schemes can raise serious horizontal equity issues, since more prosperous areas can finance the same service as poor areas at lower tax rates, or better services with the same tax rate.

For this reason, nations that have gone the route of fiscal decentralization have often found it necessary to establish interregional equalization funds. The countries with the longest-standing systems of this type, like the Scandinavian countries and Colombia, now rely heavily on national taxes to supplement local sources.

Constructing an equalization scheme, however, can be quite complex, since it must do more than consider need (population, illness, and income). It also has to create incentives to prevent poor regions from lowering their own tax effort and free-riding on the collective efforts of their neighbors. Decentralizing taxing decisions also runs the risk of creating a race to the bottom, as regions compete in attracting business by lowering taxes. Richer (and more politically powerful) regions often object to the creation of an interregional system of redistribution, precisely because it threatens to eliminate their own advantages.

There are also administrative issues in using smaller areas as a tax base for health financing. The question of where income is earned or spent (and therefore who gets the tax proceeds) becomes steadily more complex. This is one reason that local governments often tax nonmoveable assets like land: at least everyone knows in which jurisdiction it is located.

Risk pooling

The effects of general tax revenue on risk pooling depend on how the government allocates the tax revenue among different health programs. In low-income countries, the government's health budget mostly goes to finance public hospitals and clinics where patients can receive free or subsidized health care. This approach *de facto* pools the costs for the patients who use the public hospitals. The better public hospitals, however, are often located in the large cities, and their services are also often used more intensively by non-poor urban residents. Under these circumstances, the risks are not pooled for those with more limited access, like the rural poor.

Economic effects

The economic effects of using general tax revenue to finance health care will depend on which specific taxes are employed and their levels. In theory, a high-income tax rate should reduce upper-income individuals' willingness to work. In fact, however, studies tend to find that for upper-income individuals, labor supply is insensitive to marginal income tax rates (Feldstein 1995). High labor costs can also decrease a country's international competitiveness, and slow the pace of investment and economic growth. As capital markets become increasingly international, the importance of such considerations is liable to increase.

We note here a somewhat obscure issue about taxes—an issue of great concern to some economists—the concept of *excess burden*. When taxes are imposed on goods, buyers pay a higher price than they would otherwise, and sellers gets less. The tax drives a wedge between what is paid and what is received. As a result, less is bought and sold than otherwise would occur in a perfectly competitive market with zero tax. From an economic perspective, this loss of output poses a problem, because customers would have been willing to pay more than the cost of producing the goods that are no longer produced. Yet, thanks to the tax, they no longer are able to enjoy this gain. And the larger the adjustment in output due to the tax, the greater the loss will be, as measured by the difference between the willingness-to-pay of customers and the cost of producing the lost marginal output. This difference is called the excess burden of a tax (Musgrave and Musgrave 1989).

In response, some economists argue for taxes that lead to the smallest changes in outputs. This turns out to imply higher taxes on goods where customers care so much that they continue to buy nearly the same amount, even as prices rise. Economists call such demand "inelastic." Ironically, such goods are also often the ones that people purchase because they are very important to them—like medical care and basic food. Taxing goods whose demand is inelastic is thus likely to violate our concern with vertical equity—which does not stop some economists from advocating such an approach (Myles 1995).

Summary

General tax revenue is a major source of financing for health systems in both rich and poor countries. International experience shows that as a country becomes more affluent, its tax base becomes larger, and as the government's ability to collect taxes increases, a larger share of the health expenditures is often funded out of general revenues. General revenue financing is also politically controllable and account-able. This source of financing can be, but does not have to be, tailored to meet both horizontal and vertical equity concerns. Finally, it has good long-run growth potential as well as the capacity to pool health risks across a wide population.

On the other hand, the controllability of general revenue can make it unattrac-tive when the political system is weak and subject to corruption and favoritism. When government functions badly, there can be problems with public acceptabil-ity and hence the collectibility of tax revenue, especially in nations with limited administrative and enforcement capacity or an especially cynical or tax-avoiding citizenry.

Certain kinds of services (public health and preventive services, or care for the poor) are often tax-supported, even when other methods dominate a nation's health-care financing system (Scheiber and Maeda 1997). This is because taxes can be redistributive, and can be raised from a broad base. In countries with well-functioning economies and strong administration, tax financing can generate sub-stantial funds for the health sector. But these conditions are not met in all countries. This helps explain the widespread interest in our second financing option: social insurance.

Social Insurance

Three characteristics distinguish social insurance from private insurance. First, social insurance is *compulsory*—everyone in the eligible group must enroll and pay the specified premium (contribution). This contribution is most often speci-fied as a percent of the wage. Once someone has paid a minimum number of pay-ments, that person is entitled to the specified benefits.

Second, most social insurance premiums represent a social compact. By law the contribution rate and the benefits are not easily adjustable by mere administrative action. Instead, they are specified in law or in a difficult-to-change regulation. Social insurance thus is based on an implicit contract between those covered and the system. Citizens agree to pay a certain amount with the expectation that the funds will be used fairly and effectively to finance care for those who belong to the system.

Third, while most ministers of finance object to earmarked taxes, social insur-ance programs typically do rely on just such revenue. As a result these programs have a particular advantage. The insurance benefits demanded by the voters come with a clear price tag—they have to put their money where their mouths are.

Social insurance schemes do not necessarily cover everyone, and many coun-tries have multiple systems. Most schemes only cover workers in the formal sector. When a country decides to provide universal coverage, the government typically must use general tax revenue to subsidize pensioners, the unemployed, the poor, workers in the informal sector, and even some small businessmen and farmers.

Social insurance is generally organized in one of two ways. Under the Bismarkian model, plans are established and managed by various nonprofit organizations, divided along industrial, geographic, or occupational lines. They are often called *sickness funds*, and have only a limited capacity to compete for enrollees (Saltman and Figueras 1997). Most social insurance plans in Europe and Latin America are of this type. This multiple organizational arrangement allows for some variation in benefit packages, and some—although often quite limited—choice by customers. But it runs the risk of adverse selection and high administrative costs. To remedy these shortcomings, several nations, such as Taiwan, have the program administered by a single parastatal agency outside of the day-to-day control of the political process (Roemer 1993, Raffel 1984).

The economics literature often describes social insurance financing as indistinguishable from government tax financing, but social insurance experts vehemently disagree (Ball 2000, Meyers 1981). Economists view social insurance as a tax-financed program mainly because the contribution is compulsory. But this view ignores many major social and institutional differences that distinguish general-tax-revenue-financed insurance (e.g., Sweden) from social insurance (e.g., Germany, Japan, and Taiwan). First, contributions (premiums) paid for social insurance programs are earmarked for those programs and are separated from general taxes. The social insurance fund generally is required to maintain its solvency, and this tends to produce greater transparency and accountability in its financial affairs. At the same time, social insurance is not a right of all citizens but only covers those who are eligible and have met the minimum contribution requirements, and the benefits they receive are often related to their contributions. As a result, people perceive that they have paid a premium contribution in exchange for the right to specified benefits. In other words, the benefits are not welfare from the government.

Equity of financial burdens and benefits

The equity effects of social insurance schemes depend on their details, which vary significantly. The vertical equity of payroll taxes depends on how much income of the rich escapes the tax system because it is from capital, and on whether there are any contribution limits. Horizontal equity will depend on whether some groups (e.g., small businesses and farmers) escape paying fair tax burdens due to legislative favoritism or simple evasion. Horizontal equity will also be diminished if there are many social insurance plans, and some (because of a more favorable mix of members) can offer lower tax rates or better care for the same price. This is likely to be the case because plans with upper-income workers not only have more revenue, they are also likely to have smaller sick populations, given the correlation of economic and health status. Thus in Germany, until inter-sickness fund transfers were imposed in the 1990s, payroll tax rates for plans for white-collar workers were well below those of plans for blue-collar workers.

Both economic theory and empirical observation suggest that over the medium term of a few years, workers pay for the largest share of health insurance premiums (either directly through their premiums, or indirectly in the form of lower wages)—even when employers nominally contribute a significant share. In economic terms, the premium cost is being *shifted backward* to the workers. The ability of employers to shift the cost to workers, rather than having it *shifted forward* in the form of higher prices, depends on conditions in the labor market, including how strong any labor unions are.

Risk pooling

Social insurance only pools the health risks of its enrollees. Since most schemes only cover the workers in the formal sector, only their health risks are pooled. If the government wants to limit the risks of those who are not covered, it needs to pursue additional financing measures, such as using tax revenue, to provide insurance coverage for the poor, elderly, rural populations, etc.

Economic effects

Do social insurance costs have an impact on economic growth? If total labor costs are not significantly affected by premium changes, then the answer should be "not much." Real labor markets, however, are full of rigidities and imperfections. In countries with strong unions and high payroll taxes, the real cost of labor can be raised by higher social insurance premiums. If some of the cost is shifted forward into higher prices, this could reduce a nation's capacity to compete internationally and encourage international companies to expand production where labor costs are lower. Moreover, high labor costs could discourage employers from adding workers, even in an expansion, causing an increase in unemployment over the medium to long run.

Implementability

Implementability is a major attraction of social insurance schemes. In many industrial economies, large enterprises employ a significant share of the workforce, and even small businesses have reasonable employment records. Moreover, the social-contract structure of social insurance can increase citizens' willingness to pay, because a dedicated fund with distinct administration is more trusted to deliver something of value to members. Citizens think, "At least those dishonest politicians cannot get their hands on 'my' money."

On the other hand, the hopes for social insurance are not always fulfilled. The social insurance system can be seen as just another government function and may be associated with past illegitimate regimes. In some post-communist countries, for example, tax evasion is widespread in the social insurance system (Schneider 2002).

In Hungary, both small and large businesses have tried to evade payroll taxes. The former claimed they were making only the minimum wage, while large businesses shifted as much employee compensation as possible from cash, which is taxed, to in-kind support (e.g., cars, houses), which is not (Preker et al. 2002). In addition, the government has been reluctant to fund its "share" for pensioners and others. The resulting social insurance system therefore lacks both the fiscal capacity and the popular acceptance its advocates hoped for.

Private Insurance

Private insurance is distinguished by buyers' voluntarily purchasing insurance from independent, competitive sellers (either for-profit or nonprofit) who charge premiums that reflect the buyer's risks rather than their ability to pay. Insurance purchases can be made on either an individual or a group basis.

In recent years, there has been increased interest around the world in various forms of private insurance as a mechanism for health-sector finance, due to two main lines of argument: The first is that private insurance will mobilize additional resources. Since nonpayers do not get coverage, the problems of tax evasion can be minimized. Advocates of private insurance also argue that when people can choose a plan and a carrier, they will feel more empowered and more willing to pay for health care.

A second contention is that those with different attitudes and values, including those at different income levels, will prefer different health insurance plans. It is claimed that a competitive market for private insurance will respond by offering a differentiated range of products, something a publicly controlled social insurance monopoly would have neither the incentive nor the inclination to do.

Private insurance often increases as an economy grows, because it appeals to the self-interest of insurance buyers. Employers want to keep their workforce healthy, gain greater loyalty from the workers, and avoid workers' pleas for financial assistance when they have unaffordable medical bills. Employees often want insurance to prepay their health-care expenses, for risk protection, and for the financial advantages of private group insurance that costs less than comparable social insurance due to economies of scale and risk pooling only with other healthy workers. For these reasons, in some middle-income countries, there is substantial pressure from the best-paid workers to opt out of social insurance schemes, and in the name of free market-competition to take their premiums and use them to buy private insurance—as the system in Chile now allows.

The most serious failure of competitive private insurance is the problem of *risk selection*. In a world where illness increasingly means chronic disease, health-care costs have become more predictable on a year-to-year basis. Those who are sick this year are likely to be sick next year. The 5% or 10% of the people in any insurance pool who are the sickest often account for 60% to 70% of the total cost (Hsiao 2000). These facts create enormous incentives for competitive insurance companies to sell policies only to healthy people. Or, if they do sell to the sick, to charge high enough rates to yield a profit, even from the poor.

The latter practice, of course, creates strong incentives for the sick to lie about their health to insurance companies. If regulators require companies to sell insurance to all customers at the same rate, then healthy people are likely not to buy insurance, because it will be unattractively expensive, as their lower risk of disease will make the coverage not worth it. This can lead to an *underwriting death spiral*. As good risks leave an insurance pool, losses mount, rates have to rise, and even more of the healthy drop out, leaving only the sickest and most expensive in the pool.

The reverse problem also arises. Insurance companies work to attract policy-holders who are especially healthy, while seeking to exclude the sick. They may refuse to sell to the sick, exclude coverage for existing conditions, cancel or refuse to reissue policies to those who become sick, or charge very high rates. Together these practices are known as *risk selection* or *cream skimming*, and they mean that those who most need insurance may well wind up uncovered in a system of private insurance.

Equity of financial burdens and benefits

The equity implications of private insurance are generally unfavorable. Premiums that do not vary at all with income are highly regressive. Indeed, given the inverse relationship between economic status and health status, risk-based premiums typically lead the poor to pay *more*. Even regulated uniform rates that do not vary with income are more regressive than other funding options. Similarly, from a risk protection viewpoint, competitive private insurance markets leave a lot to be desired, because those with low incomes cannot afford insurance. In short, those most at risk financially from serious illness are those least able to afford private insurance.

From the viewpoint of horizontal equity, the question is, What comparisons do we care about? Private insurance markets with risk-based premiums imply that those in high-risk groups pay more. It is a matter of philosophy and policy as to which differences in circumstance we want to influence individuals' health-care costs.

Risk pooling

Because private insurance pools risks across smaller groups than social insurance, this method typically offers less risk pooling than social insurance—and much less than general revenue financing. In addition, groups with the highest risks and costs (especially the chronically ill and retirees) are typically excluded. In response, some nations have regulated private insurance markets either to require uniform rates to all (*community rating*) or limit the range of allowable price differences (*rating bands*). As we discuss in Chapter 11 on regulation, however, these approaches require substantial administrative sophistication and a general attitude of rule-following on the part of insurance companies. They can also be politically unpopular, since they try to re-impose some of the risk pooling that purchasers of private insurance, especially in low- and middle-income countries, are trying to avoid.

Economic effects

One argument for private insurance is the claim that competitive insurance markets lower health-care costs. Insurers eager for customers will cut prices, and to make money, they will pressure providers to reduce their fees. Providers faced with lower revenues will then reorganize their work to reduce costs. The collapse of communism, the prestige of market ideology, and the advocacy of well-funded zealots have all reinforced the trend toward pro-market perspectives (Rodrik 1997).

The only health-care market that provides anything close to a test of this claim is the United States—which has primarily relied on private employer-purchased, competitive group insurance for the last 50 years. In the 1990s, as competition among insurance plans increased, there was some impact on health-care costs, as predicted by economic theory. But consumers became very unhappy with the limits on their ability to obtain care from the managed-care plans that came to dominate the market. As a result, insurers have in recent years decreased their efforts to control providers, and costs in the United States have begun to increase at a rate of 10% to 15% per year. Moreover, in part because of the very high transaction costs of a fragmented private insurance system, the United States does have the highest overall health-care costs of any nation in the world—by a substantial margin.

Implementability

In creating a private insurance financing system, nations confront a series of critical design issues. The first issue is whether contracts will be sold on an individual or group basis. The U.S. market is heavily based on employer groups. This is done in order to limit the incentives for, and possibility of, individuals' opting into or out of various risk pools and thereby destabilizing the system. Even where groups are small, there has been experimentation with various kinds of collective purchasing to at least lower transaction costs (Zelman 1996).

The second design issue is the nature of the insurance entities, especially the choice between for-profit or not-for-profit. If the companies are not-for-profit, are they state enterprises, independent NGO-type entities, some kind of union or community-sponsored cooperative, or some other form?

A third set of choices deals with government's role. What forms of regulation and licensing will sellers be subject to? For example, will governments insist on certain levels of financial reserves, regulate premiums, or set terms for minimum coverage?

A final set of design questions concerns the relationship between insurance companies and health-care providers. Does government exercise any regulatory control over the relationship between insurers and providers? For example, can providers and insurers be combined in some sort of arrangement like an American health maintenance organization (HMO)? Are such options forbidden, required, or optional? Will government regulate how insurance plans pay providers, as the United States government regulates the relationship of insurance plans to the providers with whom they contract?

More broadly, there is the role of government in shaping the competitive structure of these markets. How many firms do they allow or encourage? What geographic areas or population groups can each competitor appeal to, or operate within?

The private insurance option thus does not remove the government from the business of operating the system of health financing. Rather, it poses a complex set of regulatory and management issues to the government that may be quite new and different from those the government confronted if it previously relied on direct provision and general tax financing.

Unfortunately, governments may not be well equipped to undertake these new responsibilities. Does the government have the capacity for underwriting and financial analysis to set reasonable reserve requirements? Does it know enough about the dynamics of competitive insurance markets—a phenomenon that may be new to the country when companies try to attract the good risks—to create and control such markets effectively? Can it recognize and regulate cream-skimming behavior? Will it be able to control prices and/or the terms on which policies are sold? Experience with insurance regulation in the United States suggests that high levels of analytical competence and political integrity are required to perform these tasks successfully.

Under private insurance, the quantity of insurance purchased remains a decentralized decision in the hands of individual businesses and consumers. The declining rate of private insurance coverage in the United States demonstrates that as premiums rise, many consumers stop purchasing insurance. There are limits on what the government can do about this. Of course, the government can offer subsidies to encourage private insurance purchases, as occurred in Chile (World Bank 1995). But giving a subsidy amounts to moving away from insurance to tax-based financing. Controlling insurance rates has its own difficulties. If rates are set too low, then companies will flee the business, as have many U.S. insurers who no longer offer special policies to retired citizens (Buchmueller 2000). If rates are set too high, then insurance becomes unaffordable for many people.

Advocates of private insurance believe it is a solution to the health sector's financing problems. The lure of the market and the enormous sums generated by private insurance firms in the United States have made allies of an unlikely group, ranging from ruthless entrepreneurs to free-market advocates to cash-starved physicians. But this approach poses substantial problems in terms of its high administrative costs and poor performance from a risk protection and an equity point of view. The need for sophisticated regulation presents a major challenge that many countries considering such schemes cannot realistically meet.

Out-of-Pocket Payments

A fourth financing method is to have individual patients pay providers directly out of their own pockets and to have these expenditures not be reimbursable by third parties, such as insurance plans. User fees are a sub-category of out-of-pocket payments, and refer to payments when these are made for public-sector-provided services.

Health-sector reformers have been interested in such financing approaches for two reasons. First, especially in low-income countries, user fees are often seen as an administratively feasible way to raise additional revenue for institutions and activities at the periphery. The idea is that money collected locally will be spent locally. This, it is believed, will diminish leakage due to graft, corruption, and overhead expenses, as local collection and disbursement increase accountability and transparency. It is hoped that patients will be more willing to pay for care, if those payments contribute to a better quality of service in their local facilities.

The second argument, often made by economists, is that giving away health services for free encourages allocatively inefficient overuse. Their analysis rests on the subjective utilitarian premise that the purpose of the health-care system should be to maximize customer satisfaction, as measured by willingness-to-pay (Pauly 1990). When services have zero price, economists argue, customers will use these services even when the value to them is less than the cost of their production. As a result, more total customer satisfaction could be provided if those low-valued services were not produced. Then the resources used to produce those services could be used elsewhere in the economy to produce something of more value to customers. User fees, and their analogy for insured patients (namely, co-payments), are viewed as desirable because they avoid the worst misallocation by discouraging customers from consuming the services with the lowest value to them.

Notice that these two arguments are not fully consistent. Those who favor user fees for revenue-raising purposes want to put prices on highly valued services, arguing that their utilization will not change much when fees are introduced. Such advocates may also support the notion of helping those at low income pay for such fees; otherwise, their consumption might be heavily affected.

Advocates of pricing-for-efficiency, in contrast, want to raise prices for services that are both expensive to produce and of low value to customers. For them, declines in usage, as a result of instituting direct payments from patients, are not an objection to their scheme. Rather, such declines are seen as a sign of the appropriateness of the decision to institute fees in the first place.

There is another complexity. The possibility of *supplier-induced demand* means that some health-care services may be consumed that are not of much clinical value to patients. Where that occurs allocative inefficiency will persist, even with user fees. Indeed, whether allocative efficiency increases or decreases will depend on two offsetting effects. One is the impact of fees on discouraging patients from purchasing services of low value. The other is the incentives such fees give for providers to increase inappropriate use. The magnitude of the latter effect will depend on a variety of factors, including the professional norms of providers, their training, and the ways in which fee income flows to clinical decision-makers.

The amount of money currently being raised through direct patient payments in a country is often difficult to determine. The cost of collecting good data can be substantial, since sophisticated household-health-expenditure surveys may be the only way to do so. It is also not easy to control such spending since so much of the private market is unregulated and because of the widespread existence of informal or unofficial payments in state-run systems, where they are implicitly or explicitly illegal.

Informal payments often arise when budget support for the health-care system is diminished by difficult macroeconomic circumstances and providers are desperate to preserve their incomes. Local traditions also matter. In some countries, such fees are expected to ensure good care, not only by doctors but by nurses as well. They tend to be higher for providers working in fields seen as the most active or heroic—such as surgery and obstetrics/gynecology. These payments go under different names in different countries, including "gratuities," "under-the-table payments," "black money," and "gray money." From an economic point of view, these payments are a form of out-of-pocket financing since they have similar effects on demand and on the financing burden that legal user-fees have.

Recent studies of National Health Accounts (NHA) suggest that there may be substantial willingness to spend, and ability to spend, on outpatient care, even among relatively poor people, in many poor countries—especially if informal payments are included (Berman 1997). This finding raises the possibility of creating mixed systems where fees play a non-trivial role in certain settings.

On the other hand, in general the demand for acute care tends to be less price-sensitive than the demand for routine and preventive care, and the effect of price on use is higher among low-income people—as we discuss in the next chapter. This means that fees set to discourage low-valued uses will also lead customers to curtail use in ways that negatively affect their health. This suggests the need to find ways to encourage the use of public-health and prevention services. Unfortunately, in a world of chronic disease, many such encounters are not distinguishable from ordinary clinical care, since much prevention occurs *after* some disease has developed. Such activities are called "secondary prevention," for example, getting someone who has had a heart attack to quit smoking. And mechanisms to provide subsidies for the poor, to offset the use-discouraging impact of user fees, are not easy to implement.

Direct payments can be a useful supplement to tax funds as a source of institutional support. But it is doubtful that out-of-pocket payments can serve as the major fiscal basis for modern inpatient care for any but the very rich. Such care is so expensive, and the demand for it sufficiently infrequent, that countries confront substantial pressure to develop risk-pooling financing (i.e., some form of insurance), especially once a country has reached a certain level of political and economic development.

Equity and risk protection

From both risk protection and equity perspectives, out-of-pocket payment is the worst possible system for health financing. Those who are both sick and poor face the risk of either untreated disease or impoverishment—or some combination thereof. From the viewpoint of vertical equity, direct payments are highly regressive, especially given the correlation of poor health and low income. They are even worse than private insurance, which at least offers some risk-pooling possibility when there is group purchasing or when rates are regulated.

In many countries, practitioners using fee-for-service engage in some forms of price discrimination, charging the rich more than the poor. While such practices advance equity, they also help maximize the incomes of providers. By charging the rich more and the poor less, providers encourage the poor to purchase more total services, and generate more income for physicians than would otherwise occur. This produces a net gain to any seller who has excess time available and whose marginal cost of providing additional service is less than the fees charged to the poor.

Medical savings accounts

One particular method of direct payment, *medical savings accounts,* has received special attention in health-reform discussions internationally. The prototypical example is found in Singapore (Hsiao 1995). That scheme involved a conscious strategy to build up reserves, in anticipation of an increase in the elderly, high-care-using population. The policy introduced compulsory savings (based on a percentage of wages) deposited into dedicated individual savings accounts, which can then be used to pay for inpatient services.

Several features of the Singapore policy deserve comment. The system is first and foremost a savings scheme designed to compel workers to save now in anticipation of large medical expenses in later years, and hence to shift current income into the future. Until substantial balances build up in individual accounts and while people are still young, subscribers are actively discouraged from using their accounts to pay for care. Instead, great effort is made to encourage them, or their families, to pay for medical expenses out-of-pocket. Since the available balances to an individual or family are those they have paid in, there is little risk-pooling across the population as a whole.

Second, to make it possible for people to pay out-of-pocket yet afford basic hospital services, hospitals provide multiple levels of service, from "C" class multiple-bed wards, to "A" class single-bed rooms. The lowest class of service is heavily subsidized by tax revenue, making it available to people with modest incomes (medical services are not supposed to vary, only amenities). This is intended to deal with the adverse equity aspects of an out-of-pocket payment scheme. Singapore discovered, however, that many were unable to pay for inpatient services, even on subsidized wards. In 1990, the country therefore revised the savings scheme by adding a catastrophic insurance plan, in which workers pay the premiums by withdrawals from their medical savings account (Lim 1998).

Third, Singapore also has a system of case-by-case subsidies, when social workers determine that neither individuals nor their families can pay what is required, again to deal with both equity and risk-pooling concerns.

This complex scheme has been modified over a decade, evolving to address the equity problems of direct payment. Singapore's relatively unique sociocultural situation is widely acknowledged to play a major role in the scheme's functioning. It is a geographically small, relatively wealthy, largely Chinese society, in which both thrift and family responsibility are deeply engrained values. The country also has a competent and sophisticated government fiscal system. It is not clear that such a complex scheme, which relies heavily on particular cultural norms, can be transferred to other settings—despite all the international attention it has received.

Implementability

The greatest advantage of out-of-pocket payments is in the realm of implementability. Because sellers can refuse to serve nonpayers, it forces buyers to actually pay. Transactions occur on the spot, and can use ordinary commercial processes (e.g., checks, cash, credit cards) that do not generate any added record-keeping burden. From the perspective of government, this payment system is essentially self-implementing and does not require substantial public budget resources to operate. But when user fees are set very high, and sellers cannot refuse to serve patients (as is the case for American hospitals treating an emergency for someone who is uninsured), the costs to sellers of collecting the fee after the fact can be substantial (Creese 1997).

Fees do also create incentives for providers to encourage overuse, which can lead to substantial countervailing government regulatory efforts. These costs are properly considered part of the cost of the direct payment scheme. Many quality initiatives (like regulating and licensing providers) as well as price-regulatory activities have developed to address the incentive problems of direct payment financing systems. Efforts have also developed to limit the number of providers and to license institutions in order to constrain potential overuse, as we discuss in Chapter 12 on regulation.

Summary

Direct patient payments are easy to administer and a potentially effective source of revenue. They do raise serious questions from the perspective of vertical equity and risk pooling. They can also encourage inappropriate utilization through their incentive effects on physicians and other providers, even while they discourage inappropriate overuse by consumers. Direct payments also lack the capacity to finance universal coverage of expensive services. Yet, patient payments clearly have been attractive to many countries because of their power to mobilize resources otherwise unavailable to the health sector.

Community Financing

In this financing method, communities operate and control the provision of their own primary care and secondary services through locally based prepayment schemes. Under typical community financing plans, the financing and delivery of primary care are integrated, but separated from secondary and tertiary services. Providers are either individuals hired by the community or nonprofit NGOs.

Many of the world's low-income countries have despaired of finding ways to finance and deliver rural health services reliably at the village level. It is often difficult to get physicians to staff government-operated clinics. The doctors evade or refuse, do not attend regularly, or provide poor-quality customer service that is culturally insensitive. At the same time, rural residents often have little confidence in the services and facilities that do exist. As a result, they make extensive use of traditional healers and folk medicine practitioners and when acutely ill, they travel to district or regional hospitals.

In many poor countries, it is also difficult to raise additional revenue from general taxation. Corruption and inefficiency may be widespread, record-keeping poor, and tax evasion common. These conditions have contributed to increased interest in recent years in community financing. The essential idea is to raise and spend money for primary care locally, at the village level. The theory is that local control will produce transparency and accountability. This will, in turn, help ensure honest, efficient, and culturally competent services.

The hope is that such financing and administrative arrangements will prove to be attractive and credible to local people and increase their willingness to contribute financially. Advocates of community financing note the substantial sums spent by relatively poor local people on traditional healers, alternative medicine practioners, and private practice Western physicians. They are attracted by the possibility of getting access to those funds to support basic public health and primary care activities.

A model community-financing scheme involves a combination of local political accountability, community-operated primary care, and nearly universal prepayment. The concept is of a community-based, mini health-maintenance organization with salaried doctors. Secondary (hospital) care is also contracted by some of these schemes, although it can be expensive and requires a large catchment area to be economically viable. Universal (i.e., compulsory) membership is designed to get around free-riding by the well and adverse selection by the sick. Community resources may also be mobilized in other ways; for example, by labor to construct buildings.

Many experiments in raising local funds to finance primary health care have implemented only certain parts of the ideal scheme described above. It is not un-common for membership (and payment) to be voluntary; the range of services covered can be quite limited (e.g., a locally financed, revolving drug fund); and the financing can be heavily fee-for-service rather than prepayment, or can come from national tax sources, not local contributions.

Effective rural health services have sometimes been provided by centralized tax finance and public services. Sri Lanka, Cuba, and Kerala (in southern India) all have well-above average health status relative to their income levels and dense networks of effective public providers, even in rural areas. Advocates of community financing respond that such examples show that exceptional historical, political, and cultural circumstances are required for success via the centralized state route.

One limit of a local fiscal base is that it can be difficult to sustain in adverse economic times. A single rural area typically has a less diverse economy than the nation as a whole. Malaysia, for example, has relied, in succession, on tin, tea, palm oil, petroleum, and high-tech manufacturing for its growth over the last thirty years. Commodity price cycles that have seriously injured some parts of the country have been offset by growth elsewhere. An individual village, however, does not usually have the benefit of this kind of portfolio diversification.

Equity and risk protection

Where community financing is both prepaid and compulsory, it can offer a certain amount of risk protection. Unless they are subsidized by general revenues, however, community financing schemes can mobilize only modest resources, since most households involved are low-income. Moreover, the limited coverage of second-ary care means that community financing has to be supplemented by other schemes (e.g., tax-supported hospitals) if citizens are to be protected from the fi-nancial risks of serious illness. Non-compulsory schemes, where there is adverse selection by the sick into the covered pool, offer even less risk protection. Given the relatively small and geographically concentrated nature of the populations covered by such schemes, they cannot do enough risk spreading to provide insur-ance against localized adverse events like epidemics or natural disasters.

From a vertical equity view, a critical question is the nature of the pre-payment system. In particular, does the premium vary with income? Per-capita or per-family fee schemes will exclude the poorest of the poor, unless there are some exemptions or subsidy mechanisms. From a national perspective, serious fairness issues are raised in forcing relatively poor local people to pay for their own care while con-tinuing to subsidize health services for the nation's elite. On the other hand, if the scheme makes available to poor communities services that would otherwise not exist, the participants may gain more than they pay.

Horizontal equity here is paradoxical. Areas with more local administrative and organizational capacity and community leadership do better when it comes to creating and operating such schemes. In a sense, those with the most complaints will be people living in areas where such schemes are *not* created, or where they function badly, and who therefore enjoy less service. In countries with significant variations in local culture and capacity (e.g., across ethnic or cultural groups), these differences can be an issue, because community financing will work much more effectively in some places than in others.

Implementability

As with any decentralized scheme, implementability will depend on capacity and leadership at the local level. This implies a need to invest in capacity building at the periphery. On the other hand, when local people gain confidence in the community-based scheme, collection of premiums can become easier.

Some local areas may not be able to adopt community financing. Villages can be full of internal struggles and divisions by clan, family, ethnicity, religion, and economic status. In these situations, creating a collective community effort may be difficult or impossible. Central governments thus need to consider the limits of the organizational and technical capacity available locally when designing such schemes. They may well need to supply the missing expertise, and provide organizational support either temporarily or permanently, depending on a realistic assessment of each particular situation.

Summary

The main advantages of community financing are in the credibility and sustainability that those initiatives can produce, and the modest, but valuable, level of risk protection they can offer. Some of the biggest gains may occur not in the financing realm, but in the increased efficiency and responsiveness of services when providers are subject to effective local control. The relatively good record of tax-financed, community-controlled health services for Aboriginal communities in parts of Australia shows the importance of this aspect of the scheme.

Once again, however, the specifics of implementation matter. Attention must be paid to building the needed institutional prerequisites—both technical and political. Otherwise, such initiatives amount to shifting a problem that the central government has not been able to solve onto the shoulders of less-well-off and less-well-equipped regional and local authorities. Attention also has to be paid to the communities that get left behind when "demonstration projects" are undertaken. Far too often, the successful sites are areas that are better off—politically and economically—while places with the least capacity and most need (e.g., tribal areas in India, tea estates in Malaysia) get the least attention.

Foreign Aid as a Financing Source

Many poor countries rely significantly on foreign aid as a financing source for their health sectors. Such aid often comes with a price—namely, the donors' commitment to specific objectives. Such commitments are motivated by a combination of donor concern, donor values, and donor politics. For example, national aid agencies are responsible to their national legislatures, while WHO executives are responsible to the World Health Assembly.

In recent years, donors have become less focused on supporting health-sector reform and more on specific programmatic objectives with measurable outcomes— vaccination, disease elimination, and safe childbirth. The extent to which donor preferences alter or distort national policies depends greatly on a nation's own fiscal capacity and its dependence on donor funds. The poorest nations, and societies in post-conflict situations, are often the most vulnerable in this regard.

We would urge recipient nations to deal actively with bilateral and multilateral donors. The importance of local conditions implies that local leaders and experts have much to contribute to any discussion of policy options. The inappropriate enthusiasm of international experts for "one-size-fits-all" solutions has been often demonstrated in the past. At the same time, international experience can be a valuable source of guidance and advice about reform alternatives. Local reformers need to recognize that not every reference to international experience represents disrespect or "intellectual imperialism." Health-sector reform is so complex and difficult that self-critical openmindedness is an obligation of all who take the process seriously.

A Final Comment on Financing Methods

Before we move on, note *what is not part of our categories*. In particular, we have tried to separate financing from other aspects of the system. For example, the general revenue category, in our typology, does not require direct public provision of services—although that is often the case. Instead, this category includes different methods of service provision: independent providers (Canada), a mix of private doctors and public hospitals (Sweden), as well as systems that are largely publicly operated services (U.K.). Similarly, the private-insurance category includes both for-profit and nonprofit entities (like American Blue Cross plans) and insurers that pay providers in all possible combinations of methods. Insurers can even employ doctors and operate hospitals to provide care directly. For example, the Kaiser Health Plan, which sells health insurance in the United States, is both a nonprofit and a direct care provider. Yet we include them under the private insurance alternative. We have constructed our categories this way to leave issues of payment and organization as decisions under other control knobs. The breadth of these categories thus illustrates the range of choices on nonfinancing matters still available, even after decisions on financing have been reached.

Resource Allocation and Rationing

Once funds are raised, how they will be used, and for whom, matters greatly in determining who has access to, what types of health care, and the quality and quantity of that care. How a nation does on these intermediate performance measures, in turn, influences health outcomes and financial risk protection, as well as the allocative efficiency of a nation's health system and its total costs. In this section, we discuss resource allocation within the health sector. (The broader issues of intersectoral resource allocation are too complex to be treated here and are beyond the scope of what we can consider.)

The need to allocate resource arises from a dismal fact: Human wants far exceed the resources available. Governments, private firms, and individual households all have to make painful choices about allocating scarce resources. We have to choose how much to spend for health care versus other desirable goods; and decisions must be made on how to spend our money to achieve the best possible results. Governments make these choices at two levels. First, there is the tradeoff between spending in one sector and spending in another. Second, within a given sector, there is the tradeoff between one program and others. For example, more money for primary care means less for inpatient hospital services (Bitran y Asociados 2000).

Allocative decisions alone, however, even when made "correctly," will not by themselves produce the desired outcomes. Money itself does not produce health care. Funds have to be transformed into health care through a complex set of production processes. How that occurs is influenced by the system's incentive structures, organizational patterns, and regulatory activities. Too often, the argument is made that if resources are allocated appropriately, health outcomes will be improved. For example, the 1993 *World Development Report* adopted just this kind of simple approach to health improvement. Yet while sensible resource allocation is not enough to produce better outcomes, it can still be very helpful in doing so. But how do we know whether a nation's pattern of allocation is sensible? That is the topic for this section.

Definitions

The apportionment of health resources in many cases is a multilevel process. Governments first decide how to distribute resources across broad groups or categories of uses—say, by region or disease type. These funds are then further allocated to institutions or individuals. The economics literature on resource allocation often talks of resource allocation as if it were a unitary process. This may be a reasonable treatment when markets allocate goods and services directly to individuals. But under national-health-service systems, funds for health care are often allocated first by formula to communities, then by other means to institutions and individuals. Health insurance also uses a two-level approach. The design of the benefit package is used to allocate funds first to types of services. Then other means are used to ration services to individuals. In this book, we distinguish how resources are apportioned to a population group or for selected types of services (such as primary care and hospital services) and call this *"resource allocation."* We term the distribution of scarce health care to individuals *"rationing"* (Ubel 2000, Klein 1993).

Alternative Ways to Do Resource Allocation and Rationing

Even if everyone agrees that health-care resources have to be allocated and rationed, there is little agreement on the criteria that should be used for doing so. Nonetheless, some nations are more explicit in setting the rules than others. Europeans often debate health-care rationing (Klein 1993, Doyal 1997), while the United States almost never does.

On the other hand, conflicting values make it difficult to reach consensus on principles for rationing health services (Maynard 1996, Barnum and Kutzin 1993). One reason may be that clear rationing rules literally involve life-or-death decisions for *identifiable* individuals. Another difficulty in establishing rationing rules is disagreement about whose values should dominate: patients, doctors, payers, politicians, public health experts, etc.

Many criteria have been used to allocate funds at the population level to communities or to classes of service. For example, the United Kingdom and Canada allocate funds to communities based on income and health status. Other schemes focus on outcomes. For example, the World Bank argues for the selection of health services in insurance benefit packages based on their relative cost-effectiveness.

Once funds are allocated to population groups or types of service, health care still has to be rationed to individuals. No nation can afford to provide enough health care to meet all possible needs and wants. Instead, various methods are available to ration care (i.e., to limit use). *Price* is a common measure used for health-care rationing, but it has serious equity implications. As an alternative, many nations make selected health services free (or nearly free) and rely on waiting time to ration the limited supply. The United Kingdom is a good example. Sufficient preventive and primary care services are produced to meet patients' wants at zero price, but certain expensive surgical and laboratory services are not. These services are rationed by having non-urgent patients wait an extended period of time for care. Other means are also used to ration limited health resources to individual patients, for example, by (perhaps unintentionally) making certain services less attractive and thereby discouraging demand. Such practices include offering no choice of physicians, providing poor amenities at health facilities, offering care with a lack of professional courtesy or culturally appropriate treatment, or a lack of physical availability that imposes long travel times on patients.

Different rationing methods affect various patient groups differently. For example, price rationing impairs poor households' access to health care more than the rich. Poor service often has similar distributive effects, since upper-income people are likely to be more persistent or gain access through informal payments.

Waiting time at a clinic has two offsetting impacts. High-wage workers lose more pay than low-waged workers. Yet the latter may be less able to tolerate the resulting income loss.

The Principles and Politics of Resource Allocation

Many of the ethical perspectives we reviewed in Chapter 3 would suggest that governments give priority to basic health services and prevention programs—especially for groups with poor health. These services are often cost-effective from an objective utilitarian point of view, and raising the health-care status of the worst-off is especially attractive from an egalitarian liberal perspective. In addition, some subjective utilitarians are aware of the limits of individual sophistication about health choices. They would favor prevention education efforts and public funding for vaccination to correct market failures and improve individual decisions.

Yet many countries make quite different choices. When left to their own devices, citizens often exhibit a great willingness to pay for acute hospital care—especially in the case of life-threatening illnesses. Citizens then urge governments to save them from their own choices by subsidizing hospital care. This can lead to a major difficulty in apportioning public resources between primary care and hospital services. Allocating resources to pay for primary care is more cost-effective in improving health status but does not provide financial risk protection. Meanwhile, allocating resources to pay for inpatient hospital services offers financial risk protection but is less cost-effective in improving health status. This is a major dilemma for low- and middle-income countries that lack funds to pay for both.

The World Bank and WHO have urged governments to use cost-effectiveness criteria to allocate public funds and design social insurance benefit packages. But the public clearly wants and demands financial risk protection from expensive medical services. Consequently, most countries have not followed the recommendations from these international organizations. Instead, when countries discover they lack the public resources to fund both primary care and hospital services, most decide to continue to pay for hospital services at a level not justified by cost-effectiveness considerations. Table 8.2 shows the large share of public health budgets spent for hospital services for selected countries.

The design of health financing policy, like all other policy decisions, is a profoundly political process. The process is affected by strong stakeholders in the health sector—organized medicine, labor unions, and the insurance and pharmaceutical industries. Each possesses political resources that—as we discussed earlier—determine their relative power in shaping health financing policy.

Political scientists such as Marmor and Barr (1992) and Reich (1994) have long argued that politics plays the critical role in deciding who pays the costs and

TABLE **8.2.** Share of Government Budget Allocated to
Hospitals for Selected Countries

COUNTRY	HOSPITAL SHARE
Bangladesh	61%
Burundi	66%
China	61%
Côte D'Ivoire	46%
Ethiopia	49%
Jamaica	72%
Mexico	58%
Philippines	71%
Somalia	70%
Turkey	63%
Zimbabwe	54%
OECD mean	54%

Source: Barnum and Kutzin 1993.

who receives the benefits of health care. Even in poor countries, the economic and political elite often want to support a few world-class tertiary hospitals utilizing costly equipment (frequently imported) and serving their needs. It is common for these national and regional centers (which are often also teaching hospitals) to absorb a large share of the nation's overall health budget. Furthermore, the most prestigious institutions often have substantial political connections and influence that allow them to defend their interests effectively.

Resource Allocation and Equity

In addition to the tradeoffs in allocative efficiency between health gains and financial risk protection, many governments also seek to achieve equity gains through health financing decisions. Such governments seek to subsidize those who are poor and those who have the greatest health needs but lack the ability to pay. To achieve these gains, a government can target its resources to intended beneficiaries through various means. It can target its subsidies by income group, by the health and socioeconomic status of a community, by class of hospital ward, and by types of services. Alternatively, a government can directly provide free (or nearly free) services to poor communities and the most vulnerable population, such as the disabled and elderly.

As a result of the political pressures discussed above, in practice many nations are not allocating their health resources equitably. Even nominally free tax-supported public services, intended to assure equal access for the poor and low-income households, often lead to inequitable consequences. In particular,

TABLE 8.3. The Incidence of Public-Health Spending in Selected Countries

		Share of subsidy (%)	
		POOREST QUINTILE	RICHEST QUINTILE
Sri Lanka	1979	30	9
Jamaica	1989	30	9
Malaysia	1989	29	11
Brazil	1985	17	42
Egypt	1995	16	24
Kenya	1993	14	24
Vietnam	1992	12	29
Indonesia	1989	12	29
Ghana	1992	11	34
Jamaica	1989	30	9
Malaysia	1989	29	11

Sources: Alailima and Mohideen 1984, Demery et al. 1995, Grosh 1994.

tax-financed health services can be disproportionately utilized by the urban middle and upper classes. This is especially so for costly services like the more sophisticated forms of hospital care. Incidence analyses indicate that public expenditures on health do tend to benefit the rich disproportionately in Ghana, Indonesia, Vietnam, and Brazil (see Table 8.3), and studies in India have yielded similar results.

This inequitable distribution of public-health-care resources highlights a fundamental difficulty facing rational resource allocation in the health sector. Unlike public health programs, personal health services provide direct and immediate benefits to identifiable individuals. Those who are ill can be expected to lobby hard for access to services. And those with higher economic and social status are likely to have the skills, resources, and connections to capture the most valuable benefits for themselves. Their personal tradeoffs tend to be very different from the statistical calculations of public officials seeking to maximize total health benefits for the population.

Conditional Guidance

Financing policy is complicated, because the multiple objectives typically sought in health systems require painful tradeoffs. Inevitably, then, decisions on financing will depend on each nation's social values.

Our review of the financing control knob and the five health-financing methods leads us to three main conclusions. First, there is no perfect financing method. Each option has pluses and minuses. Some are more equitable or more feasible or sustainable than others in a particular context. But there will always be tradeoffs. Second, the optimal choice for a country will depend on how the country addresses a set of fact and value issues. How important are vertical equity and redistributive financing? How much administrative capacity is there to collect taxes or social insurance contributions? How cynical and free-rider-inclined are citizens when it comes to community-financing schemes? Third, whatever combination of methods is chosen, the details and implementation matter. For example, the horizontal equity of a social insurance system will depend on how small businessmen are treated. The vertical equity of a system that relies on regional taxes will depend on the kind of interregional equalization mechanism that is created.

Nations that want to mobilize a significant percentage of their GDP for health care must develop a coherent and rational financing strategy. The appropriate combination depends on each country's particular context—including its social values, economic condition, industrial structure, and administrative abilities. The capacity of each source in a particular context will depend on many local features of the situation. Still, that does not mean that what everyone is doing is appropriate. It is possible to do better or worse. It is possible to use international experience and theoretical insight to reach plausible conclusions about what is appropriate for your context. And such judgments are required, if the financing control knob is to be adjusted most effectively.

Specific Suggestions

Here are some specific suggestions, based on our review of international experience and the relevant political and economic theories:

- Poverty itself imposes a basic financial constraint. Poor households cannot afford to pay for health care. They have to be subsidized by the government if they are to have access. If equity is to improve, therefore, public spending must be targeted to the poor—which is not the case now for most low- and middle-income countries.
- For the world's two billion poor people who live in rural areas, many goals would be advanced if private out-of-pocket spending were substantially replaced with prepaid community financing schemes. Such schemes could use the current spending more efficiently and effectively, improve the quality of health care, and pool some of the risks to reduce impoverishment due to large medical expenditures.
- User fees have generated additional funds for public facilities in some countries, and induced customers to be more careful of their utilization of previously free services. Many user fee schemes, however, have not produced net additional funds for health care because of high administrative costs, and when additional funds were produced, they did not necessarily lead to the better services desired by patients. Moreover, many user fee systems have not succeeded in assuring the

poor adequate access to public health services, although they have often been designed to remedy this potential problem. In short, user fee systems require careful design and capable administration before they can produce the desired outcomes.

- To the extent that they are affordable, social insurance schemes have the greatest potential for providing effective risk protection. In low-income countries, such schemes are likely to be limited to workers in the formal sector. As national income rises, governments can expand such coverage by providing subsidies from general tax revenues. In high-income countries, compulsory universal systems are likely to be cost-effective.
- Private insurance has high administrative costs and tends to decrease risk-pooling. From an equity perspective, adverse effects are minimized if it functions in a supplementary role (to social insurance) to cover otherwise uncovered services and to provide higher levels of service quality. In high-income countries, upper-income individuals are likely to demand such coverage, because they want better care than public arrangements typically provide.
- Basic public health and preventive care will generally have to be tax-supported if a nation wants to have a cost-effective pattern of resource allocation to maximize health status. Out-of-pocket payment or insurance schemes are likely to under-provide such services from an allocative efficiency viewpoint.
- These observations in turn lead us to a view about the appropriate financing strategy for countries at different income levels.

    Low-income countries: Social insurance for the formal sector; community financing in rural areas—with modest subsides from general revenue; public services for the poor, perhaps user fees for public hospital care, with low-income exemptions, if these can be properly implemented.

    Middle-income countries: A similar overall strategy with more subsidies for expanding the social insurance system and extending community financing to secondary care. Public services need to be organized in a way that is accessible to the poor.

    High-income countries: Universal social insurance with general tax revenue subsidies for low-income groups has much to recommend it. Private insurance is likely to play a role for upper income groups.

Financing and Equity

Equity has been a continuing theme of our discussion of all financing options. Our conclusions about user fees, private insurance, and community financing are all driven in part by our equity concerns. So, too, was the discussion we offered of the fairness aspects of resource allocation.

From an egalitarian liberal perspective, the key departure point is that a fundamental level of health is a necessity for human well-being. Our ability to learn, work, achieve our potential, and enjoy life clearly depends in part on our health. A just and fair society, then, should provide sufficient funds to assure that everyone has access to the health care they need to relieve suffering and reach a certain level of functioning. Governments should accept responsibility for mobilizing the necessary funds so that every citizen, rich or poor, has an appropriate level of health care.

We recognize, of course, that there are other points of view. Objective utilitarians, for example, do not believe citizens have positive rights to health care, or to anything else. A country run on objective utilitarian principles could conceivably decide that what really advanced well-being was maximizing economic growth. Such a government would only provide funding for the health-care services that contribute most to such economic growth. Equal access to health care and equal health status would not be a priority.

As we discussed in Chapters 3 and 5 (on ethics and performance criteria) each nation has serious decisions to make about its own equity position. Our point is that it is not possible to develop a coherent financing and resource-allocation strategy without engaging these equity issues directly. The international community's recent focus on poverty reduction does introduce a new set of pressures and opportunities into each nation's decision processes. But health-sector reform cannot and should not avoid confronting this issue explicitly.

Summary

In summary, we believe that every nation considering health-care reform should conduct a systematic review of how health care is financed, and prepare a coherent and realistic financing strategy for public deliberation. The strategy will inevitably use a combination of financing methods to mobilize funds from different population groups. In our view, the strategy should take into account the conclusions derivable from previous international experience that are reviewed above, if the society is to foster equity of access and cost-effective resource allocation to improve health status.

As we will see in subsequent chapters, important complementary efforts need to be made in payment, organization, regulation, and behavior if any financing strategy is to succeed. To put it simply, raising more funds alone does not insure they will be well spent, and there is little point in focusing on fund-raising without also paying attention to how the delivery system functions.

Finally, nations and their political leaders and technical experts need to be realistic about their financial situation. As we stated initially, all resources come from somewhere; all have an "opportunity cost." Only honest leadership can help nations face the difficult choices that the reality of limited resources imposes on us all. Unrealistic promises or unrestrained pursuit of narrow interest-group gains will only sow the seeds of long-run conflict and citizen disillusionment.

References

Atkinson, Anthony; and Joseph Stiglitz. 1980. *Lectures in Public Economics.* New York: McGraw-Hill.

Ball, Robert. 2000. *Insuring the Essentials: Bob Ball on Social Security.* New York: The Century Foundation Press.

Barnum, Howard; and Joseph Kutzin. 1993. *Public Hospitals in Developing Countries: Resource Use, Cost, and Financing.* Baltimore, MD: Johns Hopkins University Press.

Berman, Peter. 1997. "National Health Accounts in Developing Countries: Appropriate Methods and Recent Applications." *Health Economics* 6(1): 11–30.

Bitran y Asociados. 1998. *Targeting Public Subsidies for Health.* Washington, DC: Economic Development Institute, World Bank.

Buchmueller, Thomas C. 2000. "The Health Plan Choices of Retirees Under Managed Competition." *Health Services Research* 35(5): 949–76.

Creese, Andrew. 1997. "User Fees." *British Medical Journal* 315(7102): 202–3.

Doyal, Lenh. 1997. "The Rationing Debate: Rationing Within the NHS Should Be Explicit: The Case For." *British Medical Journal* 314(7087): 1114–8.

Feldstein, Martin. 1995. "The Effect of Marginal Tax Rates on Taxable Income: A Panel Study of the 1986 Tax Reform Act." *Journal of Political Economy* 103(3): 551–72.

Hsiao, William C. 1995. "Medical Savings Accounts: Lessons from Singapore." *Health Affairs* 14(2): 260–6.

———. 2000. *What Should Macroeconomists Know About Health Care Policy? A Primer.* IMF Working Paper No. 136. Washington, DC: Fiscal Affairs Department, International Monetary Fund.

Klein, Rudolf. 1993. "Dimensions of Rationing: Who Should Do What?" *British Medical Journal* 307(6899): 309–11.

Köeck, C. M.; A. Minnick; M. J. Roberts; K. Moore; and N. Scholz. 1998. "Use of Administrative Personnel in Hospitals: A Three-Nation Comparison." *Wiener Klinische Wochenschrift* 110:789–95.

Lim, Meng-Kin. 1998. "Health Care Systems in Transition II. Singapore, Part I. An Overview of Health Care Systems in Singapore." *Journal of Public Health Medicine* 20(1): 16–22.

Marmor, Ted; and Michael S. Barr. 1992. "Making Sense of the National Health Care Reform Debate." *Yale Law and Policy Review* 10(2): 228–82.

Maynard, Alan. 1996. "Rationing Health Care." *British Medical Journal* 313(7071): 1499.

Meyers, Robert J. 1981. *Social Security.* 2nd edition. Bryn Mawr, PA: McCahan Foundation.

Musgrave, Richard A.; and Peggy B. Musgrave. 1989. *Public Finance in Theory and Practice.* New York: McGraw-Hill.

Myles, Gareth D. 1995. *Public Economics.* New York: Cambridge University Press.

OECD. 2002. *OECD Health Data 2002: A Comparative Analysis of Thirty Countries.* Paris, France: OECD.

Pauly, Mark V. 1990. "Financing Health Care." *Quarterly Review of Economics and Business.* 30: 63–80.

Peters, David H.; Abdo S. Yazbeck; Rashmi R. Sharma; G. N. V. Ramana; Lant H. Pritchett; and Adam Wagstaff. 2002. *Better Health Systems for India's Poor: Findings, Analysis, and Options.* Health, Nutrition, and Population Series, Human Development Network. Washington, DC: World Bank.

Preker, Alexander S.; Melitta Jakab; and Markus Schneider. 2002. "Health Financing Reforms in Eastern and Central Europe and the Former Soviet Union." In: Elias Mossialos, Anna Dixon, Josep Figueras, and Joe Kutzin, eds., *Funding Health Care: Options for Europe*. Buckingham, England: Open University Press.

Raffel, M. W., ed. 1984. *Comparative Health Systems: Descriptive Analysis*. University Park, PA: Pennsylvania State University Press.

Reich, Michael R. 1994. "The Political Economy of Health Transitions in the Third World." In: Lincoln C. Chen, Arthur Kleinman, and Norma C. Ware, eds., *Health and Social Change in International Perspective*. Boston, MA: Harvard School of Public Health.

Roberts, Marc; and Thomas Bossert, 1998. *Health Care Options for Polish Municipalities: The Implications of International Experience*. Working Paper. Boston, MA: International Health Systems Program, Harvard School of Public Health.

Rodrik, Dani. 1997. *Has Globalization Gone Too Far?* Washington, DC: Institute of International Economics.

Roemer, Milton I. 1993. *National Health Systems of the World, Volume 2*. New York: Oxford University Press.

Saltman, Richard B.; and Josep Figueras, eds. 1997. *European Health Care Reform: Analysis of Current Strategies*. Copenhagen, Denmark: World Health Organization.

Scheiber, George; and Akiko Maeda. 1997. "A Curmudgeon's Guide to Financing Health Care in Developing Countries." Prepared for the Conference on Innovations in Health Care Financing, March 10–11, Washington, DC.

Schneider, Friedrich. 2002. *The Size and Development of the Shadow Economies of 22 Transition and 21 OECD Countries*. Discussion Paper No. 514. Bonn, Germany: Institute for the Study of Labor.

Ubel, Peter A. 2000. *Pricing Life: Why It's Time for Health Care Rationing*. Cambridge, MA: MIT Press.

World Bank. 1993. *World Development Report 1993: Investing in Health*. New York: Oxford University Press.

———. 1995. *Chile: The Adult Health Policy Challenge*. Washington, DC: World Bank.

Zelman, Walter A. 1996. *Changing Health Care Marketplace: Private Ventures, Public Interests*. San Francisco, CA: Jossey-Bass.

9

Payment

The second of our five control knobs is the payment system. In the previous chapter, we discussed the ways in which money is raised. Now we have to discuss how that money is paid out. All organizations that mobilize funds for the health sector (governments, social and private insurance plans, and community financing schemes) have to decide which organizations to pay, what to pay them for, and how much to pay them. These decisions create powerful incentives that influence the actions of all the organizations and individuals in the health-care system. In this chapter, we look at the incentives that payment schemes create for both buyers and sellers and how these incentives can be adjusted to further the goals of health-sector reform.

Empirical evidence consistently shows that financial incentives are among the most important influences over organizational and individual behavior in the health sector (Cutler and Zeckhauser 2000). Unlike regulation, which relies on the power of the state to coerce individuals to comply through the "stick" of threatened punishment, financial incentives rely on the "carrot" of monetary reward to induce changes in behavior.

These incentives have many effects on the health-care system. They influence both the quantity and quality of services. Pay more for new technology, and hospitals will rush to acquire MRI machines. Pay hospitals more for each day a patient stays, and lengths of stay go up. Pay more for Caesarian sections, and their rate goes up and the rate of normal deliveries will go down. Put doctors on salary, they see fewer patients. Pay them for each visit, and they will see more patients. Indeed, as we discuss in Chapter 10 on organization, payment has a large impact on which kinds of providers exist in the system. It also has a direct impact on the health system's cost, since the total expenditure for health care is the price per unit of service times the volume of service summed for the whole country.

Not only does payment affect the organization of the system, but the reverse is also true—the organization influences payment options. For example, when financing organizations (governments or insurance plans) directly own and manage providers (hospitals and clinics), certain payment methods, like global budgets for hospitals or having doctors on salary, are clearly relevant. When financing organizations and providers are independent and deal with each other at arm's length, then other payment methods become relevant, such as fee-for-service or capitation.

Our discussion throughout this chapter recognizes the intensely political nature of policy decisions about payment—exactly because it has such powerful effects. And the resulting conflicts will be ongoing. Once a payment method has been chosen, the level of payment has to be decided and adjusted to reflect inflation, changes in production costs, budget pressures, and other factors. Setting those levels typically becomes a matter of great contention between buyers and sellers. Providers want payments to be as high as possible—to increase their income. Payers, on the other hand, want payment levels as low as possible to keep down their costs.

This chapter on the payment control knob is organized in five sections. We first briefly explain how financial incentives affect health-system performance. The next section discusses the four key factors to be considered when designing a payment system. We then describe and analyze the principal payment methods. And lastly, we present some conditional guidance for reformers about which payment methods to use.

The Impact of Payment on Outcomes

The incentive effects of payment systems depend in part on what economists call *moral hazard,* on both the demand and supply sides (Arrow 1963, McGuire and Pauly 1991). For example, on the demand side, if patients do not have to pay for health services they will demand a greater quantity of services. The price patients pay also influences where and when they seek care. Even when there are no alternative providers, high fees can lead patients to avoid doctors and self-treat minor illnesses.

On the supply side, the payment system elicits complex responses from physicians and hospitals. Incentives from payment can induce physicians to change the total number of hours worked and the number of patients treated per hour, where they work (in the public sector, the private sector, or both) and even how they treat a specific patient (e.g., whether they perform surgery). Payment also affects the behavior of hospitals. Hospitals have been known to alter lengths of stay, admission rates, and the quantity of services they provide in response to payment changes.

The impact of payment on the volume of care occurs because physicians can induce demand for their services. Because their medical knowledge is far superior to that of patients, physicians can positively or negatively change utilization by advising patients on when to come back for another visit, what drugs to take, what specialists to see, and what laboratory tests or surgical treatments to undergo. Providers can use this power to increase their income, improve their professional standing, reduce their workload, or whatever suits their interests—given the payment system.

The changes that payment creates in the behavior of both buyers and sellers have an impact on both the intermediate performance measures and the performance goals we discussed in Chapters 5 and 6. For example, the price that patients pay influences the volume of services they use. This in turn affects their health status. This is one reason why poor people in countries where patients have to pay for care out-of-pocket often have worse health status—because they cannot afford to pay for needed care. Alternatively, if care is free, patients may demand drugs or treatments that are not cost-effective. Here, satisfying the patient's demand reduces technical efficiency and raises health-care costs. The public may also become less satisfied with the health system when it is especially costly. Thus, there are many links between payment and health-sector performance.

The impact of payment on the quality of care can be equally profound. If quality is defined as the *quantity of care* (see Chapter 6), then payment systems, like fee-for-service, will increase quantity and hence quality. Conversely, paying hospitals a fixed fee per admission will lead them to discharge patients "quicker and sicker." Using payment to influence clinical quality (skill and judgment) or service quality (amenity, convenience, and care) is more difficult. Medical knowledge is limited in general, and its application to a particular case is often quite uncertain—since patients vary so much in response to any given treatment. This makes it difficult to pay for quality based on either decision-making or results—since these are often both controversial and unpredictable. Moreover, service quality is highly multidimensional. And the relative importance of any given aspect of service, as judged by the patients themselves, is likely to vary from individual to individual. Thus, despite all the discussion of linking payment to quality, this practice is still in its infancy.

Different payment rates for different payers can have significant effects on patients' access to health care. For example, some countries have several insurance plans that pay different amounts for the same service. Providers then have a reason not to serve patients insured by plans that pay lower rates. In countries where government-employed physicians have private practices, they typically charge high prices, which lower-income households cannot afford. And this, too, can create profound differences in access—even to public services—when public doctors give favorable treatment to their private patients.

Access to care will also be heavily influenced by the relative prices paid for different services. If some activities are more profitable (high prices relative to costs) than others, the profitable services are much more likely to be available. If capitation rates are set higher (relative to costs) for some patients than others, the unprofitable patients may find it difficult to get doctors to accept them as patients—an experience common to the poor women covered by the Medicaid insurance scheme in the United States and minority Roma women in Bulgaria. Research on the response of German physicians to price changes shows that profitability is not the only factor determining what they do. Risk to the patient also matters—reflecting the intersection of economic factors with the physicians' professional values. But the incentive effects of relative prices are also clear in this work (Mattke 2001).

In sum, prices and payment levels give crucial signals to both consumers and providers. On the supply side, payment influences how many providers enter the market and how services will be produced. On the demand side, patients decide what to purchase and how much to consume, based on the amount they have to pay. Payment is a key mechanism to ration scarce economic resources—it determines the production, distribution, and consumption of health services, drug utilization, and the pattern of capital investments. Payments and their incentives thus play a critical role in determining health-system performance.

Design Decisions

In designing a payment system, health reformers must keep in mind the powerful effects of incentives on the behavior of both buyers and sellers. Attention needs to be paid to both the distribution of financial rewards and the levels of risk bearing. Getting the relative payment levels right also has to be a matter of continuing concern. In this section, we turn our attention to the basic decisions that have to be made in designing a payment system.

Payment Methods

The first question in designing a payment system is what payment method to use. Each payment method has an associated unit of activity that the method uses, as shown in Table 9.1. How we choose the unit of activity for payment affects the supply, efficiency, and quality of health services. For example, when services such as tests, drugs, and procedures for a given disease are bundled together into a single unit of payment (such as per admission or per day), hospitals have a reason to provide fewer services. This could lower costs, but there also is the risk that some services might be under-provided.

Eight options for payment method and the associated unit of service are summarized in Table 9.1. The incentives created by each payment method and their impacts are presented below.

TABLE **9.1.** Payment Methods for Physicians and Hospitals

PAYMENT METHOD	UNIT OF PAYMENT	PHYSICIANS AND OTHER HEALTH PROFESSIONALS	HOSPITALS AND OTHER PROVIDER INSTITUTIONS
Fee-for-service	Units of service	X	X
Salary	Time	X	
Salary plus bonus	Time plus performance	X	
Capitation	Persons registered	X	X
Per diem	Days		X
Per admission	Admissions		X
Case-mix adjusted admission	Admissions by disease category		X
Line item budget	Budget line		X
Global budget	Hospital expenditure		X

Payment Rates

Once a payment method has been chosen, the next task is to determine the rate or level of payment. The effects of a payment scheme on health-sector performance are heavily influenced by how rates are set. High rates can lead to higher costs, incomes, and profits. Low rates can discourage supply or undermine quality. Reflecting the complexity of actual financing and payment systems, most countries use a mixture of rate-setting approaches. They typically choose among five basic techniques: charges, costs, past practice, negotiation, and bidding. In practice, these decisions reflect both technical and political considerations.

The most obvious and technically simple method is to pay providers according to posted *charges*, since these are typically easy to observe. Economists argue that if markets are competitive, these charges will reflect the costs of production. Moreover, competition will force providers to keep those as low as possible. But since most health-care markets are not particularly competitive and suffer from various market failures, these arguments are not especially compelling. For this reason, most governments or large social insurance funds do not base payments on charges. In some cases, however, private insurance funds do pay charges—perhaps because they lack the technical capacity or economic power to do otherwise. Moreover, paying charges allows them to reduce conflict with the provider community.

When payers do pay charges, they have a choice about whether to use each doctor's or hospital's rate or to use a uniform figure for each geographical area. For example, the U.S. Medicare system began by using the "usual and customary" rate for physician services in each region. Indeed, payers can even use a rate below the average price in the market—in the hopes of containing costs. This is how some national payment systems for pharmaceuticals, the so-called reference pricing systems, operate. The most extreme example of these is New Zealand, which uses the lowest available price for each group of drugs (Woodfield 2001).

An obvious alternative to charges, one designed to help avoid excess provider profits, is to base payment rates on the *costs* of each service. Here again, there is a choice between using each provider's own costs and some sort of regional or group average.

The two largest objections to cost-based reimbursement are its technical difficulties and its incentive effects. Doctors and hospitals provide a wide range of services, and the accounting problems involved in determining the costs of each service are formidable. Ideally, a cost-based system requires uniform accounting systems in each hospital, as well as uniform rules for classifying treatment activities and disease states. Few hospitals in low- or middle-income countries have such expensive and complex data systems.

From an incentive point of view, cost-based reimbursement is also a problem, since providers that are less efficient and have higher costs receive more funding. This creates a strong incentive to increase costs. Cost-based systems often try to limit this possibility by only paying "reasonable" costs—for example, by using some sort of regional or group average (plus an allowed degree of variation) as a ceiling.

Since determining costs is so difficult, and to minimize the incentive to increase costs, nations have sometimes used costs in a base year adjusted annually by an inflation factor. Indeed, this adjustment can be kept below the rate of general inflation for cost-control purposes (as has been done periodically in Canada and Australia).

Another way to try to contain costs is to set cost-based rates prospectively—so that reimbursement does not necessarily cover all incurred costs. This gives the government greater predictability and reduces provider incentives to be inefficient— especially if the "cost" being used is some group or regional average. Otherwise, if this year's costs become the basis for the next year's rates, providers know they will recover their costs eventually, albeit with a one- or two-year lag.

The third major approach to rate setting is *past practice* (also typically modified by some annual adjustment factor). Again, it is relatively simple to use. But the incentive and distributive effects depend critically on how the base-year rates were set. For example, if they were based on historic costs, historically inefficient hospitals are rewarded for their poor past performance. Such an approach is also poorly equipped to respond to changes in cost, technology, utilization, or consumer demand. It is most frequently used in connection with various budget systems, where current year allocations are derived mechanically from prior years' disbursements.

In the three methods discussed so far, the rate-setting process is relatively mechanical. The next two options, in contrast, are more interactive and process-oriented. They are especially applicable in the context of a contract approach to paying for services—as discussed in Chapter 10. First, some large and sophisticated payers use *negotiation* to set rates. These talks may occur with individual providers or, as in the case in Germany and Japan, between payers and the medical society and other key stakeholders—in which case the sellers in effect act as a cartel. To avoid that contingency, buyers will often try to deal first with a low-cost provider to set a rate they can use as a benchmark in later negotiations.

An alternative to negotiation is to use *competitive bidding*, which is also inter-active. While competitive bidding can theoretically lead to rates that are close to the bidders' actual costs, providers often object strongly to this approach because the less efficient among them would lose. Furthermore, competitive bidding may not produce satisfactory results unless the process is well designed and appropri-ate information is given to all potential bidders. Moreover, when the government manages competitive bidding, politics can intrude as sellers manipulate the pro-cess to their own advantage.

As a result of these difficulties, many nations have tried to find payment systems that require them to set a smaller number of rates. In particular, many have moved away from the fee-for-service payment method because of the enormous number of distinct items. For example, the insurance programs in the United States offi-cially recognize more than 9000 service items for payment (AMA 1994). In con-trast, capitation methods to pay for physician services and per-admission payments for hospital services require many fewer rates to be set.

The problem of rate setting is made more complicated by the difficulty in find-ing an objective basis to resolve the inevitable disagreements. Economists typi-cally argue that the right level of payment for physicians, for example, is one that would balance supply and demand. But because health-care markets are so im-perfect, this theory is difficult to apply in practice. Consider, for example, the case of countries with physician surpluses—often because medical education is free. Setting free market rates is likely to produce a decline in physicians' incomes that would be quite unacceptable to the provider community.

One option is to have payment rates set by an autonomous agency, insulated from political influence as much as possible. Yet even then politics will almost always play an important role. Hence, our advice to health-sector reformers is to think about implementation and politics *before* you select a plan. Will you have the technical skill and political support to implement the proposed payment scheme? In the long run, it is difficult to use a politically controversial method because stakeholders will work to overturn its operation.

Payment Methods and Provider Incentives

In this section, we examine the incentive structures that payment systems create for health-care providers and patients. We present each payment method commonly used around the world and summarize how each method affects the behavior of provider organizations and health professionals. We examine how each method affects the technical efficiency and quality of health services and summarize recent empirical evidence on the strength of these incentives. In the next section, we do the same for the financial incentives that influence patients.

We analyze the incentive structure for the eight payment methods presented in Table 9.1 above. In practice, societies rarely use just one payment method. Instead, two or more forms are combined and tailored to the particular situation and to the requirements of the specific health-care system.

In this discussion, we must keep in mind how payment systems create and share different kinds of financial risk among payers and providers. For example, if physicians are paid on the basis of capitation (a fixed fee for each enrolled patient), they bear the risk if patients are sicker then anticipated. In contrast, when doctors are paid through fee-for-service, the payer bears that risk.

Payment Methods for Physicians and Other Health Professionals

Over the last decade, a growing interest has emerged in the role of financial incentives in health-care organizations. Inspired by other industries, health-care managers have designed financial incentives in order to induce more cost-reducing behavior by physicians. (These financial incentives, however, often run counter to other professional and legal constraints.) Recent research on health services and organizational theory has highlighted the importance of three factors in the design of such incentives: proximity, intensity, and interaction (Harshbarger 1999).

Proximity refers to how direct the link is between a physician's decisions for a patient and their economic rewards. Capitation, for example, is a high-proximity incentive structure. Physicians' incomes are directly linked to their practice of medicine. *Intensity* represents the magnitude of the incentives facing the individual physician. For example, the broader the scope of services included in the capitation rate, the larger the maximum potential loss or gain for the physician. (Pearson et al. 1998). The last factor, *interaction*, refers to the behavioral dynamic among physicians. To what extent do my payments depend on others' decisions?

Fee-for-service (FFS)

In this arrangement, the unit of payment consists of individual visits or clinical activities such as injections, laboratory tests, and X-rays. This payment method gives providers an incentive to perform more services. This is the only form of payment under which the provider does not have any incentive to select healthier patients; in fact, the opposite is true. Under FFS, the provider bears no risk for the cost of treatment. The payer, the insurer, or the patient is entirely at risk for the cost of care. Theoretically, patients and third-party payers have a reason to question the need for additional services and negotiate lower payments. In reality, however, patients and third-party payers can seldom negotiate effectively due to the professional power of physicians.

Studies in many countries, both developed and developing, have found that a fee-for-service payment system promotes an excessive use of services and an increase in costs (Barnum et al. 1995). Comparing resource utilization under two provider-payment methods (FFS and capitation) in Thailand, Yip et al. (2001) found a significant difference in the average length of stay, drug charges per admission, and lab costs per case. Under FFS, resource utilization by providers was consistently greater. A study in the United States (Krawelski et al. 2000) found similar results. Costs were significantly lower under medical group practices paid by capitation than those paid by FFS.

Although both theory and evidence point to the cost-increasing impact of FFS payment methods, it is still the most widely used method in developing countries to pay private-sector hospitals and individual practitioners. This can be explained by the fact that most governments in developing countries have taken a benign neglect position toward private-sector providers. Thus, providers establish their own unit and level of payment, and choose FFS, since it is the easiest, most profitable and most flexible method.

Capitation

Under capitation, the unit of payment is defined on a per-person basis. A payment is fixed to pay for all services that a person may use during a period of time, such as a month or year. The most common capitation payment is a fixed rate paid to a general practitioner for each patient registered with him for that month, regardless of the services required by or rendered to the patient. This payment can vary by the patient's age, sex, and health status. Capitation has been used to pay for primary care (capitated to general practitioners), for specialist services (capitated to multi-specialty clinics), and for inpatient services (capitated to hospitals). It is also possible to bundle the primary, specialty, and inpatient services into one capitation rate that is paid to a single entity that takes responsibility for all services.

Capitation payments transfer most of the financial risk to providers. These risks vary according to the specific contract terms and organizational arrangements. For example, many Colombian insurance plans contract with general practitioners for primary care services and pay them by capitation. In comparison, social insurance plans in Thailand contract with hospitals for all primary care, specialist, and inpatient services, and pay them a capitation rate. The hospitals then contract with general practitioners for primary care and pay them a capitation rate. The incentives under the capitation method vary according to the specific services covered. In the Thailand example, hospitals have an incentive to limit not only primary care and drugs but also diagnostic, specialist, and inpatient services in order to be financially solvent or earn a surplus at the end of the year.

Numerous studies show how incentives under capitation have affected provider behavior. Iversen et al. (2000) evaluated the impact of capitation on Norwegian GPs' referral decisions. They found a 42% increase in the rate of referral from general practitioners to specialists after Norway introduced a new, experimental payment system in which GPs are contracted only for primary care and are paid by capitation. Under this arrangement, Norwegian GPs referred patients more frequently to specialists, reduced the average number of visits per registered patient, and increased the number of registered patients in their panel. In another recent study, Bitran (2001) found that in response to rising health-care costs, Argentinean social insurance plans have been moving away from direct provision and towards the purchasing of health services via capitation. After shifting to capitation in 1997, one insurance plan experienced a drop in the number of hospitalizations per 100 beneficiaries from 2.83 in 1997 to 2.6 in 1998.

Under capitation, providers may choose to accept only healthy and less complicated patients, a practice known as *risk selection*, to minimize their exposure to risk (Frank et al. 1998). Newhouse (1996) examined managed care plans in the United States and concluded that capitation payments encouraged providers to become more efficient in their use of resources but that they also created risk-selection problems.

Salary

This unit of payment is based on a time period that employed physicians are at work, regardless of the number of patients seen, volume of services, or cost of services provided. Physicians paid by salary bear little financial risk but may alter their decision-making to minimize the time and effort they expend at work. In developing countries, the employer, often the government, bears the financial risk and to maximize efficiency may ask each physician to see a certain number of patients per hour.

A recent study reviewed 23 published papers on salary payments and their effects on providers' behavior in developed nations (Gosden et al. 1999 and 2001). The authors found some tentative evidence that salary payment is associated with lower productivity when compared with fee-for-service and capitation payment methods. Specifically, they found an association between salary payments and *(1)* a reduced number of services per patient; *(2)* a reduced volume of patients per physician; *(3)* longer patient visits; and *(4)* greater degrees of preventive care compared to fee-for-service. Other anecdotal evidence indicates that salary payment does not encourage physicians to be responsive: the lack of financial incentive dampens their enthusiasm for satisfying the concerns of patients and fellow physicians (Harshbarger 1999).

Salary plus bonus

Because a straight salary system has so few productivity incentives, many health-care organizations that use salary payment supplement it with bonuses of various kinds. In China, for example, hospital-based physicians may receive a bonus based on the number of patients seen or on the revenue they generate for the hospital by their prescribing and test-ordering behavior. In the United States, health plans that employ physicians have a variety of bonus plans based on such factors as individual productivity, patient satisfaction, or financial results (for either a particular practice or the plan as a whole).

Bonus schemes increase the level of administrative costs, and the *pay-for-performance* movement in industry and health care certainly has its critics (Colliver

TABLE 9.2. Payment Methods for Physicians: Financial Risks and Incentives

	Risk Borne By		Provider Incentives To			
PAYMENT METHOD	PAYER	PROVIDER	INCREASE NUMBER OF PATIENTS TREATED OR REGISTERED	DECREASE NUMBER OF SERVICES PER CHARGEABLE UNITS OF CARE OR CONSULTATION	INCREASE REPORTED ILLNESS SEVERITY	SELECT HEALTHIER PATIENTS
FFS	All risk borne by payer	No risk borne by provider	yes	no	yes	no
Salary	All risks	No risk borne by physician	no	N/A	N/A	no
Salary and Bonus	Salary portion	Bonus portion	yes	N/A	N/A	yes
Capitation	Amount above "stop-loss" ceiling	All risk borne by provider up to a given ceiling (stop-loss)	yes	N/A	no	yes

Sources: Hsiao et al. 1999, modifying data from WHO 1993, Bodenheimer and Grumbach 1994.

2002, Kohn 1999). Nonetheless, many provider organizations around the world are adding a bonus component to salary-based systems.

Summary

Each payment method for physicians and health professionals creates a particular set of risks and incentives for providers. In Table 9.2 we summarize the payment methods and show how each method produces a financial reward or risk for the physician and the payer, and the likely responses of physicians to the different payment methods.

Payment Methods for Physicians: Financial Risks and Incentives

Per admission

The first payment method for hospitals and provider institutions uses an admission as the unit of service. A fixed amount is paid to cover all the services during a particular hospital stay regardless of the actual services provided. This method transfers a portion of the financial risk to the provider. Generally, as the number of services bundled together increases, the financial risk borne by providers increases as well. With this system the incentive for the hospital is to reduce the length of stay and the amount of care given to each patient. The per-admission method also gives hospitals an incentive to select patients with less severe illnesses and to admit as many patients as possible, as long as they can find patients whose added cost to the hospital of care is less than the fee received for each patient.

Case-mix adjusted per admission

To remedy some of the shortcomings in per-admission payment, case-mix adjusted payment separates patients into disease and treatment categories and pays more for those who cost more to treat. In this way patients in categories that on average cost more to treat generate more revenue for the hospital. The diagnostic-related grouping (DRG) method has become the most widely used approach for doing this kind of case-mix adjusted per admission payment.

Under such systems, hospitals have an incentive to shorten lengths of stay, provide less care and admit more patients. They also have an incentive to focus on patients who are profitable. These are the patients within each category who are relatively healthy, and patients in those classifications where payments, on average, are high compared to the costs of care.

In a recent study evaluating the impact in Italy of DRG-based payment, Louis et al. (1999) reported a 21.1% decrease in hospital bed days after the introduction of this payment system. Another study in the United States (Gilman 2000) found evidence that hospitals selected profitable patients to treat. These findings are consistent with the findings of an earlier synthesis study on the impacts of DRG-based payment (Ellis and McGuire 1993).

Per-diem

Payment on a per-day basis is commonly used for hospitals. A fixed rate is paid per day of hospitalization regardless of the actual services given or their costs. This fixed rate per day gives hospitals incentives to reduce costs and reduce tests and procedures. The hospital also has an incentive to keep patients in the hospital longer—especially since days of care tend to be less costly toward the end of a stay. As a result, per-diem payments encourage hospitals to have a high occupancy rate and expand their bed capacity. Prudent payers find it necessary to perform utilization reviews to control unnecessarily long hospital stays.

Studies have found strong statistical correlation between per-diem payment and average length of stay (ALOS). For example, Rodwin and Okamoto (2000) examined the impact of per-diem payments introduced by the Japanese authorities and found that the average hospital length of stay in Japan is three times longer than that in the United States for the same diagnostic categories. In the case of appendicitis, the ALOS in Japan was 9.8 days, while in the United States where hospitals are often paid on a per-case basis, the stay was 3 days. Similarly, in Slovakia, Langenbrunner and Wiley (1999) reported an ALOS of 7.5 days for childbirth under a nationwide per-diem payment system, versus about two days in the United States under the DRG system.

Line-item budget

In this widely used payment method, the unit of payment is an expense category (e.g. salary, supplies, transportation, drugs) for an organization. The amount budgeted is typically based on some mix of the facility's caseload, the number of staff, and past budgets. Once the funding agency (the ministry of finance) has approved the budget, the provider (hospital or clinic) has little discretion to switch funds across budget categories. This type of budgeting provides an incentive for hospital directors to overestimate budgetary needs and spend the entire budget. Hospitals have little incentive to admit more patients—unless that indicator plays a major role in the budget process. The result is often a high level of technical inefficiency, especially when budget categories are very narrow so that managers cannot shift resources to respond to changing conditions.

Langenbrunner and Wiley (1999) studied the impact of line-item budget payment systems in Eastern Europe—systems that are now being abandoned throughout the region. They concluded that: *(1)* little incentive existed for facility directors to be cost-conscious and innovative; *(2)* facilities tended towards under-providing health services; *(3)* little attention was paid to health outcomes and patient satisfaction; and *(4)* no real incentive existed to downsize the level of fixed resources (i.e., staff and facilities).

Global budget

This payment method sets an all-inclusive operating budget in advance. Often the organization must meet certain output targets, like a number of bed days or outpatient visits, or face a penalty. A global budget represents the broadest scope of bundling services. Every service performed on every patient during one year is aggregated into a single payment (Ashby and Greene 1993).

Under a global budget system, managers have an incentive to control their expenses while attaining their production targets, although the potential always exists to distort decisions to reach those targets (Bishop and Wallack 1996). For example, German hospitals operate on the global budget payment system with bed days as the production target. Germany, as a result, has among the longest lengths of stay of all industrialized nations.

Many global budget systems pay a hospital more when it exceeds its production target and penalize it when it fails to reach that target (Fan et al. 1998). If such payments are based on average costs, the hospital can increase profits by expanding days since its marginal costs will be below its average costs. Paying or penalizing the hospital based on its marginal costs can help solve this problem, and that in fact is how the German system of the early 1990s operated.

In Table 9.3 we summarize the payment methods for hospitals, the incentive structures created for the payers and the hospitals, and the likely responses of hospitals to the various payment methods.

TABLE 9.3. Payment Methods for Hospitals: Financial Risks and Incentives

PAYMENT MECHANISM	Risk Borne By		Provider Incentives To			
	PAYER	PROVIDER	INCREASE NUMBER OF PATIENTS	DECREASE NUMBER OF SERVICES PER PAYMENT UNITS	INCREASE REPORTED ILLNESS SEVERITY	SELECT HEALTHIER PATIENTS
Fee for Service	All risk borne by payer	No risk borne by provider	yes	no	yes	no
Case-Mix Adjusted Per Admission (e.g., DRG)	Risk of number of cases and case severity classification	Risk of cost of treatment for a given case	yes	yes	yes	yes
Per Admission	Risk of number of admission	Risk of number of services per admission	yes	yes	no	yes
Per-Diem	Risk of number of days to stay	Risk of cost of services within a given day	yes	yes	no	no
Capitation	Amount above "stop-loss" ceiling	All risk borne by provider up to a given ceiling (stop-loss)	yes	yes	N/A	yes
Global Budget	No risk borne by payer	All risk borne by provider	no	N/A	N/A	yes

Sources: Hsiao et al. 1999, modifying data from WHO 1993, Bodenheimer and Grumbach 1994.

Payment Systems and Patients

Payment systems affect patients as well as providers by determining how much patients must pay for services. There are two cases to consider—those in which the
government directly operates the care system, and those where it acts indirectly on
prices (e.g., through its operation or regulation of the insurance system). Almost all
consideration of patient incentives, however, arises in the context of fee-for-service
payments, since patients typically pay for care primarily in this way.

Most nations that directly operate health-care systems use tax revenues to subsidize the cost of health care provided at public facilities. This practice reduces
the price faced by patients, resulting in increased demand. As we discussed in the
last chapter, the result can be allocative inefficiency and "excess burden" from a
subjective utilitarian point of view. Patients use care where the value to them is
less than the cost of production, because that care is free. For this reason, some
nations have imposed user fees for their public services to reduce inappropriate
utilization (and to generate increased revenue).

Many nominally free public systems, however, are not actually free to patients.
Often supplies and drugs must be provided by patients (and bought by them in the
marketplace), and various kinds of bribes, gratuities, and informal payments may
be expected by providers. In addition, the time and travel costs of seeking care
can be substantial. All of these costs can lessen the magnitude of the efficiency
distortions created by nominally free care.

Where governments do not directly provide extensive public care, the existence
of insurance affects the payments that patients must pay, and hence their incentives and behavior. There are two interacting phenomena here. First, all insurance
plans in effect lower the prices customers pay at the time they get sick. As a result,
such schemes raise the same allocative efficiency problems as directly provided
(and subsidized) care.

In addition, in much of the world, health insurance is not purchased on an individual basis, but rather through tax-supported social insurance schemes. These typically
include a substantial element of redistribution or cross-subsidy from general revenue.
This arrangement encourages citizens to push for coverage that is more generous
than many of them would be willing to pay for out of their own pockets. Government
subsidies for the purchase of private insurance have a similar effect. As a result,
nations that finance health care through insurance often incorporate deductibles,
co-payments, coinsurance, and payment ceilings. All of these pricing schemes are
intended to create incentives for patients to reduce their use of inappropriate care.

Deductibles are payments made by the patient before the insurance policy begins
to cover incurred expenses. The deductible level is set for either individuals or
families and is sometimes based on the level of income.

Co-payments are fixed payments made by the patient for each physician visit or
each hospital day.

TABLE 9.4. Financial Risks and Patient Incentives Under Various Pricing Schemes

	Risk Borne By		Incentive For
	PAYER (E.G., INSURANCE OR GOVERNMENT)	PATIENT	PATIENT
Free	All	None	Increase demand
Full User Fee	None	All	Reduce demand
Deductible	Amount above deductible	Amount up-to-total deductible	Reduce demand until deductible amount reached, then increase demand
Fixed Copayment Per Visit	Full charge minus copayment	Co-payment	Reduce demand for visits
Coinsurance (% of Charges)	$(1–X)\%$ of charges	$X\%$ of charges	Reduce demand (depending on percentage of coinsurance)

Source: Hsiao et al. 1999.

Co-insurance refers to patients being responsible for a certain percentage of their costs.

Payment ceilings are a maximum amount of money an insurer is liable to pay per patient per year.

Table 9.4 summarizes the distribution of financial risk and the incentives that affect patients under various pricing schemes. As shown in the table, under free care, the insurer bears all the risk, while the opposite is true under a full user fee. Other benefit designs divide the risk and generally tend to reduce the amount of health care demanded by the patient. Deductibles and co-payments have their largest effect on routine care, while co-insurance and ceilings can have an impact on more expensive hospital care. Payment ceilings in particular impose a significant risk on patients if a catastrophic illness occurs.

Assessing the empirical importance of these price effects on patients requires an evaluation of the *elasticity of demand*. The phrase "elasticity of demand" refers to the percentage change in demand for a good or a service in response to a percentage change in the price of that good or service. On average, the price elasticity of demand for health care is not high, which implies that the distortions may not be serious. In other words, changes in prices do not generally result in large changes in demand for health care. As Table 9.5 shows, however, studies in developing countries consistently show that price elasticity is higher for lower-income households and for children. Thus user fees have a greater adverse impact on the care, utilization, and well-being of those groups.

TABLE 9.5. Elasticity of Demand for Health Services: Selected Results

STUDY (YEAR PUBLISHED)	LOCATION (YEAR OF DATA)	Results		
Jimenez (1989)	Ethiopia (1985)	Overall:	−0.05 to −0.50	
Jimenez (1989)	Sudan (1985)	Overall:	−0.37	
Yoder (1989)	Swaziland (1985)	Overall:	−0.32	
Gertler & Van der Gaag (1989)	Côte d'Ivoire (1985)	Rural hospitals Income quartile	Adults	Children
		Lowest	−0.47 to −1.34	−0.65 to −2.32
		Second	−0.44 to −1.27	−0.58 to −1.98
		Third	−0.41 to −1.18	−0.49 to −1.60
		Highest	−0.29 to −0.71	−0.12 to −0.48
Gertler & Van der Gaag (1989)	Peru (1985)	Rural Hospitals Overall:	−0.57 to −0.50	−0.41 to −0.81
		Income Quartile	Adults	Children
		Lowest	−0.57 to −1.36	−0.67 to −1.72
		Second	−0.38 to −0.91	−0.48 to −1.20
		Third	−0.16 to −0.37	−0.22 to −0.54
		Highest	−0.01 to −0.04	−0.03 to −0.09
Sauerborn et al. (1994)	Burkina Faso (1985)	Overall:	−0.79	
		Age Groups:		
		<1	−3.64	
		1–14	−1.73	
		15+	0.27	
		Income Quartile		
		Lowest	−1.44	
		Second	−1.21	
		Third	−1.39	
		Highest	−0.12	

Source: Reddy, Sanjay and Vandenmoortele, Jan. User financing of basic social services: A review of theoretical arguments and empirical evidence. Office of Evaluation, Policy and Planning. UNICEF, New York, 1996.

Conditional Guidance

Table 9.6 shows the impact of each payment method on health-care costs and the quantity and quality of services. Empirical studies have found that payment mechanisms have measurable effects on many variables, including: *(1)* the kinds of medical care provided to patients; *(2)* the types and amounts of drugs prescribed; *(3)* the quantity of services provided; *(4)* hospital lengths of stay; *(5)* the proportion of patients treated on an outpatient basis; *(6)* the labeling of diseases and their severity; and *(7)* the frequency with which patients are referred to specialists

TABLE 9.6. The Impact of Financial Incentives

PAYMENT MECHANISM	IMPACT ON MEDICAL DECISIONS AND COSTS
Fee-for-service	Providers favor this method; quantity of service per patient and total supply increase; inflationary; quality may decrease due to over-treatment and overuse of drugs.
Per case	Improves efficiency of hospital services; increases admissions somewhat; quality may decrease because of too-short stay per admission and underuse of tests.
Per-diem	Less inflationary than fee-for-service; significantly increases length-of-stay; quantity of services per day may decrease.
Capitation	Significantly reduces unnecessary services; improves efficiency; patients maybe under-treated; risk selection by providers.
Global budget	Improves efficiency; most effective in controlling inflationary health costs; quality may decrease; quantity may increase if volume standard is tied to the budget.
Salary	Removes incentives for over-treatment of patients; quantity of output per-hour may decrease; quality of care may decrease; providers self-refer patients to their private practice.

and given laboratory tests. These effects indicate that the choice of payment method is a critical decision for a health-sector reformer.

Choosing Payment Methods

This review implies that no payment method is perfect—each has both positive and negative attributes. While nations vary in their health-system goals and circumstances, international experience suggests some conditional guidance for readers to bear in mind. Here are five critical lessons about the payment control knob:

- Decisions on payment method must be considered in the context of how the system is organized; organization and payment must complement each other.
- Fee-for-service payment encourages health-care cost increases. Nations would be wise to avoid this method unless there are strong reasons to do otherwise.
- The salary-plus-bonus payment method is superior to salary only. The former can motivate health professionals to increase productivity and improve quality of services. This advantage is especially evident for specialists, provided they are employed by organizations such as hospitals or insurance programs.
- Capitation payment for primary care has much to recommend it, especially when there are competing services in the same community.
- For high- and middle-income countries, per-admission payment and simplified DRG payment to hospitals have desirable incentive effects but also create

administrative complexity. For hospitals in low-income countries, global budgets may be preferable because of their more limited administrative requirements.

To what extent do we need to adjust these conclusions, especially where fee-for-service payment is used, in light of the effect of payment on buyers' decisions? Because the average value of the price elasticity of demand for medical services is not high, the loss of economic efficiency from low prices is not that significant—especially given all the costs that buyers do typically bear. On the other hand, requiring patients to pay some user fees when their elasticity of demand is high can reduce waste. For example, making drugs free to patients can increase wastage (raising the likelihood that drugs are taken home but not consumed). For insurance plans, of all the methods to control utilization, deductibles are easiest to administer, since the insurance plan then does not have to reimburse patients for thousands of small bills.

Setting Payment Levels

Establishing payment levels requires the reformer to consider a complex set of market and regulatory factors. If the level of payment is set too low, providers will opt out of government-financed insurance schemes or charge additional amounts to patients or seek under-the-table payments—depending on what the law allows. On the other hand, if payment levels are set too high, the result will be higher premiums or taxes and less money available for other public purposes.

Setting the right payment level is a contentious and sensitive affair. Competitive bidding has much to recommend it when there are competing providers and the process can be combined with selective contracting—as discussed in the next chapter. But this condition may not exist, or providers as a group may resist such a method. Attempting to set a reasonable payment level based on cost data is also likely to be controversial; payers and providers will rarely accept one common set of data as truly objective. Even where they do agree on the facts, disagreements on value issues—like the socially appropriate level of provider incomes—are likely to be significant.

A fundamental tension exists in payment systems: payers want to keep the payment level as low as possible, while providers want to raise the level as high as possible. International experience shows that bilateral negotiation can produce mutually acceptable results in certain circumstances. But once governments become involved and the situation becomes politicized, governments are likely to find themselves under substantial pressure from well-organized provider groups to devote additional resources to health-care salaries. Reformers therefore need to consider in advance the political as well as the economic consequences of various payment systems—and make their decisions accordingly.

Payment Methods and Equity

Payment links to equity in two different ways, depending on whether patients pay their own bills or not. When patients do not pay their own bills, there is the risk that the payment system will not reflect the varied costs of different patients. In such situations, high-cost patients can become economically less attractive, and as a result they can encounter barriers to access. These barriers may range from the subtle to the explicit, from culturally insensitive or inappropriate service to outright refusals to provide care. This pattern has important equity implications, since patients from lower socioeconomic strata and marginalized social groups are often less healthy, less compliant with treatment regimes, and more difficult for doctors from privileged backgrounds to deal with. Thus, in designing payment systems, reformers have to be conscious of these risks. (The special problems of providing services to rural areas—one manifestation of this concern—are discussed in Chapter 10.)

A parallel issue can arise when payments for specific services, which are disproportionately used by marginalized populations, are set at a low level versus their costs. This practice can also lead to a withdrawal of providers. Even in the United States with its very high payment rates, low payments for certain emergency care and mental health services have led hospitals to close trauma centers and psychiatric wards—creating access problems that raise grave equity concerns.

The seriousness of these two concerns—payments set too low for certain patients, and for certain types of care—depends in part on the organization of the delivery system. As we discuss in Chapter 10, two key features are relevant. First, how competitive is the provider sector? Second, to what extent are providers organized on for-profit principles? Competitive, profit-making providers are likely to be very sensitive to price-cost margins, and hence governments need to be especially careful about setting equity-sensitive payment levels in such situations.

The second kind of equity concern embedded in the payment system occurs when patients pay their own bills. Because the price elasticity of demand is significantly higher for low-income households, there are strong equity reasons for user-fee schemes to include needs-based exemptions—despite the administrative costs and corruption potential of such arrangements. For the same reason, services that reformers particularly want to encourage—like vaccination and prevention—should probably not be subject to user fees at all. These services are likely to have a higher price-elasticity of demand for all income groups, than curative care. After all, given travel time and costs, forgone income, bribes, and the need to buy drugs and supplies, even "free" services are seldom really free—especially for poor people in poor countries. Indeed, because much prevention actually occurs during routine medical care, income-based exemptions to user fees may be the only effective way to deliver such services to the disadvantaged.

Summary

Economists sometimes overstress the incentive effects of payment systems, as noneconomists underappreciate their impact. As we have noted in this chapter, the effect of payment schemes on health-sector performance depends both on how they affect providers' opportunities and on the values and attitudes providers bring to their response. Some doctors and hospitals provide care for "unprofitable" patients out of a sense of social responsibility. And around the world, professional norms constrain physician's willingness to create supplier-induced demand— albcit to varying degrees in different settings.

On the other hand, not all performance dimensions that reformers care about can be easily and reliably measured, and hence not all can be easily paid for. The risks of distortion and dishonesty are always present. Still, payment systems remain one of the most powerful control knobs available to health-sector reformers. "You get what you pay for" is generally the best place to begin to understand the economics of any national health-care system. At the least, reformers would be wise not to establish payment systems that create incentives at odds with their priority goals.

References

AMA (American Medical Association). 1994. *Physician's Current Procedural Terminology*. 4th Edition. Chicago: American Medical Association.

Arrow, Kenneth J. 1963. "Uncertainty and the Welfare Economics of Medical Care." *The American Economic Review* 53: 941–73.

Ashby, John L.; and Timothy F. Greene. 1993. "Implications of a Global Budget for Facility-Based Health Spending." *Inquiry* 30: 362–71.

Barnum, Howard; Joseph Kutzin; and Helen Saxenian. 1995. *Incentives and Provider Payment Methods*. HRO Working Papers No. 51. Washington, DC: Human Resources Development and Operations Policy (HRO), The World Bank, March.

Bishop, Christine E.; and Stanley S. Wallack. 1996. "National Health Expenditure Limits: The Case for a Global Budget Process." *Milbank Quarterly* 74: 361–76.

Bitran, Ricardo. 2001. *Paying Health Providers through Capitation in Argentina, Nicaragua, and Thailand: Output, Spending, Organizational Impact, and Market Structure*. Technical Paper #1. Bethesda, MD: Partnerships for Health Reform Project, Abt Associates.

Colliver, Victoria. 2002. "Health Care Plans Sign On to Rating System for Doctors." *San Francisco Chronicle*. January 16, 2002: B1.

Cutler, David M.; and Richard J. Zeckhauser. 2000. "The Anatomy of Health Insurance." In: Anthony J. Culyer and Joseph P. Newhouse, eds., *Handbook of Health Economics, Volume I*. Amsterdam: Elsevier, 563–643.

Ellis, Randall P.; and Thomas G. McGuire. 1993. "Supply-Side and Demand-Side Cost Sharing in Health Care." *The Journal of Economic Perspectives* 7: 135–51.

Fan, C. P.; K. P. Chen; and K. Kan. 1998. "The Design of Payment Systems for Physicians under Global Budget—An Experimental Study." *Journal of Economic Behavior & Organization* 34: 295–311.

Frank, Richard G.; Jacob Glazer; and Thomas G. McGuire. 1998. *Measuring Adverse Selection in Managed Health Care.* Working Paper No. 6825. Cambridge, MA: National Bureau of Economic Research.

Gilman, Boyd H. 2000. "Hospital Response to DRG Refinements: The Impact of Multiple Reimbursement Incentives on Inpatient Length of Stay." *Health Economics* 9: 277–94.

Gosden T.; F. Forland; I. S. Kristiansen; M. Sutton; B. Leese; A. Giuffrida; M. Sergison; and L. Pedersen. 2001. "Impact of Payment Method on Behaviour of Primary Care Physicians: A Systematic Review." *Journal of Health Services & Research Policy* 6: 44–55.

Gosden T.; L. Pedersen; and D. Torgerson. 1999. "How Should We Pay Doctors? A Systematic Review of Salary Payments and Their Effect on Doctor Behaviour." *Quarterly Journal of Medicine* 92: 47–55.

Harshbarger, Melanie. 1999. *Note on Physician Compensation and Financial Incentives.* Cambridge, MA: Harvard Business School.

Hsiao, William; Winnie Yip; et al. 1999. *Improving Hong Kong's Health Care System: Why and For Whom?* Hong Kong: Government Printing Department.

Iversen, Tor; and Hilde Lurås. 2000. "The Effect of Capitation on GPs' Referral Decisions." *Health Economics* 9: 199–210.

Kohn, Alfie. 1999. *Punished by Rewards: The Trouble with Gold Stars, Incentive Plans, A's, Praise, and Other Bribes.* Boston, MA: Houghton Mifflin.

Kralewski, J. E.; E. C. Rich; R. Feldman; B. E. Dowd; T. Bernhardt; C. Johnson; W. Gold. 2000. "The Effects of Medical Group Practice and Physician Payment Methods on the Cost of Care." *Health Services Research* 35: 591–613.

Langenbrunner, John C.; and Miriam M. Wiley. 1999. "Paying the Hospital: Payment Policies and Reforms in Eastern Europe and the Former Soviet Union. Issues, Options, Early Results." Washington, DC: World Bank (unpublished draft).

Louis, D. Z.; E. J. Yuen; M. Braga; A. Cicchetti; C. Rabinowitz; C. Laine; and J. S. Gonnella. 1999. "Impact of a DRG-based Hospital Financial System on Quality and Outcomes of Care in Italy." *Health Services Research* 34: 405–15.

Mattke, Soren. 2001. *The Effect of Financial Incentives and Institutional Arrangements on Provider Rehavior.* Doctoral dissertation. Boston, MA: Harvard School of Public Health.

McGuire, Thomas G.; and Mark V. Pauly. 1991. "Physician Response to Fee Changes with Multiple Payers." *Journal of Health Economics* 10: 385–410.

Newhouse, Joseph P. 1996. "Reimbursing Health Plans and Health Providers: Efficiency in Production versus Selection." *Journal of Economic Literature* 34:1236–63.

Pearson, Steven D.; James E. Sabin; and Ezekiel J. Emanuel. 1998. "Ethical Guidelines for Physician Compensation Based on Capitation." *New England Journal of Medicine* 339: 689–93.

Rodwin, Marc A; and AtoZ (Etsuji) Okamoto. 2000. "Physicians' Conflicts of Interest in Japan and the United States: Lessons for the United States." *Journal of Health Politics, Policy and Law* 25: 343–75.

Woodfield, Alan E. 2001. "Reference Pricing: Theory and Evidence from New Zealand." In: Guillem López-Casasnovas and Bengt Jönsson, eds., *Reference Pricing and Pharmaceutical Policy.* Barcelona, Spain: Springer.

Yip, Winnie C.; Siripen Supkankunti; Jiruth Sriratanaban; Wattana S. Janjaroen; and Sathirakorn Pongpanich. 2001. *Impact of Capitation Payment: The Social Security Scheme of Thailand.* Major Applied Research 2, Working Paper 4. Bethesda, MD: Partnerships for Health Reform Project, Abt Associates.

10

Organization

In Chapters 8 and 9, we discussed options for how money for the health-care system can be raised (financing) and alternative mechanisms for distributing those funds (payment). Now we consider how government can influence the organization of the health-care delivery system. Each of the five control knobs has an organizational aspect. For example, how should we organize a social insurance system, or should the medical society be given the responsibility for disciplining physicians? In this chapter, we focus on the narrower question of the organization of health-care provision.

We use the term "organization" to refer both to the overall structure of the health-care system, and to the individual institutions that provide health-care services. In the second sense an "organization" is a distinct entity that uses "inputs" (people, buildings, equipment), within a defined authority structure, to produce various goods and services. Some health-care organizations closely match this concept; e.g., an independent private hospital. A traditional healer who operates from her home is also an "organization" in this sense. Other providers raise real definitional issues. Is a primary health-care center run by the ministry of health an "organization," or should that term be reserved for the whole national public delivery system? For better or worse, the boundaries of many particular "organizations" are ambiguous, and all we can do is try to be clear about our meaning as we proceed.

A reformer who wants to "turn" the organization control knob has to focus on four major characteristics of the health-care system.

- The mix of organizations that provide health-care services.
- The division of activities among these organizations.
- The interactions among these organizations and their relationship with the rest of the political and economic system—especially how they get the resources they need to continue to exist.
- The internal administrative structures of these organizations.

In some cases government can act directly to change these features of the system: for example, by creating a new system of community health workers or by reorganizing its hospitals' governance to increase hospital autonomy. In other cases, a government may act indirectly through the other control knobs. For example, governments could make new payments available to private investors to foster the emergence of private hospitals. Or it might use regulation to require private providers to offer certain services, for example, immunization. As we noted in Chapter 2, there are often linkages between control knobs, with actions in one either needing or affecting actions in another. But these linkages are especially important here, because the organization of health-care is affected by many different types of policy interventions. At the same time, many of the incentive effects of payment and the coercive effects of regulation depend on eliciting or producing organizational changes—especially of a managerial sort—if they are to have their desired impact.

Alternative Strategies

Understanding the organization of the health-care system in this way leads us to identify three types of interventions that "turn" the organization control knob.

- *Who-does-what strategies*: The first set of interventions focuses on the first two characteristics identified above: that is, on changing the mix of organizations or the division of tasks among them. These interventions might result in changes in the public-private mix in ownership, or in the scale and scope of new or existing organizations. As always, our interest is not in the organizational characteristics themselves, but in their effects on system performance.
- *Incentive strategies*: The second option is to operate on the third characteristic described above—namely, on the incentives created by the connections between health-care organizations and the rest of the system. We will explore two specific approaches designed to change these incentives: efforts to increase competition, and efforts to use contracting to affect the delivery of health-care services.
- *Managerial strategies*: These interventions involve our fourth characteristic above; namely, changing what happens *inside* organizations. When government

operates the delivery system, it can simply impose such changes. When it does not, it has to rely on the other control knobs to produce such changes. Corporatization, total quality management, and efforts to improve public-sector management are examples we will discuss. We include decentralization strategies in this category, because they involve changes in the way parts of government relate to each other, much like changes in the internal organization of a large multinational corporation.

As we have already noted, reformers can adopt various *mechanisms* to achieve these changes. For example, a government can use payment to shift functions among different kinds of providers. It can use regulation to influence incentives by increasing competition (through anti-trust policy) or to require changes in the management of private hospitals, or it can use its direct authority to make such changes in government hospitals. It is not these mechanisms, however, but the changes in organization that these mechanisms can produce that constitute the interventions we are considering.

Health-care services are delivered by various "front-line workers": the doctors, nurses, technicians, and others who see the patients, run the X-ray machines, and do the vaccinations. How these people do their work is what ultimately determines how health care is delivered. So we always have to look at how organizational changes affect the incentives, opportunities, and obligations these workers face, as well as their skills, attitudes, and motivation. And when it comes to determining those features of the front-line workers' world, managers are key. For it is the managers who buy the equipment, organize the work, and recruit, reward, and sometimes inspire the workers.

The central role of workers and managers allows us to clarify the relationships among the three broad classes of strategies we have identified. Incentive strategies are based on the belief that *if* enough pressure is put on organizations, they will make the managerial changes needed to improve performance. There is the additional Darwinian vision that organizations that don't change will shrink or die, while those that adapt will survive and grow. Changes aimed at altering who-does-what also presume that the organizations gaining functions will have the managerial capacity to deliver higher quality and lower costs. This is, for example, what private-sector advocates claim (Herzlinger 1999). For any nonmanagerial intervention to succeed, therefore, change at the managerial level has to occur.

Unfortunately, key managerial aspects of proposed organizational reforms are often left unspecified, so their consequences are hard to predict. Will "corporatized" hospitals have lower costs than the existing public system? Will decentralizing control of health centers to the village level improve service quality? In other words, will these changes produce more competent and responsible managers? Will they lessen patronage and corruption? The answers to such questions will depend on how reforms are carried out. Hence, we will stress throughout this chapter that "the devil is in the details" when it comes to predicting the impact of organizational change on system performance.

Changes in external incentives and in internal management are powerfully complementary. Giving managers incentives without also giving them the skills, authority, and resources they need to respond to those incentives is likely to be quite ineffectual. The same is true in reverse. Increased managerial authority is not likely to lead to improved care if managers have no incentive to do so. This is why various writers on organizational reform in health care have seen a need for "consistent" change (Harding and Preker 2002). It is not aesthetics that lies behind their observations, but rather the need to combine *reasons* to do better with the *capacity* to do better—in the same reform package.

Some reforms do combine external incentives and internal managerial changes (e.g., many decentralization or privatization efforts). But for analytical clarity, we will consider the various aspects of such mixed reform efforts separately.

To highlight the linkage of all reform efforts to the managerial level, we will repeatedly explore how reform affects what we call the "Six Keys to Organizational Performance" (see Table 10.1). These six factors determine how and why incentives for the organization filter down to managers and workers. They also tell us to focus on the skills and attitudes that workers and managers rely on when they respond to those incentives.

The Effects of Alternative Strategies

What can reformers hope to accomplish by changes in the organization control knob? How might such changes affect the performance of the system in terms of the categories we developed in Chapters 5 and 6?

To improve access and risk protection, reformers can change who-does-what. For example, to improve access and equity in rural areas, various nations have worked to develop community-based health workers. In Indonesia in the 1980s, for instance, it was found that more dispersed lower-level facilities—such as sub-centers—were more effective in reaching the rural poor than larger, more fully-staffed health centers (Berman et al. 1987, Berman et al. 1989).

Incentive strategies like competition can lower costs (improve technical efficiency) and improve service quality and customer satisfaction. Contracting can also be used to increase efficiency and improve quality. Decentralization advocates hope it will have similar effects (Bossert 1998). Managerial initiatives, too, focus on producing lower costs and better quality. If any of these interventions work, health status and satisfaction might both be improved. (Whether cost savings are translated into more service and hence into health-status gains—or used to produce non-health benefits—depends on the political system.)

We will see, however, that these changes come with risks and tradeoffs. Excessive competition can lead to supplier-induced demand, allocative inefficiency, and

TABLE **10.1.** The Six Keys to Organizational Performance

Incentives for the Organization

What does the organization have to do to acquire the resources it needs to survive and grow?

What other constraints or opportunities does it face from competitors, customers, regulators, budget makers, grant givers, etc.?

Incentives for Managers

How are managers rewarded or punished?

How is this tied, if at all, to the performance of the organization?

What channels of reporting, supervision, and accountability exist?

What is their potential career path outside their current organization?

Skills and Attitudes of Managers

What do managers bring to their work in terms of skills and attitudes?

How are these shaped by education, selection, training, and work experience?

How do managers see their job? What is their view of their responsibilities?

Authority of Managers

What decisions can managers make, both internally and externally, about products, prices, production processes, purchasing, personnel, etc.?

Can they hire and fire, make investment decisions, choose strategies, etc.?

Incentives for Workers

How, if at all, do the rewards workers enjoy vary with their performance and/or that of the organization as a whole?

What determines pay, employment, promotion, etc.?

Do they have any significant nonmonetary incentives?

Skills and Attitudes of Workers

What do workers bring to their work in terms of skills and attitudes?

How are these shaped by education, selection, training, and work experience?

How committed are workers to the "product" of the organization as a desirable activity?

---

health-status declines. It can also make providers unwilling to subsidize the poor, thereby diminishing their access and health status. Similarly, altering who-does-what to produce a dense network of unspecialized providers, in the name of improved access, can lead to diminished technical quality.

We will also see that these strategies are not "self-implementing." The results of decentralizing control to the local level will depend on local administrative and political capacity. Contracting can be used, not to improve efficiency, but to hand out political patronage. The "within strategy" variations in outcomes—which depend on detailed design and implementation—are perhaps largest for this control knob. With this awareness, then, what strategies are available to reformers who want to change the organization control knob?

Changing Who-Does-What

The first strategy is to change the mix of organizations and how tasks are divided among them. Such changes are often what people think of first when they consider organizational reform. What reformers don't always consider carefully is how changing the role of providers will affect health-sector performance. For example, does it matter if new high-tech services are provided by public hospitals or private entrepreneurs? Is it better to have primary care provided by independent general practitioners (as in the United Kingdom) or by clinics with multiple specialists (as was the case until recently in much of Eastern Europe)? Are immunization programs best organized separately—or as part of the general primary care system? We address three general characteristics of organizational design: ownership, scale, and scope. We also discuss the particular organizational problems of providing service in rural areas. Throughout, keep in mind that changing who-does-what can influence performance through both supply- and demand-side effects—for example, through the cost of services and through the attractiveness of care to various patients.

Over the years, various organizational fads and fashions have appeared in international health-reform debates: to take two examples, integrated primary care and comprehensive reproductive health programs. We want to warn health-sector reformers not to become overly focused on such strategies. Too often, such reorganization does little to change the capacities, incentives, or motivation of front-line workers—or their managers. As a result, there may be less effect on performance from such changes than their advocates hoped for. Indeed, reorganization can seem attractive exactly because it *avoids* the difficult problem of making meaningful incentive or managerial changes. It substitutes, instead, the deceptively easy task of rearranging the ministry of health's organization chart or the mix of actors in the private sector.

Privatization

One widely advocated organization reform strategy involves shifting services to private-sector providers. But the world is full of examples of good and bad performance in both the public and the private sectors. One study in Malaysia found that preventive care offered by private doctors was of worse quality and more limited than that provided in public clinics (Aljunid and Zwi 1997). Conversely, private mission facilities in The Gambia were found to provide higher-quality care, resulting in greater demand and geographic coverage (Newbrander and Rosenthal

1997). To devise effective reforms, therefore, we need a better understanding of how ownership influences the behavior of health-care organizations.

Why do public and private-sector hospitals and clinics often behave differently? Refer back to the Six Keys (Table 10.1). The first point involves incentives. The private sector largely depends on markets. To make profits, competitive sellers have to please customers by offering reasonable quality and cost. They have no interest, however, in providing care to those who cannot pay—like the poor.

Public-sector organizations that get their funds from government budgets could try to provide great service and hope their customers will lobby the government to increase those budgets. An alternative "patronage" strategy involves relying on employees to be a pressure group on, and political resource for, the government. Since employees are easier to identify, influence, and organize than customers, the patronage strategy is by far the more common pattern. The result is often excess staff, high costs, political involvement in hiring and purchasing, and mediocre-to-poor customer service (Osborne and Gaebler 1993, Barzelay and Armajani 1992).

There are also public–private differences in the incentives of managers. Private-sector managers often find that their compensation and employment depend on profits. Private companies may give managers stock options to increase their firm's profitability. Indeed, some managers are owners and earn profits directly. Public managers, in contrast, often come from politics or the civil service and are given few performance-based incentives (Shaw 1999, World Bank 1997).

Public managers also generally have less authority than private managers. Restrictive purchasing and personnel systems are often put in place in the public sector to prevent public managers from using their power for political ends. But, as a result, they often cannot create strong incentive systems for their workers. In Tanzania and Zimbabwe, for instance, a study found that private-sector hospital administrators enjoyed wide flexibility to hire and fire staff as well as shift funds between line items, whereas government managers were bound by time-consuming bureaucratic rules and regulations (Gilson et al. 1997).

Public and private managers also often differ in skills and values. Well-run private organizations recruit managers who have the training, temperament, and interest to do managerial work. Many public-sector health managers are doctors without managerial training who are not especially interested in a management career. They see management as a diversion from their "real work," and often don't even know what they don't know about how to be an effective manager. In India, for instance, medical officers are promoted to block- or district-level administrative positions and expected to supervise—without specific managerial training—extension workers and primary-care interventions (Martínez and Martineau 2002).

Finally, there may be differences between public and private employees. In some cases, the public sector attracts people committed to social goals, while the private sector appeals to people seeking their own economic gain. On the other hand, the public sector, by providing secure if unexciting jobs, can attract people who are relatively rigid and risk-averse. Private businesses, which reward the entrepreneurial, are more likely to attract those who find uncertainty and opportunity more congenial.

We also need to stress that health-care ownership choices are more complex than the classic public-private dichotomy suggests. There is often a "third way" in the form of nonprofit, non-government organizations. Such NGOs often combine incentives to and accountability of managers with a board of directors that is not solely profit-oriented. At their best, such NGOs can produce greater "technical efficiency" (including efficiency in the production of quality) than rigid public organizations. Moreover, they can recruit staff with different skills and motives than either for-profit business or classic bureaucratic public agencies (Gilson et al. 1997).

In summary, the public sector often exhibits higher cost and less customer responsiveness than the private sector. The private sector, in contrast, is often more flexible and ruthless and less socially responsible. And private ownership only produces efficiency and quality when competitive markets force managers to make such efforts. At the same time, the variation in performance within each category is substantial. There are high-performance public agencies and poorly managed private ones. There is no theoretical reason why good service and low cost cannot be achieved by well-run public providers. Observed differences are mainly the result of specific structures and practices, rather than being determined by the ownership of providers per se. Details and implementation are critical. How, then, should health reformers choose between using the public and private sectors to deliver services?

We believe this decision should depend on several features of a nation's circumstances and of the particular activity under consideration.

- *Regulatory capacity*: A government with greater technical expertise, a relatively law-abiding citizenry and a well-functioning legal and administrative apparatus can more easily control the excesses of private-sector providers.
- *Reform priorities*: Markets do better on efficiency but worse on equity. The choice of ownership may well depend on the relative importance of these goals.
- *Public-sector managerial capacity*: The more expert, better-managed and less patronage-ridden the public sector, the less compelling the case for privatization.
- *Customer sophistication*: The more sophisticated the customers, the easier it is to rely on private markets. Customers can judge dentistry more easily than brain surgery.
- *Professional self-discipline*: Health-care markets function better when sellers accept professional norms that limit patient exploitation and when there are effective formal discipline systems to help enforce such behavior.

This review suggests, first, that nations will often want a mix of private and public provision—depending on their goals in a particular area, buyer sophistication, professional behavior, and other factors. Second, this review reveals the deep irony that the nations least-equipped to make their public sector function effectively are often those least able to discipline private markets to achieve public ends. This should serve as a warning to reformers who see the inadequacy of current public organizations but have not analyzed what will happen if for-profit, private providers come to dominate instead.

Scale and Health-Sector Performance

A second system-design choice that reformers face is the scale of various provider organizations. Scale affects performance in several ways. First, larger scale can lower costs. Larger hospitals, for example, can fully utilize specialized equipment and personnel (X-ray machines or laboratory blood analyzers—and their associated technicians; Feldstein 1993). Administrative costs (e.g., the director's salary) can also be spread over a larger patient base. Such advantages vary for different health-care activities. Hospitals seem to benefit from lower costs up to about 300 to 400 beds. Primary care is likely to get little or no cost advantage from having many physicians working together in the same facility.

Larger scale can facilitate clinical quality. Doing more of something—at least potentially—can make one better at it. These "practice effects" operate at both the individual and the team levels. Clinical skill depends on both the current rate of "throughput" (how many cases are seen per month) and providers' total cumulative experience with a particular type of case. These advantages have become larger in recent years, as medical knowledge has expanded and medical equipment and techniques have become more esoteric. Since many illnesses are uncommon, a large population base is required to provide enough cases to support a highly specialized care unit or a highly specialized physician.

The problem is that having a few large referral centers leads to access barriers, for those outside major metropolitan centers, particularly poor and rural people, and those in marginalized groups. Thus, the search for clinical quality can lead to lower health status among groups with the poorest health status (World Bank 1993). Without pressure from competitors, such centers also may not achieve their potential cost advantages, because they will not work hard enough to do so. There are also political pressures that run counter to regionalization. Providers and political leaders in towns that are not chosen to be regional centers have been known to resist such arrangements strenuously.

Moreover, there can also be diseconomies of scale, where costs increase as size increases. Large institutions often suffer from a lack of coordination and find it difficult to motivate staff. Employees feel insignificant and hence not responsible for actual outcomes. In addition, workers have to travel longer distances in a system with fewer large centers, so labor costs can increase.

Similar issues arise at the primary-care level. A choice among individual family doctors, small clinics with three to five practitioners, and larger clinics with twenty or so doctors, is also a scale issue. And some of the same tradeoffs arise among clinical quality, service quality, and effective availability.

We have no simple advice on the scale of facilities to create. The advantages and disadvantages of large scale will depend upon each country's particular situation. Densely settled urban environments can provide enough population to support a number of competitive large-scale providers. The same will not be true in rural areas, or even in modest-sized cities. Uruguay is not Uzbekistan. The availability of transportation services, the degree of sophistication among rural people, the burden of disease in a country, and its overall level of economic development will all influence the consequences of centralized versus dispersed services. Politics, too, will vary. In part, the question depends on which performance criterion (health status versus customer satisfaction) matters more, since scale may improve clinical quality while decreasing equity of access and satisfaction.

Moreover, the potential gains from larger-scale operations will not be automatically realized. What actually happens will depend (as always) on how managers react. The possible negative effects of larger scale on market competition and organizational incentives, therefore, have to be borne in mind. For countries with limited budgets, however, the cost and clinical quality advantages of larger scale should, we believe, remain a serious consideration.

"Scope"—the Effect of an Organization's "Product Line"

Governments often manipulate the set of activities each provider undertakes. To what degree is their product line specialized rather than diversified (i.e., they do many different things)? For example, should society support specialized maternity or cancer hospitals, or general hospitals that care for all kinds of patients? Specialized "vertical" disease-prevention programs or an integrated "horizontal" primary-care system? Family medicine doctors or primary care teams of multiple specialists?

Diversification can lower costs if, for example, it allows a hospital to use X-ray, laboratory, and operating room facilities to care for more patients. Similarly, a primary-care center that already has facilities, refrigerators, and nurses can provide immunizations less expensively (as an addition to its product line) than a wholly separate service with its own costs.

Broader scope also reduces the necessary population base for a provider and hence allows for a denser (and more accessible) set of providers. A small town may not provide enough volume for an obstetrician, but it might be able to support a family doctor who also performs deliveries. The epidemiological shift to chronic disease increases the importance of this point, since the effective management of chronic conditions requires relatively frequent patient contact.

On the other hand, diversification risks losing some of the gains of specialization. Industrial experience suggests that diversified companies may end up not doing any one thing well. An organization with a narrow product line, in contrast, can attract workers with a particular interest in, and commitment to, a particular activity. The organization can develop an "esprit de corps" and well-defined performance goals based on a clear and narrow mission. A well-run specialized heart institute or disease-control program can benefit from such focus in a way that a general hospital or a general primary-care system often cannot (Herzlinger 1999).

What advice can we offer to health-system planners about the appropriate scope of different providers? For primary care, where access is critical, broad scope (and hence a smaller population base) has much to recommend it. In rural areas, this is typically the only option at the primary level. On the other hand, the goal of improving clinical quality through an increase of specialization explains why so many countries have regional or national referral institutions for more difficult cases. But each nation has to make these tradeoffs in light of its own settlement patterns, transportation system, and priorities. And it may well make sense to make different decisions for different regions or services.

Reformers need to remember, however, that changes in scope change what is *possible*, not necessarily what will *actually* happen. The unit cost of an X-ray machine might fall if a broader scope of service produces enough cases for it to be fully utilized. But this will *not* occur if the machine is badly maintained, or the hospital runs out of film, or the technician is incompetent or frequently not on duty. Managerial effectiveness is thus essential if the potential benefits of reforms are to be realized.

Providing Services to Rural Areas

In many countries, a particular who-does-what problem arises in providing services in rural areas. Often, the ministry of health operates a network of health centers (with a few inpatient beds and physician staff) and subcenters (with non-physician staff and no beds). Yet the same complaints are commonly heard. Doctors don't want to go to remote areas, and if assigned they don't fulfill their responsibilities. Drugs are lacking, equipment is not maintained, and the resulting poor quality discourages utilization (Griffin and Shaw 1995, Akin et al. 1995).

The reasons for all this are apparent. Often physicians in the public sector (officially or unofficially) supplement their incomes with private practice (Ministry of Health, Egypt 1994–95). In Indonesia, for example, private practice enables urban doctors to earn one and a third as much as doctors posted in rural areas. This differential exists even though rural providers earn a substantially higher public-sector salary (Chomitz et al. 1998). Poor rural areas offer few such opportunities, as well as little in the way of educational or social opportunities for physicians and their families. Supervisors seldom visit remote posts, and there is little monitoring of the quality of care. Building more facilities—which will still be understaffed, under-equipped and underutilized—is seldom an effective answer. There are countries where the ministry of health is able to provide service in rural areas, like Sri Lanka and Cuba (Hsiao 2000). But these are special cases: small nations, with relatively dense rural populations and a high degree of ideological motivation in the public sector.

The private sector often fills in the resulting gap in services—if only by default. Many of the practitioners in question are not fully qualified by Western standards. Some are traditional healers. The best of these may have been trained in formal programs of the sort that exist in India and China, but others have only an apprenticeship background. Still others have had some Western-oriented training—as pharmacists, practical nurses, or aides (Fried and Gaydos 2002, Kakar 1988, Shankar 1992). Since these practitioners operate with little regulation and on a fee-for-service basis, local citizens have little or no protection against poor quality or financial risk when they use such services (Berman 1998, Claquin 1981).

In response, many governments offer incentives for doctors to serve in rural areas. Some Indian states give preference for admission to specialty medical training to those who do so, and they offer selective "location" or "non-practice" bonuses that don't involve changing the formal uniform-salary scale. Countries as diverse as Canada (for Arctic communities) and Uzbekistan have created differential pay levels to attract doctors to rural areas (in Uzbekistan by paying a doctor more than one salary; Lassey et al. 1997). In rural areas of Kerala, in south India, local governments are allowed to supplement the statewide salary scale to attract doctors.

An alternative is to change the kind of provider, on the theory that those with less education and status, and from a similar cultural background, will be easier to locate in rural areas. Poor countries have relied on nurses or community health workers in such contexts. In many former communist countries, care in rural areas was provided by *feldshers* (Roemer 1977). These providers (akin to physician assistants in the United States) have substantially less training than fully prepared physicians but are often counted as "doctors" in some national statistics.

Yet the political difficulties of closing facilities or services can mean that programs that were begun as substitutes—to lower costs—can end up as supplements, so that the hoped-for budget savings do not materialize. The new program then can fail because, in a competitive fiscal environment, the initiative does not get sufficient funds. This fate has befallen some programs for community health workers, for example.

Some countries (e.g., Mexico) use weekly or biweekly visits by well-staffed mobile vans to supplement the routine care offered by local nursing staff (Health Secretariat Mexico 2000). Australia and Botswana both supplement care in remote areas (offered by a resident nurse) with a "Flying Doctor" service, which is both an evacuation system and a mechanism for bringing in doctors to run periodic clinics in remote areas (McDonald 2002, O'Connor 2001).

Another alternative is to contract with non-public organizations to deliver care. In Andhra Pradesh and other Indian states, governments have selectively contracted with NGOs to operate rural health centers. In many East African countries, church-affiliated organizations receive government funds to run hospitals that substitute for government-run district hospitals (Gilson et al. 1997). In aboriginal communities of Australia, public funds once used to operate state-run medical services are now sometimes turned over to local NGOs (supervised by community boards) to operate locally controlled medical services (Percy 1999).

To take advantage of these options, reformers must realize that a uniform system may not be the best approach in a socially and geographically diverse country. Defending uniformity on equity grounds, when the approach produces inequitable care in practice, simply confuses rhetoric with reality.

Who-Does-What and the Supply of Inputs

To alter who-does-what in the delivery system, a government may find it useful—even necessary—to change the inputs into the system. A decision to rely on capitated family doctors, for example, is unlikely to work unless the government produces more family doctors. Conversely, restricting access to critical capital equipment can also be an effective way to provoke system change.

Where doctors and nurses are trained in government schools, the number and mix of personnel trained can be changed administratively. For example, in Australia, to expand the number of doctors in rural areas, medical school places were reallocated to a new institution focused on preparing physicians for such roles (Wronski, 2001). In other situations, private medical and nursing schools may be licensed by the government, or they (or their students) may rely on government financial aid. These mechanisms can be used as a tool to alter the mix of graduates.

Training more physicians may lead to increased price competition or to supplier-induced demand. An excess supply of doctors can lead to enormous political pressures for overstaffing the public system, as occurred in Egypt in the mid-1990s (Berman et al. 1997). Unfortunately, health system consequences are often not paramount when governments decide on training capacity, because of the political pressures that surround such decisions.

Governments can also alter which providers have access to specific kinds of capital equipment. Governments can introduce these rules directly in their own facilities. In addition, in some countries government is a major source of capital even for private providers. In Germany, almost all hospital capital investment—even for independent hospitals—comes from the state governments, and they can help shape which institutions grow in which clinical areas (White 1995). In a number of middle-income countries, such as Thailand, Colombia, and the Philippines, governments have initiated subsidized lending programs to encourage private health facility development (Herrin 1997, Griffin 1992). Where the private sector is self-financing, a variety of regulatory and payment tools is available. For example, hospital purchases of new equipment require provincial consent in

Canada, and high-technology equipment—such as MRI machines—is limited mainly to academic medical institutions (Patel and Rushefsky 2002).

Incentive Strategies

Incentive strategies take advantage of the fact that every organization has to acquire financial resources to continue to operate. To change the behavior of organizations, therefore, reformers can change what must be done to obtain such resources. Health-sector organizations generally obtain resources in three ways, from markets, by budget processes, and from gifts. Competition, the first strategy we explore, operates in the context of markets. Contracting, the second strategy, can function within any context. These strategies are *not* mutually exclusive. For example, contracting can be a tool to increase competition or change the provider mix. We identify and analyze the linkages between the two strategies as we proceed.

Fostering Market Competition

As noted in Chapter 1, there has been much interest in recent years in using markets to provide health-care services. The problem for reformers is to ensure that such markets provide the right incentives—which means ensuring that they are reasonably competitive.

In a classical market situation, customers (i.e., patients) choose what to buy and from whom, and they pay for their purchases. This occurs in the large private ambulatory-care sectors in many countries. Other health-care providers confront situations with some, but not all, of the features of a classic market. For example, public hospitals in many countries have budgetary support but also receive significant income from user fees and informal payments. This combination subjects them to some market incentives. Indeed, for some public hospitals (as in China today, and in most public hospitals in the United States), such fees constitute most of their revenues, so they are very much in a market-dependent situation (Yip and Hsiao 2001).

Competition is desirable because it pushes sellers to keep down costs and prices and respond to customers in order to attract additional business. The managers of firms that might not survive have a powerful incentive to work hard and take risks. Indeed, firms managed by their owners are often more successful—and take bigger risks—exactly because managers have so much to lose, and gain, from their company's success (Berle and Means 1991).

Competition also creates incentives for workers. As the English essayist Samuel Johnson wrote, "The prospect of hanging serves wonderfully to concentrate the mind." Workers know that a failure to adapt in a competitive marketplace could result in the loss of their jobs. This may make them more willing to work hard and accept changes designed to increase the firm's prospects.

As noted in Chapter 3, economists often favor competitive markets because of their theoretically desirable properties in fostering allocative efficiency and Pareto Optimality. But in the real world, competition's greatest value may be in holding down costs and improving service quality. In the medium run, competition also encourages innovation, both new forms of medical care (e.g., new drugs) and new models of service delivery.

Even when patients do not pay directly for care, competitive incentives can arise from financing and payment arrangements. Hospitals may compete to serve patients covered by insurance. General practitioners may find themselves competing for patients when paid a capitated fee by government. Even budget-supported hospitals will face some market pressure if budgets are set in a way that reflects the volume of care they provide. The key to the incentive effect of a market is whether buyers have choices and whether the money follows the patient (or the customer)—regardless of where the money comes from.

Many real health-care markets are what economists call "oligopolies"—they have only a few sellers, who can potentially coordinate their behavior to raise prices and limit competition. At the extreme, there may be only one seller— a monopolist who escapes market pressures to control costs or provide good service because patients have no other source of care.

Many forms of quality regulation in health care—including training and licensing requirements—have the unfortunate side-effect of limiting competition. Professional associations can act both formally (through pricing agreements) and informally (through social pressure) to limit competition (Brennan and Berwick 1996; Starr 1982). In some cases, governments have given medical societies the ability to restrict the entry of new practitioners, a move with obvious anti-competitive implications.

Economists have explored how *industry structure* influences the level of competition in a particular market (Boner 1995, Caves 1992, Hoekman 1997). "Structure" refers to the number and size-distribution of sellers, and the presence or absence of "barriers to entry." Such barriers include legal limits (such as patents), control over scarce resources (such as having the only X-ray machine in town), a seller's reputation that guarantees business ("product differentiation"), and problems that would-be entrants have in acquiring capital. Competitive outcomes are more likely when there are more sellers and when it is easier for new sellers to enter a market. Where there are only a few, well-protected firms, they are more likely to be able to collude successfully. Government, therefore, can follow several strategies to overcome entry barriers, increase the number of sellers, and increase competition:

• *Decrease regulatory barriers*: Governments can relax licensing or patent laws, issue additional permits for facilities or equipment, or deprive professional societies of their exclusionary powers.

- *Support new producers*: Governments can use loans, grants, direct investments, or long-term contracts to help new entrants raise capital or ensure they have customers. For example, a local vaccine producer, started with government loans, can exert helpful price discipline on foreign suppliers.
- *Enforce antimonopoly laws*: Many countries have antimonopoly or pro-competition statutes that typically forbid collusion on prices and outlaw explicit agreements to divide markets. In some cases, they limit anti-competitive mergers. Making sure these laws are enforced, and that they can be applied to professional societies, can enhance competition.

How far governments should go to increase competition in health care, however, is complicated by several features of the sector. First, when providers are paid a fee for service, increased competition can lead them to exploit patient ignorance and create supplier-induced demand (Yip 1998). There is a real risk, therefore, that pro-competition policies will increase the volume of inappropriate care. Relaxing licensing laws can also raise concerns about clinical quality if less-well-trained producers enter the market. Moreover, as noted above, there can also be a tension between competition and the advantages of economics of scale.

Contracting

Under the payment systems discussed in the previous chapter, some government agency (e.g., the ministry of health or a social insurance fund) establishes a price schedule, and all qualified providers are paid accordingly. While this is the most common approach to paying for health care, there is an alternative. Selective contracting for services can be used to provide incentives even where markets are imperfectly competitive—although increasing competition can be a complementary strategy (England et al. 1998).

A "contract" is a written agreement between a buyer and a seller. The seller agrees to provide certain goods and services, and in return the buyer agrees to give the seller a certain amount of money. The contract sets out the terms of that agreement: what the seller provides, what the buyer pays, delivery and payment dates, the time period of the agreement, renewal provisions (if any), penalties for nonperformance, and processes to resolve disagreements. A contract can provide a more detailed and flexible set of incentives than a payment system. In effect, it combines some of the coercive features of a regulatory scheme with the incentive effects of a payment system.

For example, a ministry of health could contract with hospitals to pay a fee to cover certain fixed costs plus a volume-based payment to cover variable costs. The size of each payment could be based on each hospital's particular financial situation. This combination would both create productivity incentives and offer the hospital some protection against financial risks if volume declines. Such a philosophy of supply-side cost- and risk-sharing guides government contracting with hospitals in the Kyrgyz Republic, where hospitals are reimbursed on a per-patient basis, incorporating adjustments depend on the diagnosis at entry (analogous to the diagnosis-related group or DRG mechanism discussed in Chapter 9; Gauri 2001).

Contracting may be particularly helpful where public hospitals have significant autonomy and independence. The incentives provided by contracts can help fill the gap created by diminished direct supervision. For example, a contract could specify that a hospital has to provide a certain volume of free care to poor patients. In the Philippines private hospitals must reserve at least 10% of bed capacity for charity patients (Herrin 1997). The outputs delineated in a contract can further ensure that these hospitals work towards the public sector's goals and not disregard them. The autonomized Kenyatta National Hospital in Kenya is an example of the latter. Since being given greater freedom, it incurs higher costs than previously, apparently does not provide more services, and has reduced services to the inner-city poor. It is difficult to know if this hospital has or has not met the government's goals, because it has no specified role according to a governmental contract (England 2000).

Contracting can also be used to implement changes in who-does-what. For example, a social-insurance fund could decide to pay for certain services only in selected regional "centers of excellence"—and write contracts only with those centers (Becker et al. 1999, Walter 1999). Or a ministry could use contracting to shift care from one set of providers (hospital outpatient departments) to another (family doctors).

Contracting can also be used to alter management practices: for example, to require hospitals to hire managers with certain qualifications, or to provide certain staffing levels. Similarly, as part of a contract, a hospital might have to agree to set up processes to review all patient deaths, or to create a review board to ensure that all research projects meet certain standards. The hope is that such review processes will generate new incentives for doctors—if only the desire to avoid embarrassment for poor decision-making in front of their peers (Bosk 1979).

The relationship created by a contract may be a simple arm's-length one, or it can be more extensive. A simple contract may specify that the seller will deliver so many doses of vaccine of a specified potency to a particular place by a certain date, and will receive a specific sum on delivery. Or the agreement can involve a complex merging of risks and responsibilities—as when an NGO agrees to run a number of health centers staffed by some government personnel with government responsible for some functions (building maintenance) but not others (drug supply).

Complex contracts require a degree of mutual trust between buyers and sellers. The two parties need to exchange information and work together to solve problems in an ongoing relationship (England 2000). In such situations, the narrowly defined written terms cannot cover all the unanticipated contingencies that may arise. Dealing with unforeseen developments—e.g., the contractually-operated health centers are hit by floods—requires some reciprocity, based on a commitment by each party to take the other's interests seriously.

The processes for putting contracts in place can vary substantially. Sometimes there is a formal competitive "tender offer" process in which the low bidder wins. Sometimes bids are evaluated on quality as well as price, and a "score" is assigned. Sometimes potential bidders submit their qualifications, and only those deemed qualified are allowed to bid. Sometimes negotiations are conducted as a "sole source" process—or perhaps with two or three potential contractors in an informal competition.

Experience suggests that formal procedures work best with standardized (easy-to-describe) outputs. More discretionary processes may be the only way to deal with complex or unique situations. Since these processes involve a greater risk of favoritism or corruption, they are best accompanied by a device like an outside review panel, to preserve both the appearance of and the reality of fairness.

Contracting outcomes depend on the level of competition in the market. Competition helps contracting function more effectively, since buyers can threaten to go elsewhere. Thus, fostering competition can help support a contracting strategy. Moreover, the larger the buyer, the more favorable terms they can demand from the seller.

When a buyer is the sole customer—e.g., a national insurance fund—the dynamics can change. For then, if the buyer is too demanding, the seller might go bankrupt. Faced with such a prospect, sellers will mobilize politically to protect themselves and use the threat of bankruptcy to get tough contracts renegotiated. When both buyers and sellers are monopolists (what economists call "bilateral monopoly") the outcome is difficult to predict (Feldstein 1993). Then the buyer needs the seller (e.g., the only hospital in a region) as much as the seller needs the buyer (the only purchaser of services).

The question of competition is particularly relevant when governments use the form of contracting sometimes called "quasi-markets" or "purchaser-provider-separation." In this strategy, a public agency that previously both financed and provided care is divided into two entities. In short, financing is separated from provision. A buyer agency is created and is empowered to contract with various sellers—including the service-providing units of the former unified structure (England et al. 1998, Flynn and Williams 1997). When the new seller has a monopoly, it can effectively resist the purchaser's efforts at cost control. This happened in New Zealand, when newly created regional health boards went to negotiate with the newly independent (but locally monopolistic) public hospitals (Crown Health Enterprises 1996).

Countries that plan to use contracting need to consider the capabilities required to implement this successfully. Do they have the expertise to develop specifications, make contracting decisions, write contracts, and oversee compliance? Contracting does not end the role of a ministry of health, but it substantially changes that agency's role (and the associated needs for skills and personnel; Bennett and Mills 1998).

These tasks can be especially challenging when the "deliverables" in the contract are complex. Then, the processes of negotiating and administering the detailed contract are particularly important to outcomes. Sometimes an agency inappropriately focuses on the process of awarding the contract—on who "wins." Yet, what the winner wins (the terms of the contract), and how the winner is dealt with over time, are likely to be critical to the impact of contracting. Remember, for-profit contractors have every incentive to cut costs (and services), raise prices and lower quality, unless contract administration or the threat of nonrenewal leads them to do otherwise.

Zambia and Ghana have both tried to implement elements of the quasi-market approach to contracting, dividing their ministries of health into a funding or "commissioning" agency and a health-care delivery organization. Both countries have discovered that this type of change requires much greater management capacity than the traditional budget-driven government department (Gilson et al. 1997, Mills and Broomberg 1998). Similarly, an evaluation of contracting out the running of rural hospitals in South Africa found mixed results, in large part because the government was poorly set up to write, award, and manage contracts (Broomberg et al. 1997).

Apart from performance concerns, contracting has other disadvantages. The substantial work in contracting processes raises administrative costs above those of a simple uniform payment system. In addition, the discretion involved creates risks of patronage and corruption. Thus, the applicability of this strategy depends in part on the skill and probity of the relevant agencies. Moreover, unless the managers of the organizations being contracted with have the authority, motivation, and skills to respond to the incentives created by contracting, the potential benefits from this setting on the organization control knob may not be realized.

Incentive Strategies: Summary

To summarize, how can the incentive strategies we have explored affect the performance of the health-care system?

Competition serves primarily to lower costs and increase responsiveness to customer preferences, because that is what competitors have to do to be successful. These changes should increase satisfaction with the health-care system. Whether health status also increases depends, however, on how providers react and on how government chooses to use any cost savings. For example, competition that provokes inappropriate over-utilization will diminish clinical quality and raise costs. Costs for marketing or for care that patients judge to be desirable but that does not contribute to improved health status could also increase. The pressure to avoid financial losses could also decrease access and risk-protection for the poor.

The impacts of contracting depend on how it is implemented. Done well, it can improve technical efficiency (by provoking cost control), allocative efficiency (by redirecting resources), and clinical and service quality (if the contract includes measurable performance goals). Contracting to improve access by requiring a volume of free care—and thereby improve the equity of system performance. As noted, contracting does raise transaction costs—the expenses of writing, awarding, and managing contracts—which must be considered. Resources for these activities are critical, since badly done contracting is not likely to achieve its potential gains.

Managerial Interventions

The consequences of changing external incentives or who-does-what depend on how these interventions influence the delivery of health-care services. And that depends critically on the management of health-care organizations. This section looks at policy changes aimed at managerial practices—the third set of strategies under the organization control knob.

We first explore two interventions that involve "restructuring" the public sector: decentralization and corporatization. We then examine changing managerial practices without restructuring, and at the applicability of total quality management and contracting out as ways to advance the goals of health-sector reform.

Restructuring the Public Sector 1: Decentralization

So far, we have discussed incentives for private or quasi-public providers. What options are available to reformers who want to increase the accountability and improve the performance of providers but leave them in the public sector? One increasingly popular answer around the world is decentralization.

The underlying argument is that centralized national systems cannot (or at least often do not) provide effective supervision of local service delivery, especially in a large and diverse country. Unhappy citizens face too many bureaucratic obstacles in making their complaints heard. With many facilities to monitor, managers at the center cannot keep track of—or have much reason to be interested in—performance deficiencies in individual hospitals and clinics. Moreover, district or regional managers are seldom held accountable for the quality of services in their area (in part because performance is often not monitored). So, these managers also do not provide effective control over, or accountability for, local managers.

The kind of decentralization we consider here is sometimes called "devolution." It involves the transfer of authority to subnational units of government. For primary care, this often means shifting authority to the local level. Larger geographic units (e.g., districts) more frequently take responsibility for hospital care. Changes that simply give more authority to the regional offices of a centralized structure, often called "deconcentration," are really a different kind of managerial reform (Mills et al. 1990).

Proponents of decentralization argue that local control will improve service delivery. Poor performance will be more visible, and managers will feel more pressure to respond. Patronage and corruption will be more visible, and the price they extract (in the form of poor performance) will be less acceptable. Citizens will have someone accountable to receive their complaints, someone who will have a reason (electoral success) to respond to their concerns. Managers, in turn, will be held accountable by local or regional political institutions for their performance. All this, it is claimed, will lead to lower costs as well as better clinical and service quality (Ostrom et al. 1993, World Bank 1993).

In principle, national bureaucracies can respond to varied local conditions. But decentralization advocates contend that, in practice, bureaucracies often ignore such variation. Decentralization, in contrast, will increase responsiveness to local circumstances and preferences. For example, more money will be spent on malaria control in malaria-prone areas, or the mix of services will adjust to fit the preferences of local people.

Most decentralization involves a mix of incentive and managerial reforms. For instance, managers often face added accountability in the form of local management boards that will hire, fire, and compensate them based on their performance. In addition, managers are given more power over personnel, contracting, and purchasing—what Bossert calls their "decision space" (Bossert 1998). Our view is that these changes need to go together. Incentives without the capacity to respond are unlikely to be effective. But getting the center to relinquish control is not easy. Indeed, in Chile the government first decentralized and then recentralized salary-setting, under pressure from the public-sector unions.

Health-sector decentralization also can serve non–health-sector goals. These might include invigorating local governments by giving them more responsibilities, or shifting financial responsibilities away from a hard-pressed national government. In such cases, governments may accept lower health-sector performance to achieve these other objectives.

Decentralizing health-care financing can raise serious equity problems. Richer regions can finance the same services with lower taxes (or more service with the same taxes) than their poorer counterparts. Unless an interregional redistribution mechanism is established, poor regions can be victimized by such decentralization—as happened in Bosnia (Fox and Wallich 1998). On the other hand, when sufficiently strong redistributive efforts are made, poor regions can actually gain from decentralization. As evidence from Chile and Colombia suggests, formula-based redistribution may treat poor regions more generously than prior, politically-driven, budget processes (Bossert et al. 2003). In this context, community financing, as discussed in Chapter 8, can be seen as a form of decentralization that combines authority over primary-care delivery and fiscal responsibility at a very local level.

Health-system reformers contemplating decentralization need to consider how much technical and administrative capacity exists at the periphery and how quickly that capacity can be enhanced. In countries where local political processes are non-transparent, elite-dominated and patronage-ridden, the hoped-for accountability and efficiency from decentralization are not likely to materialize. Moreover, in countries with significant intercommunity conflict, marginalized groups may find themselves worse off with local decision-making.

Local capacity-building can be successfully achieved in some situations. Consider the example of Kerala, in south India, where literacy is high and where there already was substantial experience with effective local government. Informed observers credit a massive training effort of local leaders with facilitating the successful decentralization of health-sector-budget authority to the local level in the 1990s (Isaac and Franke 2002).

On the other hand, technical education will not necessarily overcome a deficit in "social capital": the willingness of citizens to cooperate in pursuit of their joint interest in ways that involve trust and reciprocal respect (Putnam 2000 and 1993). Double-entry bookkeeping can be taught much more easily than the attitudes required for successful democratic citizenship. It can also be a mistake, however, to delay implementing decentralization until all training is "finished." That day may never come. Moreover, the pressure of implementing decentralization can produce "teachable moments." That is, the need to perform can increase the receptivity of local and regional officials to acquiring new skills and concepts.

These observations about authority, redistribution, and local capacity-building illustrate our general contention that the outcome of a policy change will depend on the details of its design and implementation. The many choices involved in decentralization need to be made in a consistent and coherent way if the potential benefits are to be realized. For example, to improve efficiency or to produce services more closely tailored to local circumstances, local decision-makers need to have authority over personnel and budgets. Otherwise, how can they hope to produce the desired results?

Once a program of decentralization is initiated, the role of the central bureaucracy changes. The center now must advise instead of control, and train instead of command. Regulatory or incentive devices may be needed to push local policy toward national goals. For example, cash transfers to subordinate levels of government can be adjusted based on the achievement of national objectives. In India, for example, the national government has provided substantial cash prizes to the states with the best population-control performance. Monitoring performance becomes especially important. Otherwise, the effects of the new arrangements will remain obscure. Needless to say, many central government units find this transformation difficult to accept.

One final point involves the differences in local conditions and capacities among different regions, especially in large countries. As a result, decentralization efforts might need to vary by region. Even in the United States, where state governments are all reasonably competent, the federal government picks and chooses which technical and regulatory tasks it delegates to which states, based on differences in technical competence.

Restructuring the Public Sector 2: Autonomization and Corporatization

Another managerial intervention involves restructuring public health-care providers—usually but not exclusively hospitals—through reforms sometimes referred to as "autonomization" and "corporatization." We reviewed earlier some of the structural features of the public sector that contribute to poor performance. These reforms seek to change those structural features in order to improve performance (Preker and Harding 2002, Walford and Grant 1998).

This view has led to the creation of new organizations that import aspects of private-sector management into the public sector. The new entities have been called "quasi-public" or "para-statal" or characterized as "public corporations." The more modest reforms are sometimes characterized as "autonomization," and the more complete changes as "corporatization." In these reforms, managers are given more authority and in turn are made accountable to a new governance structure (such as a board of directors) that is not simply an arm of the ministry of health. The organization can be freed partially or wholly from government budgetary, personnel, and purchasing rules, and can be paid in various new ways—based on patient volume or incentive contracts (Shaw 1999).

This kind of restructuring is often discussed in terms of legal or formal categories like "ownership" or "governance" that do not address critical operational details. For example, if we create a new board of directors, will members be selected in ways that encourage the board to seek out competent managers or will they play political and patronage games?

One way to understand how restructuring influences performance outcomes is to ask how the changes affect the "Six Keys to Organizational Performance" in Table 10.1. The point is that the board's decisions create incentives for managers and incentives for workers, which can help predict how the new arrangements will actually work out.

- *Incentives for the organization:* Effective reform creates strong performance-based incentives, with either patients (in real markets) or other government agencies (in "quasi-markets") able to choose providers based on their cost/quality of performance. To encourage the organization to respond to these incentives, it is typically allowed to retain much, or even all, of the profits it generates. This contrasts with the practice of turning over any surplus to the ministry of finance, as is common in many bureaucratic contexts.

- *Incentives to managers*: Effective reforms give managers strong incentives to improve performance. One option is to confer the power to hire, fire, and compensate managers to a board of directors that in turn is appointed in a way that makes its members performance-oriented. For this to occur, the details of "governance" structures are critical. Reforms that allow continuing political influence on managerial appointments weaken managers' incentives.
- *The authority of managers:* To respond to their incentives, managers need authority over personnel, purchasing, pricing, and other critical areas. Managers' discretion, however, is often limited under pressure from unions eager to protect employees or customers eager to preserve low prices.
- *Managerial skills and attitudes*: Improving managers' skills and attitudes has typically been delegated—unthinkingly—to the new governance structures. Only a few countries have thought about what government can do to produce the combination of entrepreneurship and social responsibility among managers that would advance reform.
- *Worker incentives:* Improving worker performance has largely been left in the hands of management. When managers are able to hire, fire, and alter pay scales, then they can provide performance-based incentives to employees. On the other hand, sometimes the old personnel system, and the weak incentives it creates, remains in place.
- *Worker skills and attitudes:* Reformers typically have either ignored worker skills and attitudes, or else left these issues for the new managers to handle—hoping that managers will use a combination of leadership and authority to transform the workforce.

In sum, a successful hospital restructuring requires a cadre of capable, well-trained hospital managers who have reasonable authority and are rewarded for their performance. This will require attention to the training of such individuals, efforts to increase respect for their work among physicians, and the fostering of professional societies. Only a few nations (e.g., Hungary) have begun to put in place the necessary training and credentialing infrastructure to achieve this objective (Fried and Gaydos 2002).

International evidence suggests that piecemeal changes, which leave key aspects of the hospital structure unreformed, do not produce major results (Jakab et al. 2002). Increasing incentives to the organization, without giving managers the authority and skills to respond, is not a promising approach. Similarly, giving managers authority and subjecting them to market incentives—without providing external accountability—is likely to turn them into profit-seeking entrepreneurs who slight social values. The autonomized Chinese leprosy hospital, which started a turtle farm when its primary clientele became less numerous, is an example that one of us heard about while teaching in Chengdu.

Multiple meaningful changes can have an interaction or "tipping" effect, transforming the organization's culture and functioning. Where seniority and patronage hiring continue, hospitals will attract workers who like such situations. On the other hand, new managers—with new authority—can create a new environment and attract a more motivated staff who will effectively implement productivity and service improvements.

Ironically, the greater the market pressures and the more autonomized hospitals become, the more they will act like for-profit entities. Hence the more extensive and effective the reforms, the more that reorganized hospitals will need to be regulated. Here again, we see that competition and regulation are complements, not alternatives.

Unfortunately, patronage, politics, and powerful unions may make it difficult to get critical personnel decisions turned over to managers. Politicians also may be reluctant to pay explicitly for activities that were previously supported through cross-subsidies. Thus, reformers contemplating autonomization need to assess its political feasibility early in the reform process, to avoid wasting time and effort on an approach that cannot be implemented effectively.

Implementation is especially important here. Hospital reorganization is not like a strong antibiotic that will, in a short time, cure some undesirable condition. It is more like a course of physical therapy: tough, painful work that needs to be done day-by-day over a substantial period of time and joined to other therapeutic interventions, if it is to improve health-sector performance.

Improving Public-Sector Performance

When political opposition makes either decentralization or autonomization unfeasible, the question arises whether public-sector performance can be improved without such structural changes. The answer has to be a qualified "maybe," in part because improving public-sector performance depends on changes just as controversial as any reform of ownership or control.

The required changes are so obvious that only widespread political difficulties and a lack of ministerial expertise can explain why they are not more widely instituted. One reason may be that reform inside the public sector can deprive ministers of the handy excuse "I didn't do it," which can be used if a private or autonomized entity offends powerful interests. Moreover, ministers themselves often lack managerial experience or the stomach for the long-term and politically difficult effort that managerial reform entails. Once again, we can use the categories from the "Six Keys" to organize our discussion.

- *Organizational incentives*: Funding can be tied to performance in various ways. For example, budgets can be varied based on the quality and quantity of services provided. Incentives (e.g., prizes) can be given to regions or agencies that do better on measured performance goals. Performance reports and rankings can be made public, and certification provided to high-performing organizations.

- *Managerial incentives*: The role of politics and patronage can be limited and managers selected, promoted, and compensated based on their skill and performance as managers. Systems of reporting and supervision that create real accountability can be established—which is especially important if managers are to be given increased authority.
- *Managerial skills and attitudes*: Formal management-training programs can be developed and made a prerequisite for certain jobs. Managerial career tracks can be developed. The prestige of managerial roles can be enhanced with various awards and publicity efforts. Able candidates can be encouraged to pursue management careers.
- *Managerial authority*: Managers can be allowed to make more decisions about budgeting, purchasing, pricing, personnel, and production methods.
- *Worker incentives:* Personnel systems can be changed to reward performance and limit political influence and patronage.
- *Worker capacities and attitudes*: Recruitment patterns, training systems, and personnel practices can be revised to attract and retain motivated employees.

These changes could significantly improve the performance of many public-sector agencies. Countries that resist such measures—that give managers little authority, allocate budgets based on past history, and rely on patronage for hiring—should not be surprised if their public-sector health system continues to perform badly.

Other Specific Managerial Innovations: TQM and Contracting Out

What are options for improving organizational performance that empowered managers, in any setting, should consider? The first option is called "Total Quality Management" or "Continuous Quality Improvement" (Berwick et al. 1991, Crosby 1979, Dever 1997, Palmer et al. 1995). This approach has been increasingly attractive to health-care managers around the world in recent years.

These ideas are fully compatible with the framework we are using. "TQM-CQI" experts all advocate performance measurement, managerial accountability, worker involvement, a focus on customer service, and leadership from the top (Morgan and Murgatroyd 1994). They focus on the idea that the key to lower cost and higher quality is the careful redesign of systems of production. They also emphasize the importance of systematic objective analysis (just as we do at the health-system level) as crucial to effective reform.

A key insight from TQM/CQI is that better quality cannot come from fear or coercion. Improvement has to emerge from a system that makes it easy to do things well and hard to do things badly. Targeted quality-improvement efforts in the health sector—to improve drug ordering or inventory management—are often based on this approach. And they are often badly needed. For in the health sector, operating procedures can reflect efforts by professional groups, unions, or control-oriented civil servants to advance their own ends—as opposed to maximizing system performance. And they can persist, unchanged, because organizations and their managers have lacked the incentives or the ability to institute change.

We cannot recapitulate here the huge literature on quality improvement methods. Our point is that such programs cannot substitute for good management. On the contrary, these approaches have had their biggest positive impact in already well-managed organizations. Thus, TQM is not a substitute for the kinds of managerial reforms we discuss in this chapter. On the contrary, TQM methods are most likely to bear fruit when management capability is improved enough for the methods to be implemented effectively.

A second specific management practice often considered by health-care reformers in recent years involves contractual arrangements with private-sector firms to provide certain services for the public sector. The most common areas for this approach are is nonclinical services like food, housekeeping, and laundry. But it is also being used in clinical areas (e.g., contracts to perform certain laboratory tests, or to run specialized services like hospice care; Mills 1998).

The lure of "contracting out"—as these arrangements are called—is that specialized suppliers can take advantage of economics of scale in a particular function (e.g., laundry) that an individual hospital cannot achieve. In addition, suppliers can focus on an activity (like housekeeping) usually ignored within a medically oriented hospital. Moreover, the hope is that the bidding process will lead contract-seeking firms to offer good service at a low price. In countries where the public sector is inefficient and difficult to reform, contracting out may seem an attractive option. These hopes are most likely to be fulfilled when an experienced set of competitive suppliers seeks to obtain the business. Contracting with a monopolist, in contrast, is not likely to produce the hoped-for cost and service gains (Mills 1998).

To contract successfully, hospitals need to be able to write specifications, evaluate bids, draft contracts, and monitor performance. Moreover, unless the hospitals themselves are under pressure to improve their performance, they will have no more incentive to do contracting well than they formally had to do well at direct service delivery. Thus, hospitals and their managers need increased performance-based incentives and accountability in order to contract out effectively.

Summary on Managerial Interventions

In the context of overall health-sector performance, managerial interventions are somewhat narrowly focused. They are generally not directed at access or risk protection. They also are seldom a response to problems of allocative inefficiency

(i.e., *what* is produced). Instead, these reforms focus on *how* things are produced—on technical efficiency and improved service and clinical quality. This
makes sense because what organizations produce is primarily determined by their
external incentives, while the structure and functioning of the system of production is essentially an internal matter.

The politics of such reforms typically reflects conflicting pressures. Citizens'
dissatisfaction with poor service may support such changes, even as politicians
and entitled workers oppose them. And non–health-sector concerns like strengthening local governments can also play a role. If these reforms succeed, then costs
should be lower or health status and satisfaction should be higher. Exactly how
potential gains are split among these objectives, however, will depend on other
decisions made in the financing and payment areas.

Conditional Guidance

Attention to the organization control knob is often essential if the potential gains
from other reform initiatives are to be realized. Changing financing and payment
can change the funds available to providers and the incentives given them. But
such changes alone do not increase the capacity of the delivery system to produce
better care. And unless that capacity is enhanced, efficiency, quality, and access
will not improve—nor will overall system performance.

This conclusion has often been ignored in health-sector reform. That may be
partially a matter of ignorance. Reformers tend disproportionately to be either
economists or doctors. Economists often believe that changing money flows alone
will improve performance. Doctors focus on clinical issues and devalue what they
see as intrusion into their work by "bureaucrats" or "pencil pushers" who worry
about organizational issues. It is also a question of politics. Changing the delivery
system is always opposed by those who will lose functions and resources. Efforts
to improve the functioning of the public sector can confront grave political opposition from patronage-based politicians or entrenched unions (Walt 1994).

Despite these difficulties, reformers need to confront a basic truth about the
health-care delivery system, stated at the beginning of this chapter. *Provider organizations will not function effectively unless managers have both the incentives
to improve performance and the capacity to respond to those incentives.* If reformers are unwilling or unable to make the changes required to bring this about,
then they should not be surprised if health-system performance continues to be
disappointing.

In terms of incentives, we explored how competition and contracting can be
used to influence both private, for-profit providers and public-sector providers
who have some managerial autonomy (as in the case of quasi-markets). We also
looked at decentralization inside the public sector as a way of increasing incentives and accountability.

In terms of increasing capacity, we explored various restructuring options (auto-nomization and corporatization) and the possibilities of improved managerial capacity within the un-reorganized public sector. We also noted that two particular managerial innovations (TQM and contracting out) depended for success on increases in managerial capacity. They are complements to, not substitutes for, managers with the skills, authority, and incentives to improve organizational performance.

This same basic insight applies also to efforts to change who-does-what in the delivery system. Some efforts—like shifting activities to the private sector—rely on providing both incentive and capacity changes. Other changes, like altering the scale and scope of providers, depend on managerial actions to produce their potential gains. Too often reformers have not thought through how such changes will work themselves out at the managerial level.

Choosing Among Reform Options

When deciding what to do, reformers have to realize that with an extensive and entrenched patronage system, only significant structural reforms will lead to significantly improved performance. More modest reforms are most likely to be useful where managerial competence and staff motivation are already relatively good. Unfortunately, it is exactly where drastic reform is most needed that it is the most difficult politically.

The mix of decentralization and corporatization a nation should consider will depend on a number of variables. Is corruption and inefficiency better or worse at the local level? What is the likelihood we can get political approval for new forms of hospital governance that will lead to real managerial improvements? How effective are our payment and regulatory systems in creating the incentives and controls we will want to influence the behavior of autonomous providers?

The most radical restructuring strategies involve going all the way to privatization and a reliance on the market. As we noted, whether this makes sense for a nation depends on several issues. How competitive will the resulting market be? Private monopolies are unlikely to produce desirable results. The second consideration is the sophistication of buyers. The better buyers can judge options, the better the market will function. Third, what are the reformers' goals? Equity concerns imply less use of the market. A focus on customer satisfaction makes market provision more appropriate. Unfortunately, here we encounter yet another difficult paradox. Governments with weak public-delivery systems also often lack the financial and administrative skills to effectively purchase from or regulate private providers.

In addressing these questions, reformers must also consider the importance of maintaining professional norms within the health-care delivery system. The "agency" problem means that doctors can easily exploit patients if they choose to do so (McGuire 2000). Market competition can easily erode the professional norms that limit such exploitation. Indeed, the more competitive (and better) the market, the more pressure there is on providers to maximize their own incomes.

Organizational Change and Equity

Organizational changes can have significant equity implications. As noted previously, changing the class of providers (nurses versus doctors) or the practice setting (local dispensaries versus district hospitals) can influence the physical and effective availability of services for poor or socially marginal groups. Such changes can alter the location and travel time, or the cultural sensitivity and acceptability of service delivery.

Using private markets also has serious equity implications. Competition can decrease the funds available to cross-subsidize poor patients. Therefore, how care for the poor is paid for will determine whether it is attractive for competitive providers to provide such care. The more competitive and market-oriented the providers, the more they will respond to even small changes in price signals.

A final link between fairness and organization arises in the context of decentralization. The risk is that variations in levels of local social and economic development will be made worse by such reforms. More-advanced communities will be better able to operate services, and unless strong equalization measures are in place, they will wind up with better services or lower tax rates—or even both.

Summary

We began this chapter by defining what we mean by "an organization"—as a provider of health-care services—and what we mean by "the organization of the system." We described three kinds of interventions: changes in who-does-what, changes in incentives, and managerial changes, and discussed how they can improve overall performance.

We have stressed that these interventions need to work together. Incentive changes like decentralization or contracting will not alter outcomes unless accompanied by changes at the managerial level. Similarly, the potential cost savings and clinical quality gains from changing scale and scope will only be realized if managers take advantage of their opportunities. Ultimately, the behavior of front-line workers and their managers has to be changed to produce real improvement.

We have seen that organizational changes often require the use of other control knobs. Financing, payment, and regulation are especially important, particularly when the target organizations are not fully under the authority of the ministry of health. Korea and Japan, for example, have used regulation to separate dispensing from prescribing medicines by physicians. To help some providers grow, governments can pay them more or selectively contract with them, lend them money or guarantee their debts. All these can change the organization of the system.

Because details do matter, and they are often incompletely worked out at the policy level, implementation is critical for the successful use of the organization control knob. A persistent attention to detail and a focus on follow-through are necessary. Reformers need to consider carefully whether they will have ongoing political support when the inevitable objections arise. Changing organization is not an enterprise for the impatient or the fainthearted. Yet it also may well be essential if other reforms are to yield their hoped-for gains in health-sector performance.

References

Akin, John S.; David K. Guilkey; and E. Hazel Denton. 1995. "Quality of Services and Demand for Health Care in Nigeria: A Multinomial Probit Estimation." *Social Science & Medicine* 40(11): 1527–37.

Aljunid, Syed; and Anthony Zwi. 1997. "Public and Private Practitioners in a Rural District of Malaysia: Complements or Substitutes?" In: Sara Bennett, Barbara McPake, and Anne Mills, eds., *Private Health Providers in Developing Countries: Serving the Public Interest?* London: Zed Books.

Barzelay, Michael; with the collaboration of Babak J. Armajani. 1992. *Breaking Through Bureaucracy: A New Vision for Managing in Government.* Berkeley, CA: University of California Press.

Becker, E. R.; D. C. Morris; S. D. Culler; P. D. Mauldin; L. J. Shaw; J. D. Talley; and W. S. Weintraub. 1999. "The Changing Healthcare Market and How It Has Influenced the Treatment of Cardiovascular Disease—Part 1." *American Journal of Managed Care* 5: 1119–24.

Bennett, Sara; and Anne Mills. 1998. "Government Capacity to Contract: Health Sector Experience and Lessons." *Public Administration and Development* 18: 307–26.

Berle, Adolf A.; and Gardiner C. Means. 1991 (c1932). *The Modern Corporation and Private Property.* New Brunswick, NJ: Transaction Publishers.

Berman, Peter. 1998. "Rethinking Health Care Systems: Private Health Care Provision in India." *World Development* 26: 1463–79.

Berman, Peter A.; Davidson R. Gwatkin; and Susan E. Burger. 1987. "Community-based Health Workers: Head Start or False Start Towards Health for All?" *Social Science & Medicine* 25(5): 443–59.

Berman, P.; A. K. Nandakumar; M. El-Adawy; J. J. Frere; S. El-Saharty. 1997. "Egypt: A Strategy for Primary Care Reform." Bethesda, MD: Partnerships for Health Reform Project, Abt Associates.

Berman, P.; D. G. Sisler; and J. P. Habicht. 1989. "Equity in Public Sector Primary Health Care: The Role of Service Organization in Indonesia." *Economic Development and Cultural Change* 37: 777–803.

Berwick, Donald M.; A. Blanton Godfrey, and Jane Roessner. 1991. *Curing Health Care: New Strategies for Quality Improvement*. San Francisco, CA: Jossey-Bass.

Bosk, Charles L. 1979. *Forgive and Remember: Managing Medical Failure*. Chicago: University of Chicago Press.

Boner, R. A. 1995. "Competition Policy and Institutions in Reforming Economies." In: C. Frischtak, ed. *Regulatory Policies and Reform: A Comparative Analysis*. Washington, DC: World Bank.

Bossert, Thomas. 1998. "Analyzing the Decentralization of Health Systems in Developing Countries: Decision Space, Innovation and Performance." *Social Science & Medicine* 47: 1513–27.

Bossert, Thomas; Osvaldo Larrañaga; Ursula Giedion; José Jesus Arbelaez; and Diana M. Bowser. 2003. "Decentralization and Equity of Resource Allocation: Evidence from Colombia and Chile." *Bulletin of the World Health Organization* 81: 95–100.

Brennan, Troyen A.; and Donald M. Berwick. 1996. *New Rules: Regulation, Markets, and the Quality of American Health Care*. San Francisco, CA: Jossey-Bass Publishers.

Broomberg, J.; P. Masobe; and A. Mills. 1997. "Contracting Out District Hospital Services in South Africa." In: Sara Bennett, Barbara McPake, and Anne Mills, eds., *Private Health Providers in Developing Countries: Serving the Public Interest?* London: Zed Books.

Caves, Richard E. 1992. *American Industry: Structure, Conduct, Performance*. Englewood Cliffs, NJ: Prentice Hall.

Chomitz, Kenneth M.; Gunawan Setiadi; Azrul Azwar; Nusye Ismail; and Widiyarti. 1998. *What Do Doctors Want? Developing Incentives for Doctors to Serve in Indonesia's Rural and Remote Areas*. Policy Research Working Paper 1888. Washington, DC: World Bank.

Claquin, Pierre. 1981. "Private Health Care Providers in Rural Bangladesh." *Social Science & Medicine* 15(2): 153–57.

Crosby, Philip B. 1979. *Quality Is Free: The Art of Making Quality Certain*. New York: McGraw-Hill.

Crown Health Enterprises. 1996. *Briefing to the Incoming Minister*. New Zealand: Crown Company Monitoring Advisory Unit, Government of New Zealand.

Dever, G. E. Alan. 1997. *Improving Outcomes in Public Health Practice: Strategy and Methods*. Gaithersburg, MD: Aspen Publishers.

England, Roger. 2000. *Contracting and Performance Management in the Health Sector: A Guide for Low and Middle Income Countries*. London: DFID Health Systems Resource Center.

England, Roger; Ken Grant; and Jennifer Sancho. 1998. *Health Sector Reform: Separating Public Financing from Providing Services*. London: DFID Health Systems Resource Center.

Feldstein, Paul J. 1993. *Health Care Economics*. Albany, NY: Delmar Publishers.

Flynn, Rob; and Gareth Williams, eds. 1997. *Contracting for Health: Quasi-markets and the National Health Service*. New York: Oxford University Press.

Fox, William; and Christine Wallich. 1998. "Bosnia-Herzegovina: Fiscal Federalism—the Dayton Challenge." In: Richard M. Bird and François Vaillancourt, eds., *Fiscal Decentralization in Developing Countries*. New York: Cambridge University Press.

Fried, Bruce J.; and Laura M. Gaydos, eds. 2002. *World Health Systems: Challenges and Perspectives*. Chicago: Health Administration Press.

Gauri, Varun. 2001. *Are Incentives Everything? Payment Mechanisms for Health Care Providers in Developing Countries*. Working Paper. Washington, DC: World Bank.

Gilson, L.; J. Adusei; D. Arhin; C. Hongoro; P. Mujinja; and K. Sagoe. 1997. "Should African Governments Contract Out Clinical Services to Church Providers?" In: Sara Bennett, Barbara McPake, and Anne Mills, eds., *Private Health Providers in Developing Countries: Serving the Public Interest?* London: Zed Books.

Griffin, Charles C. 1992. *The Private Sector in the Philippine Health Care System.* Washington, DC: Urban Institute.

Griffin, C. C.; and R. Paul Shaw. 1995. "Health Insurance in Sub-Saharan Africa: Aims, Findings, Policy Implications." In: R. Paul Shaw and Martha Ainsworth, *Financing Health Services Through User Fees and Insurance: Case Studies from Sub-Saharan Africa.* Washington, DC: World Bank.

Harding, April; and Alexander Preker. 2002. "Innovations in Health Care Delivery: Autonomization, Corporatization and Privatization of Public Hospitals." In: Alexander Preker and April Harding, eds., *Innovations in Health Service Delivery: The Corporatization of Public Hospitals.* Washington, DC: The World Bank.

Health Secretariat Mexico. 2000. *Acuerdo de Coordinación que celebran la Secretaría de Salud y el Estado de Puebla, para la ejecución del Programa de Ampliación de Cobertura (PAC) en la Entidad.* Mexico.

Herrin, Alejandro. 1997. "Private Health Sector Performance and Regulation in the Philippines." In: William Newbrander, ed., *Private Health Sector Growth in Asia: Issues and Implications.* New York: Wiley.

Herzlinger, Regina E. 1999. *Market-Driven Health Care: Who Wins, Who Loses in the Transformation of America's Largest Service Industry.* Reading, MA: Perseus Books.

Hoekman, B. 1997. *Competition Policy and the Global Trading System: A Developing Country Perspective.* Policy Research Working Paper no. 1735. Washington, DC: World Bank.

Hsiao, William. 2000. *A Preliminary Assessment of Sri Lanka's Health Sector and Steps Forward.* Colombo, Sri Lanka: Institute of Policy Studies, Health Policy Program.

Isaac, Thomas; and Richard W. Franke. 2002. *Local Democracy and Development: The Kerala People's Campaign for Decentralized Planning.* Lanham, MD: Rowman & Littlefield.

Jakab, Melitta; Alexander Preker; April Harding; and Loraine Hawkins. 2002. *The Introduction of Market Forces in the Public Hospital Sector: From New Public Sector Management to Organizational Reform.* HNP Discussion Paper. Washington, DC: World Bank. June.

Kakar, D. 1988. *Primary Health Care and Traditional Medical Practicioners.* New Delhi, India: Sterling Publishers.

Lassey, Marie L.; William R. Lassey; and Martin J. Jinks, eds. 1997. *Health Care Systems Around the World: Characteristics, Issues, Reforms.* Upper Saddle River, NJ: Prentice Hall.

Martínez, Javier; and Tim Martineau. 2002. *Human Resources in the Health Sector: An International Perspective.* London: DFID Health Systems Resource Center.

McDonald, Roger. 2002. *Australia's Flying Doctors.* Australia: Sandpiper Press.

McGuire, Thomas G. 2000. "Chapter 9: Physician Agency." In: Anthony J. Cuyler and Joseph P. Newhouse, eds. 2000. *Handbook of Health Economics.* New York: Elsevier.

Mills, Anne. 1998. "To Contract or Not to Contract? Issues for Low and Middle Income Countries." *Health Policy and Planning* 13: 32–40.

Mills, Anne; and Jonathan Broomberg. 1998. *Experiences of Contracting: An Overview of the Literature.* Geneva, Switzerland: World Health Organization.

Mills, Anne; Patrick J. Vaughan; Duane L. Smith; and Iraj Tabibzadeh, eds. 1990. *Health System Decentralization: Concepts, Issues and Country Experience.* Geneva: World Health Organization.

Ministry of Health, Egypt, Department of Planning; and Data for Decision Making Project, Harvard School of Public Health. 1994–95. *Egypt Provider Survey Report.* Boston, MA: International Health Systems Program, Harvard School of Public Health.

Morgan, Colin; and Stephen Murgatroyd. 1994. *Total Quality Management in the Public Sector: An International Perspective.* Buckingham, England: Open University Press.

Newbrander, William; and Gerald Rosenthal. 1997. "Quality of Care Issues in Health Sector Reform." In: William Newbrander, ed. *Private Health Sector Growth in Asia: Issues and Implications.* New York: Wiley.

O'Connor, J. 2001. "The Royal Flying Doctor Service of Australia: The World's First Air Medical Organization." *Air Medical Journal* 20: 10–20.

Osborne, David; and Ted Gaebler. 1993. *Reinventing Government: How the Entrepreneurial Spirit Is Transforming the Public Sector.* New York: Plume.

Ostrom, Elinor; Larry Schroeder; and Susan Wynne. 1993. *Institutional Incentives and Sustainable Development: Infrastructure Policies in Perspective.* Boulder, CO: Westview Press.

Palmer, R. H.; A. G. Lawthers; J. DeLozier; N. J. Banks; L. Peterson; and B. Duggar. 1995. *Understanding and Choosing Clinical Performance Measures for Quality Improvement: Development of a Typology.* Washington, DC: Agency for Health Care Policy Research.

Patel, Kant; and Mark E. Rushefsky. 2002. "The Canadian Health Care System." In: Khi V. Thai; Edward T. Wimberley; and Sharon M. McManus, eds., *Handbook of International Health Care Systems.* New York: Marcel Dekker.

Percy, Fiona. 1999. *Ethics of Care: Yarrabah Community and the Practice of Public Health.* Doctoral dissertation. Boston, MA: Harvard School of Public Health.

Preker, Alexander; and April Harding. 2002. *Innovations in Health Service Delivery: The Corporatization of Public Hospitals.* Washington, DC: The World Bank.

Putnam, Robert D. 1993. *Making Democracy Work: Civic Traditions in Modern Italy.* Princeton, N.J.: Princeton University Press.

———. 2000. *Bowling Alone: The Collapse and Revival of American Community.* New York: Simon & Schuster.

Roemer, Milton I. 1977. *Comparative National Policies on Health Care.* New York: Marcel Dekker.

Shankar, D. 1992. "Indigenous Health Services—The State of the Art." In: *The State of India's Health.* New Delhi, India: Voluntary Health Organization of India.

Shaw, R. Paul. 1999. *New Trends in Public Sector Management in Health: Applications in Developed and Developing Countries.* Washington, DC: World Bank Institute.

Starr, Paul. 1982. *The Social Transformation of American Medicine.* New York: Basic Books.

Walford, Veronica; and Ken Grant. 1998. *Improving Hospital Efficiency.* London: DFID Health Systems Resource Center.

Walt, Gil. 1994. *Health Policy: An Introduction to Process and Power.* London: Zed Books.

Walter, P. D. 1999. "Centers of Excellence: Historic Trends and Future Decisions." *Journal of Cardiovascular Management* 10: 17–24.

White, Joseph. 1995. *Competing Solutions: American Health Care Proposals and International Experience.* Washington, DC: Brookings Institution Press.

World Bank. 1993. *World Development Report 1993: Investing in Health.* New York: Oxford University Press.

——. 1997. *World Development Report 1997: The State in a Changing World.* New York: Oxford University Press.

Wronski, Ian. 2001. Personal communication. Vice Chancellor for Health Affairs, James Cooke University of North Queensland, Australia.

Yip, Winnie. 1998. "Physicians' Response to Medicare Fee Reductions: Changes in the Volume and Intensity of Supply of Coronary Artery Bypass Graft (CABG) Procedures for the Medicare and Provider Sectors." *Journal of Health Economics* 17(6): 675–99.

Yip, Winnie; and William Hsiao. 2001. "Economic Transition and Urban Health Care in China: Impacts and Prospects." Paper presented at Harvard University Conference on Financial Sector Reform in China. Boston, MA.

11
Regulation

In this chapter we discuss the fourth control knob—regulation. By "regulation" we mean the use of the coercive power of the state to change the behavior of individuals and organizations in the health sector. This applies not only to those who provide and finance health care but also to those who produce inputs like pharmaceuticals and those who educate health professionals.

One way to understand the role of regulation is to ask how it relates to the enthusiasm of Western-trained economists for using markets as a way of allocating resources. Based on a series of strong assumptions, economists argue that a system of perfectly competitive markets will produce a result that is Pareto Optimal (see Chapter 6). In that situation, no one person's utility can be increased except by making someone else worse off. Governments that want to use markets in this way use regulation to establish rules governing property rights and to guarantee that there will be honest and open exchange (North 1990, Fuller 1978). Otherwise, the most manipulative and powerful will take all (Oakeshott 1975). Even where markets work well, though, the distribution of well-being they produce may not be acceptable in terms of one or another ethical framework, and regulation is then used to achieve a more equitable outcome. Third, many markets do not work well on their own, and governments turn to regulation to improve their functioning (Heriot 1997). The fourth purpose of regulatory action arises because governments may use it to advance moral norms that markets cannot be relied upon to foster.

All of these issues arise frequently in the health sector. As a result, regulation is a major activity in all health systems and a major control knob for those who want to improve system performance. For example, using rules to specify what health services must be included in insurance benefit packages can directly improve health status and satisfaction. Rules that protect consumers against poor-quality drugs or incompetent doctors can have similar effects.

Regulation frequently has an important reciprocal relationship to the other control knobs. For the other control knobs to be effective, they often must be accompanied by appropriate regulation. For example, a country can establish a social insurance scheme, but it will probably go bankrupt unless effective regulation compels the eligible population to enroll and pay premiums. By the same token, regulation is often more effective when appropriate incentives and efforts to influence individual behavior complement regulatory initiatives (Laffont and Tirole 1993).

Regulation is not self-implementing, however. The administrative and political tasks that must be accomplished for regulation to work effectively can be daunting. Moreover, poorly designed regulation can make health systems perform worse, rather than better. Policymakers therefore must understand the strengths and limitations of regulation, and what it takes to implement regulatory initiatives, if they are to use this tool successfully.

This chapter is organized around five issues: What is regulation and why regulate? How do regulations influence the performance of health systems? What are the major determinants of regulatory success? What are the major types of regulation in the health sector? Finally, we offer some conditional guidance about how to use regulation effectively. The description of the major types of regulations is rather long, because of the myriad regulations, which differ greatly between high- and low-income countries. Readers may want to consult it selectively to learn more about the particular regulatory alternatives of interest to them.

Defining and Justifying Regulation

We use the term "regulation" to refer to the government's use of its *coercive power to impose constraints* on organizations and individuals. Under this definition, only legal rules, and not incentives or behavior change (see Chapter 12), are included under the heading of "regulation." Regulation, then, includes the full range of legal instruments (laws, decrees, orders, codes, administrative rules, guidelines), whether issued by the government or by nongovernmental bodies (e.g., self-regulatory organizations) to which the government has delegated regulatory power (OECD 1996).

Our definition of regulation excludes rules and requirements imposed on sellers by purchasers of health insurance or health-care services. For example, social and private insurance plans often constrain providers by restricting whom and how they will pay for care. These are not regulations, because they are not legal rules imposed by government, but rather contract terms negotiated between buyer and seller. This holds true even when the government itself acts as the purchaser.

We noted above that the purposes of regulation relate in various ways to perfecting or correcting the results produced by economic markets. First, any society relying on market exchange mechanisms must *ensure that exchanges and transactions are done honestly and openly* (North 1990, Williamson 1985). A basic set of rules is needed to define the legal obligations of the various players in market transactions, delineating their power, responsibility, and accountability. For example, in the health sector, governments use regulation to establish the obligations and responsibilities of both buyers (patients and consumers) and sellers (doctors, pharmacies, hospitals, and insurers) to ensure that agreed-upon transactions are honest, transparent, and reliably executed.

The second reason for regulation arises even when markets work well from an economist's perspective. In particular, *markets can't deal with unequal distribution of income and varying health needs.* For example, poor citizens get few services from hospitals organized on market principles, precisely because they are poor and cannot afford to pay. By the same token, few doctors locate in depressed rural areas because of the limited economic opportunities these areas offer. Insurance markets, too, can produce objectionable results from an equity perspective. For example, without regulation, such markets often will not cover chronically ill people, because they cannot afford the premiums. All of these situations can and have produced efforts to use regulation to promote more equal access to health care and to improve the distribution of health status.

Third, regulation arises because health-sector markets often *do not possess the requisite conditions for reasonably effective competition* (Hsiao 1995). Such *market failures* are of several different types. First, consumers may be unable to judge the quality of the goods or services they consume. Due to such problems, they may be victimized by unqualified doctors or be unable to detect drugs with impure ingredients. Governments can respond to such situations in a variety of ways. They may provide information to buyers to improve their choices; e.g., through labeling requirements. Alternatively, they may restrict what is offered in the marketplace by licensing doctors or limiting the drugs that can be sold. In the public health context, we can even limit consumers' own behavior on the grounds of their own ignorance, by requiring motorcycle helmets, for example. One especially relevant form of patient ignorance, which we discussed in Chapter 3, involves the risk that doctors will induce patients to consume too much—thereby increasing physicians' incomes. Many countries use regulation to address this problem by limiting the total number of physicians or hospital beds.

A second kind of market failure involves what economists call *external effects,* where the customer's decisions affect other people but the customer doesn't consider those benefits or costs in making their own decisions. The classic examples here include vaccination, where my immunization confers benefits to others in the community, and air pollution, where my factory's emissions harm others nearby. Many governments subsidize or require acts with positive gains and tax or forbid acts that impose costs on others. For example, requiring motor vehicles to have headlights and brakes and imposing speed limits are all ways to increase external benefits and reduce external costs to other drivers (Rosen, 2002).

A particular kind of external effect involves what some economists call *merit goods*. These are goods with widespread but difficult-to-quantify external benefits— like basic literacy and civic education—that governments often provide outside of the marketplace. Governments also often use regulation to see that these activities occur (Musgrave and Musgrave 1989).

A third kind of market failure involves the existence of a *monopoly*, a single seller, or an *oligopoly*, a cooperating small number of sellers. In such situations, competition does not force producers to lower costs and prices. As a result, some governments intervene to control anti-competitive behavior (e.g., price fixing) or limit mergers among firms to prevent monopolies from developing in the first place (Musgrave and Musgrave 1989).

Finally, regulation is promoted by some people with particular philosophical viewpoints—especially some communitarians and objective utilitarians—who object to market results for a variety of specific ethical reasons. For instance, consumers may not voluntarily purchase cost-effective preventive services, so that the market does not maximize health status. Objective utilitarians sometimes respond by urging the regulation of individual behaviors to improve health outcomes (e.g., quarantining recalcitrant HIV-infected individuals who engage in unsafe sex). Communitarians, in contrast, often want to use regulation to limit transactions that offend their moral sensibilities (abortion, the sex trade, organ sales).

In sum, our analysis of regulation does *not* presume either that the market is always best or that the economist's view of society's goals is the only way to look at health-sector reform. Instead, we want to offer a framework that encompasses the diverse ethical perspectives that inform regulatory efforts around the world. How each nation chooses to proceed, and the goals it embraces, depend on its *ethical beliefs* (see Chapter 3) as derived from each nation's particular social values (Shklar 1997) and as expressed through its political processes (see Chapter 4). (A tabulation of the ethical justifications for these four categories of regulation is provided in Table 11.1.)

Regulation and Health-System Objectives

How are different kinds of regulations connected to the various aspects of health-system performance presented in Chapters 5 and 6? First, regulations that have an impact on a population's health or provide financial risk-protection can directly affect the performance goals we have identified. For example, ensuring the safety and purity of water, food, and drugs will influence overall health status.

TABLE 11.1. Categories of Regulation and Their Related Ethical Perspective

CATEGORY OF REGULATION	RELATED ETHICAL PERSPECTIVES
Establish basic conditions for honest market exchange	Subjective utilitarianism, objective utilitarianism
Perfect what markets cannot do (such as ensure equal access to basic health care)	Egalitarian liberals, communitarianism
Correct market failures and provide public and merit goods	Subjective utilitarianism
Correct unacceptable market results (such as use of tobacco)	Objective utilitarianism, communitarianism

Similarly, compulsory enrollment in social insurance plans can ensure that all eligible persons have financial risk-protection.

Most regulation, however, affects intermediate performance measures. For example, regulations aimed at improving the quality of health services can, if successful, lead to improved health outcomes and increased public satisfaction. Regulation to correct market failures can improve efficiency, which in turn can lower health costs and make health services more affordable. This can encourage both governments and individuals to increase service use and in turn improve health status. Similarly, regulating monopolistic pricing can lower the prices of health services. This can have a positive impact on effective availability or access, and in turn on health outcomes and patient satisfaction.

The Determinants of Regulatory Success

Effective regulation is a complex and demanding process (Landy et al. 1990). First, an appropriate regulatory strategy needs to be developed—decisions made about what and how to regulate. Then agencies have to be established, including the recruitment of staff and the collection of data. Then the detailed rules have to be written. Next they have to be applied to specific cases. Monitoring processes need to be established so that violators can be identified and either persuaded to change their behavior or penalized if they do not. All of this must be done in a context in which those being regulated will protest and seek to influence the agency to treat them more leniently. Effective regulation thus requires a demanding combination of technical expertise, administrative capacity, and political support that is not always easy for nations to provide (Ayres and Braithwaite 1992).

Regulation also needs to be adjusted to local conditions. For example, because high- and low-income countries generally face different situations in their health systems, their regulatory efforts are often directed at solving different problems. Most high-income countries have enough physicians, or even a surplus. Regulation in these countries, therefore, is often directed at limiting the supply of physicians to counteract supplier-induced demand. In contrast, many low-income countries have a shortage of qualified physicians, and their regulatory efforts often focus on influencing physicians to serve in physician-scarce areas.

In addition to facing different problems, countries bring different sets of capabilities and attitudes to the regulatory enterprise. Experience with regulatory interventions around the globe suggests that successful regulatory efforts depend on three key aspects of each nation's situation: *cultural attitudes*, *government competence*, and *political support*. All of these, we believe, need to be taken into account in designing regulatory institutions.

Cultural Attitudes

Two kinds of cultural attitudes are critical to the success of regulatory endeavors— general and specific. General attitudes involve the views citizens have toward government and their overall pattern of reaction to state action. Such attitudes vary widely around the world. Countries as diverse as Denmark and Singapore have highly law-abiding citizens who see government as legitimate, trust its fairness and competence, and obey laws and rules more or less automatically. In contrast, citizens of societies as diverse as Hungary and China are more likely to look for ways to avoid rather than comply with regulation. They see the state as often unfair and illegitimate and, since rule-violation is widespread, tend to see voluntary compliance as foolish. Similarly, some governments are more willing than others to impose harsh penalties on violators, who then know that if they are caught the sanctions will be severe. These cultural factors must be taken into account in designing a regulatory program.

Reformers should also realize that specific cultural norms and social beliefs influence the effectiveness of regulation. Regulators and regulatees react differently, depending on whether they agree with the goal expressed by the regulation. When legal restrictions are compatible with social beliefs, citizens are more likely to comply; otherwise, the regulated may try to evade the regulations. Efforts to control drug and alcohol use in many countries have failed because they are not consistent with cultural beliefs. Because of such beliefs, regulation may need to be accompanied by social-marketing measures (see Chapter 12) that bring individual behaviors into greater alignment with regulatory intent.

Capacity of Government

As noted above, regulatory tasks typically raise difficult administrative and technical issues. A wide range of experts—from medicine, biology, and chemistry, to law, economics, and accounting—may be required. Extensive data and reporting systems may need to be constructed. Inspectors need to be trained and deployed and general rules applied to specific cases. Establishing and enforcing regulations can put great burdens and responsibilities on the relevant agencies. In an attempt to be explicit about what is allowed and what is not, rules and laws tend to depict reality in black-and-white terms. But many real-life situations are shades of gray, making it difficult to apply regulations in these cases. This implies that regulators have substantial discretion in the enforcement process.

The success a country has in carrying out these processes depends in part on the organizational capacity of its government. In countries with a high-quality civil service, well-functioning police and court systems, effective tax-reporting, and so on, the task of establishing a working regulatory agency is much easier.

The operations of a regulatory agency are often a focus of controversy. Because regulators are trying to change the behavior of specific groups, those being regulated have every reason to deflect or minimize the regulatory agency's effectiveness. Their efforts are likely to begin with trying to shape the design and wording of rules and administrative decisions, and continue through to all aspects of implementation. The resulting efforts range from persuasion and influence, to political pressure, to outright corruption. Inducement can come in many forms, from bribes, to gifts, to promises of lucrative post-government employment, to favors for the regulators' relatives and friends. How regulatory officials respond to pressure, persuasion, and bribery depends in part on the political structure and professionalism of the bureaucrats.

There are large variations in the nature and extent of corruption in different countries. Political cultures vary. In some societies, the failure of an officeholder to help family or clan members—or even college classmates—would be viewed as dishonorable. Even within a country there can be significant interregional or intersectoral variations. In India, Bihar is not Maharastra. In the United States, Mississippi is not Minnesota. In both cases, the second state has a reputation for much greater probity than the first. According to the Corruption Perception Index (based on bribery-taking), Canada has been consistently among the least corrupt countries, with a score of 9.2; the United States has a score of 7.8, and many low-income countries have scores of 3.5 or less, with Nigeria being the worst (Transparency International 2000). Corruption in high-income countries often takes subtler forms; for example, as contributions to political campaigns or favorable business opportunities for political leaders. Recent scandals about campaign contributions in Germany and France suggest that corruption remains a serious problem even in high-income countries.

The efforts by the regulated to protect themselves can be quite subtle, as when a regulatory agency is "captured" by those that the agency is supposed to regulate. It is not unusual for the officials appointed to lead a regulatory agency to have worked in the industry they now regulate. Sometimes this is because the industry is the only source of expertise on its own affairs. In other cases, more blatant pressure is at work. But as a result, regulators have been known to be sympathetic to, and advance the interests of, the regulated rather than those of the public (Stigler 1971).

Many low- and middle-income countries lack the technical expertise, administrative capacity, and information systems to promulgate regulations. As a result, there are fewer kinds of regulation in low-income countries, and the regulations that exist often focus on dramatic situations where bad behavior can directly impair public safety. Even then, enforcement is often uneven and hampered by corruption and favoritism. In particular, most low- and middle-income countries do little to regulate private health care or private insurance markets. Such a laissez-faire policy leaves many patients at the mercy of unregulated local doctors, private pharmacies, clinics, and hospitals. But countries seeking to correct this situation through regulation need to be realistic about whether they have the technical and administrative capacity to do so successfully.

High-income countries, in contrast, generally have the technical and legal infrastructure to effectively regulate many features of the health system, including medical quality, investments by health facilities, and the diffusion of medical technology. Moreover, where they rely on the private sector, they often can and do use regulation to try to control monopolistic prices, whether these are set by private providers or by pharmaceutical companies. Insurers, too, are regulated to assure their solvency and to reduce risk selection.

The capacity of government does not depend solely on the level of economic development—hence, neither do the regulatory options available to health-system reformers. Instead, regulatory capacity has an interactive relationship with our first variable: cultural attitudes. Countries in which citizens support government are more likely to have capable government institutions, and vice versa. Any nation that seeks to use regulation has to assess both cultural factors and regulatory capacity, and formulate its regulatory strategy accordingly.

Political Support

Regulations, whether legislated or decreed by executive order, are enacted through political processes. All nations have organized interest groups, whether formal or informal. These groups exist whether a nation is governed by a single party, a parliamentary democracy, a hereditary ruler, or a military strongman. And these interest groups can have very powerful roles in influencing regulatory decisions. Hence, in designing regulations, political skills are of great importance. These political skills include knowing who might support and who might oppose the regulation, what political alliances can be formed, what compromises may have to be made, what political strategies might work, and how regulations can be designed to be politically acceptable. (These political skills were described in Chapter 4.)

Moreover, political support is required both for instituting a regulatory process and for ensuring its effective implementation. The regulated sometimes seek to defer important decisions to the implementation phase—hoping that they will then be able to influence administrative agencies when there is less public and political attention focused on the relevant decisions. Continuing support from political leaders may well be necessary to prevent such *regulatory capture* from undermining the whole effort (Stigler 1971). This is especially so since regulations are often ambiguous when applied to specific cases, and regulators thus tend to have substantial discretion. The regulated, moreover, always press for concessions. Hence, regulatory agencies need to be well supported if they are to resist the inevitable pressures from the regulated.

The Design of Regulatory Institutions and Processes

The outcome of a regulatory initiative depends on the detailed design of regulatory institutions and processes and on how reformers respond to the attitudes, capacities, and politics characteristic of their national situation. Both technical competence and sound judgment are needed. The substance of a regulation has to be carefully crafted and worded, penalties have to be commensurate with the seriousness of harm or damage done by violators, and sanctions or incentives have to be skillfully composed to promote compliance. Otherwise, the regulation is unlikely to be effective.

Regulatory outcomes thus depend critically on the enforcement process, especially on regulators' ability to detect, penalize, and deter violators. Because regulatory agencies typically have only *limited enforcement resources,* they can only detect, apprehend, and prosecute a limited number of violators. Only if voluntary compliance is relatively widespread, and violations relatively infrequent, can these limited resources be sufficient to apprehend enough violators so that the probability of detection and prosecution will be high enough to deter potential violations (Roberts and Farrell 1978). Together, these phenomena imply that rules and sanctions that are seen as socially acceptable in a given culture are much easier to enforce.

To detect violations, *regulators need data*, which creates additional complexities. The data that are easily (and inexpensively) available are often not the data regulators would most like to have. For example, a country that wants to regulate quality can easily test new medical graduates on their knowledge of anatomy. It is much more difficult to assess how practicing physicians use their knowledge in the daily treatment of patients. Thus, regulators often face a tradeoff between the relevance of data and the cost of its acquisition. Here is one place where an assessment of a government's technical sophistication and data-gathering capacity should play a key role in devising a reform strategy.

Once violators are detected, sanctions must be imposed. Yet, if the process for imposing penalties requires long and complex court proceedings, enforcers may not have the resources to prosecute large numbers of violators. On the other hand, if enforcers can directly impose fines without lengthy court proceedings, they may abuse their power. Once police, prosecutors, or judges are involved in the process, they will inevitably find room to exercise their own discretion about how enforcement occurs. If the rules seem unfair or inappropriate to them, they will find ways to avoid enforcing them. Thus cultural attitudes affect not only regulatees but also regulators.

The question of who might most cost-effectively carry out these tasks is not easily answered. Responsibility and authority can be given to a government agency, a parastatal organization, or a private organization. Parastatal organizations have often been used because of their relative insulation from direct political influence, especially when the government is ineffective, corrupt, or dominated by interest groups. A parastatal organization has the advantages of being more insulated from politics than government agencies, non-civil service status for its employees, and greater direct accountability to the public.

Which option is most effective and efficient depends largely on the relative managerial capability of the specific organizations and on the nation's political situation. For example, many countries use their national medical society to discipline doctors because that is more acceptable to the profession. On the other hand, this arrangement raises the risk that rules will not be rigorously enforced, because the process will be "captured" by the doctors it is supposed to regulate. In response, governments can regulate the regulators by setting the rules for public representation on the review councils, transparency of review processes, and accountability of the profession to the public (Irvine 1997).

Self-regulation has been used in the health sector to assure quality that is difficult to measure or ascertain (De Geyndt 1995, Graham 1994). Indeed, health-care regulators often rely on the regulated to report on their own behavior, just as tax collectors rely on individuals and businesses to file tax returns. For example, what is the surgical complication rate or the infection rate in a hospital? In such cases, it is in the regulator's interest to ask for reports based on data already being collected by the regulated for their own purposes. Using such data lowers the cost of reporting for the regulated, making it more likely they will do so. Furthermore, it can give regulators a place to check on the accuracy of the reports they receive. To encourage accurate self-reporting, regulators have to refrain from penalizing the regulated too heavily for small violations of the rule. If they are too draconian, they will only encourage inaccurate reporting, resulting in unreliable data.

Table 11.2 provides a matrix of the organizational alternatives that can administer regulations, and some examples of these regulations.

Major Types of Regulation in the Health Sector

We divide regulatory activities into two distinct realms—regulation of the health-care sector, and regulation of the health-insurance system. We group regulatory actions into four categories, according to the four purposes discussed above. Table 11.3

TABLE 11.2. Alternative Organization of Regulatory Agencies in Relation to the Organizations to be Regulated

REGULATED REGULAR	STATE	PARASTATAL	PRIVATE
State	X	Regulation of social insurance plans such as sickness funds	Government regulation of private companies
Parastatal	X	X	Sickness funds regulate private providers; joint commission on hospital accreditation regulates hospitals
Private	X	X	Self-regulation by medical association

summarizes health-sector regulations. In the next section and in Table 11.4, we describe regulatory actions aimed at health insurance, with continued attention to the differences between high-income and low- and middle-income countries.

Establish the Basic Conditions for Market Exchange

As noted above, governments have to create a legal and regulatory framework to establish the basic conditions for market exchange. This includes a system of contract and commercial law and securities law, and the courts to enforce these. Such laws cover fraud, the failure to perform, and the system of liability and responsibility under bankruptcy. These laws and their enforcement are part of the essential institutional infrastructure of a modern market economy. While their absence can hinder the development of health-care markets, they are often not considered within the narrower agenda of health-sector reform efforts.

Another set of basic laws defines the internal structure of health-care organizations (as discussed in Chapter 10). This includes issues of governance, recourse, and responsibility for both for-profit and nonprofit entities, the role of boards of directors, and shareholder rights. There is also the need to define property rights—including intellectual property like patent and copyright protection. In contrast to more general legal institutions, these rules have drawn attention from health-sector reformers—especially in post-communist countries where market arrangements in health cannot fully develop until such organizational design issues are resolved.

In the health-care system more narrowly, there are the specific questions of patients' rights and physicians' obligations. This has been an area of much interest in advanced countries in recent years, both from the perspective of improving markets and in terms of respecting rights as a (liberal) end in itself.

TABLE 11.3. A Comparison of Regulations of High-Income Nations and Low- and Middle-Income Countries in Public Health and Health Services

CATEGORY OF REGULATION	HIGH-INCOME NATIONS	LOW- AND MIDDLE-INCOME NATIONS
Establish Basic Conditions for Market Exchange	a. Define and protect property rights and patents b. Govern solvency and bankruptcy of health-service institutions c. Protect patients' rights	a. Similar, but less enforced b. Similar c. Very little formal regulation
Perfect What Markets Cannot Do (such as assuring equitable access)	a. Assign new medical graduates to serve in under-served areas b. Assure patients' rights to emergency services	a. Similar, frequently done b. Public hospitals provide emergency services
Correct Market Failures		
A. *Deal with External Effects and Merit Goods*	Direct government provision of free or highly subsidized programs, such as health education and immunization	Same
B. *Help Consumers Make Informed Choice*	a. Labeling b. Regulate truth-in-advertising c. Restrict physicians from advertising	a. Much less regulated b. Much less regulated c. Little restriction
C. *Protect Buyers Unable to Judge Quality* (i) Regulate inputs	a. Standards for food hygiene and purity of drugs. b. Licensing of physicians, nurses, pharmacists. c. Accreditation of laboratories, hospitals.	a. Similar, but less enforced b. Similar, but may not require periodical relicensing c. Same, but may not require periodical re-accreditation

Policy	Status
(ii) Regulate process	
a. Practice guidelines	a. None
b. Patient reporting	b. Few countries have it; public hospitals rely on administrative rules
(iii) Regulate outputs	
a. Establish standard quality report cards	a. None
b. Liability	b. Most countries have no specific medical malpractice laws, but covered under other common laws (India an exception)
c. Disciplinary boards	
d. Medical malpractice	
e. Clinical audit	
D. Control Supplier-Induced Demand	
(i) Regulate manpower	
a. Limit training slots and "billing" numbers	a. Many countries have shortage of physicians, so policy is opposite of those in developed countries
b. Restrict foreign medical school graduates	b. Encourage foreign graduates
c. Disclose conflicts of interest	c. Few countries have it
(ii) Regulate capital investment	
a. Limit new technology and new facility construction	a. Most countries encourage private investment
b. Restrict imports of equipment	b. Some encourage imports
E. Counteract Monopoly	
(i) Restrict monopoly	
a. Enact anti-trust laws and restrict predatory conduct	a. Few countries have it
(ii) Regulate monopolistic prices	
a. Establish price schedule	a. Establish user fees for public facilities, but not private
b. Establish reference prices for drugs	b. Very few countries have it
Correct Unacceptable Market Results	
a. Prohibit the sale of tobacco to minors	a. Some, but not strictly enforced
b. Prohibit assisted suicide	b. Very few countries have it

In low- and middle-income countries, the enforcement of even basic business regulations can be difficult and uneven. And many specific forms of regulation (e.g., patients' rights) are frequently absent altogether.

Enhance Equity

Because free markets distribute health care based on what people can and are willing to pay, their outcome is often inconsistent with egalitarian goals. Nations, therefore, may use regulation to enhance equitable access to health services. Many low- and middle-income countries, in particular, have tried to use regulation to compel graduates of medical and nursing schools to serve for a period of time in underserved areas. For instance, Egypt, Ecuador, Nigeria, and Malaysia assign and require new medical school graduates to serve one or two years in physician-scarce areas. For similar reasons, U.S. hospitals are required to treat all emergency patients, regardless of their ability to pay.

Correct Market Failures and Provide Public and Merit Goods

This category includes all government interventions that arise because the market is not functioning properly. Health-services markets in particular often suffer from market failures because of patients' information problems (their inability to judge the appropriateness and quality of medical services) and providers' monopoly power. Regulatory interventions have been designed to counteract many of these conditions, and there is actually quite a broad range of such efforts (Feldman and Roberts 1980).

External effects and merit goods

Much regulation aims to reduce negative externalities—the adverse effects of one person's decision on others. A parallel goal is to expand the supply of goods with broad benefits to others, which we defined above as merit goods. These regulations run the gamut from sanitation requirements and rules for drinking-water quality, to quarantine and immunization, to firearms control and required health education. In each case, the theory is that markets are difficult to organize because many potential buyers are affected by a single decision, like air pollution control; or that buyers do not fully take into account all the consequences of their decision to consume the good, like taking vaccinations. Hence, the government has to intervene.

Help consumers make informed choices

Often buyers are unable to assess the content of food and drug products or to know their biological effects. In this case, regulation is needed for two purposes: to inform buyers and to ensure that products actually contain the ingredients claimed by producers. Many countries require producers to disclose the basic

ingredients contained in a product on the packaging. High-income countries devote significant resources to ensuring that products actually contain the ingredients that are claimed, and to ensure their purity. In most low- and middle-income
countries such regulations are quite lax, due to lack of resources and inadequate
administrative capability.

Similarly, because most patients do not have the knowledge to judge the appropriateness and technical quality of medical services and drugs, they are especially
vulnerable to being misled by deceptive or inaccurate advertising. As a result,
most countries regulate advertisements by physicians, pharmaceutical companies,
and hospitals. Some governments also regulate what information should be dis-
closed to patients to help improve their capacity to make such choices.

Protect buyers from poor quality

An alternative to providing or controlling information is to limit what is sold. Because the effectiveness of professional self-regulation has come into question
around the world, the governments of high-income countries are taking an increasingly active role in regulating the quality of medical services.

Using Donabedian's categories about the forms of quality control, we can think
of government as regulating the *inputs*, the *processes*, or the *outcomes* of health
services (Donabedian 1980). Regulation of inputs is easiest to establish and enforce, so it is the most prevalent. It does not necessarily ensure better outcomes,
however. Regulating the processes of care is much more difficult, and the responsibility for doing so is often assigned to the medical profession. Regulation of
outcomes may seem ideal, because outcomes are what society should be most
concerned with. But because patients may respond to treatment differently, depending on the severity of their disease and their particular physiology, sophisticated
sampling and severity adjustment is likely to be required—which is technically
very challenging. In addition, the medical profession generally resists regulation
based on outcomes as an infringement on its clinical autonomy. This resistance is
important, because to succeed, quality regulation must be acceptable to the medical profession. Since the range of these activities is quite extensive, we review
them in more detail.

Regulation of Inputs
Drug Approval
Safety and efficacy are the main motivations for drug regulation. Because of the
potential for negative side-effects, almost all countries today have regulations to
keep drugs from the market until they are proven safe. Regulatory bodies also may
require drug manufacturers to demonstrate the drug's efficacy (i.e., that it performs
as described), and in some countries, its cost-effectiveness. Manufacturers must
also provide information about possible adverse reactions and contraindications, as
well as potential reactions when combined with other drugs.

In general, high-income countries have more exacting standards and do more
extensive review of various kinds of data, from animal studies to controlled trials,

to tracking clinical experience after drugs are introduced. Low- to middle-income countries often rely on high-income nations for these analyses. They also often exempt some traditional medicines and herbal remedies from the drug regulatory regime.

Licensing and Accreditation

The main strategy for ensuring the quality of health services in low- and middle-income countries has been to rely on licensing and accreditation, in part because of the implementation and enforcement difficulties of other approaches. High-income nations in addition often have requirements for regular continuing education or re-certification.

India, Egypt, and Nigeria offer typical examples of physician-licensing practices. The graduate of an accredited medical school applies to a government board for a license to practice by showing satisfactory completion of the required courses and evidence of good character. Once the person is granted a license to practice, no relicensing is required. Authority and responsibility for ongoing regulation and monitoring rest with the medical councils (Bennett et al. 1994).

In high-income countries, the licensing and accreditation of physicians may be two independent processes. A government agency is responsible for licensing, while accreditation is often conducted through a professional peer-review system. For example, in Canada accreditation is conducted by an independent board, with representatives from the medical profession making up less than 50% of board members. This organizational structure has led to greater emphasis on education and self-development.

The licensing and accreditation of health facilities generally focuses on easy-to-observe rules about equipment or structures. Sometimes practitioners also have to have particular qualifications. In Kenya, for example, a licensed private clinic must stock essential drugs, keep an accurate record of all drugs, and be housed in a non-residential building in a good state of repair (Bennett and Ngalande-Banda 1994).

Organizational accreditation typically takes one of two forms: either the government takes a direct role in setting standards and uses them as preconditions for continued operation and funding; or an industry's self-regulating body defines standards and monitors the institutions that voluntarily choose to participate in the scheme (Kohn et al. 2000). For example, the United Kingdom has separate regulatory structures for the private and public health-care systems. The King Edward's Hospital Fund, an independent foundation in London that aims to improve the quality of management in the National Health System, has developed a partial accreditation system for the former (Scrivens 1997).

The United States relies on self-regulatory initiatives undertaken by health-care provider organizations and by the medical profession. The Joint Commission on Accreditation of Healthcare Organizations (JCAHO), an independent not-for-profit organization, evaluates and accredits over 18,000 health-care organizations and programs, and federal and state regulations largely rely on its standards (Flanagan 1997). JCAHO, however, is reluctant to deny accreditation except where there is a clear and serious deficiency, because insurance plans only pay for services rendered by accredited health facilities. Any organization that loses its accreditation faces potential financial ruin.

In general, licensing and accreditation can only assure a basic level of quality. Focused on inputs—ranging from education to capital investment—such rules do not guarantee that the inputs in question will be properly utilized. The latter task is much more difficult, as we will see in the next section.

Regulation of Process

Practice Guidelines

Practice guidelines are a regulatory device designed to influence clinical decision-making. Theoretically, guidelines should be based on a systematic review of evidence and the judgment of medical experts. Practice guidelines can be effective in creating a standard of care when physicians view them as clinically credible and face compatible payment incentives. Evidence indicates that involving groups of physicians in the development of guidelines can increase compliance (Palmer and Hargraves 1996). Indeed, many uses of practice guidelines are not truly "regulation," according to our definition, because they are done within provider organizations and not backed by the state's coercive power.

When guidelines are supplemented with incentives, they can be more effective in altering practice. For example, the state of Massachusetts sought to reduce hypoxic brain damage from anesthesia. To do so, the state issued a regulation that anesthesiologists could not be found liable for malpractice claims if they followed guidelines promulgated by the American Society of Anesthesiologists. Episodes of hypoxic brain damage decreased by over one-half in the years following implementation of these new rules (Brahams 1989, Kelly and Swartwout 1990).

Patient Assessments

Medical quality has three aspects—clinical and service quality as well as quantity (see Chapter 6). In high-income countries, patient satisfaction is a key aspect of quality evaluations, although *patient assessments* tend to focus on the service rather than the clinical component of health services. Nevertheless, patients can also provide information about what was done clinically. For instance, patients can report whether a particular examination was performed before a diagnosis was made, and whether there were follow-up laboratory tests. In the United States, patient and community involvement in assessing both the clinical and the service quality of health care has increased significantly. By providing this feedback to physicians and other health professionals, management has successfully used patients' assessments to improve the quality of services (Palmer and Hargaves 1996). Most of the experience in this area, though, like that with guidelines, does not involve formal regulation.

Regulation of Outcomes

Studies suggest that quality assurance is most effective when outcomes are monitored (Chassin et al. 1996, Palmer and Hargraves 1996, Palmer et al. 1995). Effective outcome-management systems, however, are quite demanding administratively and therefore are not easy for low- or middle-income countries to implement. They require a regulator to determine reliable outcome measures such as complication rates or unplanned readmission rates, to set performance standards for each medical procedure, and to accumulate comprehensive and reliable databases. Even then, the necessary analysis requires sophisticated algorithms. As a result, such efforts, to date, have occurred mostly in high-income countries. Moreover, in many nations where outcome data have been collected, the reports have not been disseminated because of strong physician opposition.

Standardize Report Cards

Publishing outcome results alone can sometimes improve quality. For example, the publication of New York's data on each hospital's surgical death-rate for coronary artery bypass surgery was associated with a 41% decline over four years in operative mortality. There are reports that some hospitals took direct action to reduce mortality rates in response to the publications (Hannan et al. 1989).

The Scottish Office also has published outcome data on emergency re-admissions, mortality after admission for stroke, cervical cancer mortality, and childhood incidence of measles. Though the publication was issued with a warning that no direct inference about the quality of care in particular hospitals could or should be drawn, some purchasers reported changing contracts as a result of the data release (Hsiao 1999).

In the United States, there are many other "report card" efforts. Some magazines compile lists of the best doctors or hospitals nationally or regionally. Health insurance plans are covered by the Health Plan Employer Data and Information Set (HEDIS) reporting system. Administrators in the Punjab in India have told us that hospitals there are graded by an internal auditing system. Although the results are not made public, they do encourage competitive quality improvement. The advantage of reporting is that it can prompt customer selection or managerial initiatives, without the administrative costs and hostility of penalty-based regulations.

Clinical Audit and Peer Review

The United Kingdom and its former colonies generally rely on a clinical audit system to ensure the technical quality of medical services. Most U.S. hospitals have organized peer-review processes—called Morbidity and Mortality Rounds—where groups of doctors convene as needed to review the care of patients who suffer serious complications or death in the hospital. In many states, certain classes of adverse events must be reported to state regulators. The effectiveness of these mechanisms depends critically on professional customs and attitudes—on the willingness of doctors to be critical of each other. Since such attitudes are often not present, these mechanisms have an uneven impact.

Disciplinary Boards

Many countries rely on the medical profession to discipline physicians. For example, the British General Medical Council, a statutory professional organization, is responsible for licensing physicians and for receiving and processing complaints against the medical profession (Hsiao 1999). Other countries also have created state medical licensing and disciplinary boards, empowered to process complaints against and discipline doctors. Disciplinary proceedings for professional misconduct by medical practitioners may impose the ultimate sanction—revocation of the license to practice. But this penalty, which would deny a physician the ability to earn a livelihood from medical practice, is rarely imposed. Lesser penalties (fines, suspensions, and letters of reprimand) may not have much motivational effect. As a result, the evidence suggests that most programs of professional regulation for misconduct have been ineffective, in part due to the medical profession's domination of these boards (Hsiao 1999).

Malpractice Liability

Alone among countries of the world, the United States relies heavily on the malpractice liability of physicians to control the quality of outputs. As a regulatory strategy, the system has many detractors. Studies indicate that the majority of those injured do not sue and the majority of those who sue are not injured (Weiler et al. 1993). The use of contingency fees allows lawyers to bring speculative litigation in the hope of sharing (up to 40%) in the settlement. Sympathetic (and unsophisticated) juries often award large damages—even in cases of unavoidable injury. Still, some other countries are beginning to give patients some rights to recover damages when injured—as under India's new Consumer Protection Act (Bhat 1996).

Control supplier-induced demand

Empirical studies have documented that physicians, hospitals, and pharmacists have the market power to induce patient demand for additional units of their goods and services that have little benefit for patients, but that raise total health expenditures (Yip 1998). Many high-income countries, therefore, regulate medical manpower and investment in new medical facilities and equipment, on the theory that they can limit inappropriate utilization by controlling supply.

Regulation of Manpower

There are three points at which efforts to control the physician supply can be implemented: entrance to medical school, entrance to postgraduate programs, and entrance into practice.

National governments can control the supply of physicians—both total number and specialty mix—by regulating the number of slots in medical school and postgraduate residency programs. For example, the United Kingdom Department of Health determines the total annual intake of candidates to medical schools. Since the 1940s, committees have advised on the number of physicians to be trained, alternating between reductions due to concerns about unemployment in the medical profession, and increases in order to utilize medical school capacity (Hsiao 1999).

Canada conducted a nationwide study of medical manpower needs, based on the *need ratios* of various specialists to the population. The resulting report was developed with considerable medical school input. Based on the report's findings, medical schools were asked to adjust the number of specialty slots offered and to influence medical students' choices regarding specialty and geographic location (Hsiao 1999). Singapore limits supply by restricting specialists to 40% of new physicians and training the remaining physicians to be primary-care gatekeepers (Ministry of Health 1993). Singapore also restricts the licensing of new foreign medical graduates to a very low number each year (Hsiao 1999). There are also various indirect methods to achieve these goals, including changes to the budgets for medical schools and in the amount of scholarships awarded to medical students.

High-income nations also use regulations to redistribute human resources. For example, when Canada predicted that it would have a surplus of physicians, federal authorities restricted the immigration of foreign doctors, requiring those admitted to serve physician-scarce areas (Hsiao 1999).

Other high-income countries limit physicians by restricting the numbers who can practice either in total or in a given area. In Australia, doctors need a billing number to be paid by the national insurance system. In Germany, regional medical societies can limit the number of physicians in outpatient practice. Where the production of physicians is not coordinated with available slots, substantial excess supply can result so that new graduates will have to wait several years for employment in the health system. This is now the case in several European nations.

Limiting supply, however, can reduce competition. In the United States, admission to practice in each specialty is regulated by a specialty board—run by the doctors in that specialty. In some cases, these bodies have constrained the number trained to practice in a particular specialty, such as anesthesiology, and as a result helped create an artificial scarcity, which has raised the incomes of those specialists.

In both high- and low-income nations, there is often great political pressure to expand the number of medical school training slots, because this is seen as an effective path for social and economic mobility. As a result, many nations train more physicians than they can use, even in cases where most are trained in publicly funded schools (such as Italy, Egypt, and Yemen). In other cases, the numbers of unregulated private schools have contributed to this situation (in Japan, Lebanon, and India). Such circumstances illustrate the need for political support before any successful regulatory intervention.

Regulation of Capital Investment

As capital investment and technology acquisition increase, countries often dedicate more resources to specialized care and fewer to prevention and primary care. For those concerned about the cost-effectiveness of health services (i.e., those who take objective utilitarian concerns seriously), this pattern calls for regulation of capital investments, particularly in new medical technology, to ensure that the health system uses resources cost-effectively.

Regulation of capital investment requires technology assessment. This is a process of evaluating new technologies—compared to existing practices—in order to determine the incremental costs and benefits. This analysis can be difficult for a new technology, because it takes time to conduct the relevant studies. Meanwhile, experience with the technology often accumulates rapidly, leading to expanded patterns of use. Moreover, new technologies commonly have strong advocates—including doctors who are using the new devices, and manufacturers who produce the devices. These groups will push aggressively for adoption of new technologies well before serious studies can be concluded (Bunker et al. 1977).

Technology acquisition is closely linked with manpower considerations. From a financial point of view, the annual capital cost of a new machine may be much less than the personnel and supply costs required to operate it—by as much as a factor of seven or ten to one. Many American hospitals require physicians to have specific training before being allowed to use high-tech devices such as lasers or endoscopes. Medical and professional societies in some countries have also taken a role in assessing and ensuring the appropriateness of technology use.

Under national health service systems, decisions on the cost-effectiveness of alternative spending decisions for new capital facilities, technology acquisition, and approval of new drugs can be linked with budgetary and planning processes to ensure that overall health system objectives are met. Market-driven systems, on the other hand, lack such a planning process and must therefore depend upon competitive market forces and governmental regulatory bodies to determine investment decisions. Given political and technical weaknesses in many nations, such regulation is often lacking or ineffective.

Counteract monopoly

Regulation of Monopolies

Both private and public monopolies can exploit patients—the former for profit, and the latter in ways that suit the interests of public practitioners. Monopolistic hospitals, specialty clinics, and laboratories can compromise the quality of services and charge monopolistic prices. Most high-income countries, therefore, establish and enforce antitrust regulations to curb private monopolies. As we discussed in the previous chapter, strategies to curb public monopolies have emerged in the past decade, involving the introduction of selective contracting and the creation of internal markets.

In low- and middle-income countries, both public and private monopolies are widespread since, outside of major cities, health facilities and specialists are few. Regulation in these cases has been mostly ineffective at curbing the monopolistic practices of private for-profit institutions, due to administrative and political limitations.

Regulation of Monopolistic Prices

Even though physicians' power to charge monopolistic prices has been extensively documented (Kessel 1958, Bennett et al. 1994), most nations have found it difficult or impossible to regulate these decisions directly, for both technical and political reasons. Medical practitioners provide thousands of diverse services. Regulating their fees, therefore, is extremely complicated and requires detailed information on each transaction. Bennett and Ngalande-Banda (1994) found that no African government regulates fees charged by private practitioners, and we know of no such regulation in any low- or middle-income country.

Even high-income countries find it difficult to control the prices charged by physicians. Typically, this is done in the context of purchasing, not regulation. For example, the social insurance plans in Germany and Japan negotiate a fee schedule with umbrella organizations representing practitioners. But while social and private insurance plans, acting as purchasers, can set the fees that they will pay, they have not been effective in low- and middle-income countries in prohibiting practitioners from collecting additional charges from patients.

For many low- and middle-income countries, a critical issue is the instability in the public sector caused by the higher incomes of private practitioners. Public practitioners respond to such higher earnings in several ways. Some leave for full-time private practice. Some establish a dual practice and divert wealthier patients from public clinics to their private clinics. Others charge under-the-table fees. These actions weaken or corrupt public-sector providers. Meanwhile, low- and middle-income countries can hardly afford to pay public-sector practitioners wages that compete with private-sector earnings. As a result, some low- and middle-income nations have tried to restrict private practice by public doctors to physician-scarce areas. And even where under-the-table payments are illegal, the rules are rarely enforced.

One area where most high-income countries do regulate monopoly prices is for pharmaceuticals. This regulation is often achieved by specifying what the social insurance systems will pay for drugs. One common system, *reference pricing*, sorts all compounds into classes that are deemed to be "therapeutically equivalent" (López-Casanovas and Jönsson 2001). Then some parameter of the distribution of observed prices (such as the average) is used for all in the class. These schemes require substantial technical capacity to operate, and are now appearing in many transitional economies in Central and Eastern Europe, and in other middle-income countries.

Correct Unacceptable Market Results

Results produced by competitive markets will not necessarily be acceptable to reformers who take a variety of ethical positions seriously. Those who want to maximize health status will favor regulating the consumption of tobacco and other goods that may harm people's health, and mandate the use of seatbelts and helmets to reduce injuries—even where these behaviors would not occur in a totally free market. Others might find that a variety of transactions violate community values and hence deserve regulation. Examples of such communitarian concerns include blood transfusions, the sale of organs for transplantation, abortion, assisted suicide, and the use of certain drugs.

Insurance Regulation

Now we turn from the regulation of health-care services to the regulation of health insurance. Private health insurance is a complex futures contract whereby the insured party pays a premium in return for specific compensation if certain unpredictable future events happen. The insurance policy spells out the relevant conditions, obligations, contingencies, and exclusions that define this contract. Because they are written in technical language, such contracts are difficult to understand, and consumers can easily be exploited. In countries where private insurance is widespread, governments often find it advisable to regulate the insurance industry in various ways to prevent such exploitation.

Health insurance can be provided by three types of organizations: government agencies, parastatal organizations, and private companies. Since government typically does not regulate itself, our discussion of regulation applies to the latter two categories. Most insurance regulations pertain to three purposes of regulation: setting the rules of honest exchanges; doing what market cannot do, such as promoting equity; and correcting market failures.

The regulation of health insurance differs, depending on whether the insurance is compulsory or voluntary. For compulsory social insurance, the state is often more concerned about equity issues, unfair pricing, and deceitful business practices. For voluntary private insurance, regulation is usually more stringent and extensive, because the chances for fraud and deception are larger. In most developing countries, however, private voluntary insurance companies face few regulations—exactly because the preconditions for effective regulation discussed earlier in this chapter are often lacking. This lack, in turn, has implications for the attractiveness of private insurance as a financing strategy in such situations.

Table 11.4 summarizes the different types of insurance regulations. Because insurance is seldom involved with external effects and merit goods, those categories have been omitted.

Establish Basic Conditions for Market Exchange

Regulation of insurance plan solvency

Solvency problems are more frequent in private insurance than in social insurance systems. For social insurance, inadequate funds are typically addressed through government subsidies, increases in contribution rates, or reductions in benefits. For private insurance systems, governments regulate to prevent insolvency.

TABLE 11.4. Regulation of Insurance

CATEGORY OF REGULATIONS	HIGH-INCOME NATIONS	LOW- AND MIDDLE-INCOME NATIONS
Establish Basic Conditions for Market Exchange		
(A) Solvency of Insurance Plans	a. Establish adequate minimum capital and surplus standards b. Limit investment options c. Establish financial reporting requirements d. Establish standards for long-term actuarial soundness for both private and social insurance	Modest regulation of private health insurance with weak enforcement. Huge profits usually made by companies that are able to obtain a license to sell
(B) Sales and Marketing Practices	a. Advertising b. Disclosure of commission rates, limit maximum sales and marketing expenses c. Content and form of insurance policy	Some regulations but weak enforcement
Perfect What Market Can't Do—Equitable Distribution		
(A) Risk Pooling	a. Require insurance to set premiums on a community-wide basis b. Compel eligible households to enroll in social insurance plans	Similar laws for social insurance, but weak enforcement
(B) Equity in Financing and Benefits	Premium based on a percentage of wages in social insurance.	Similar
Correct Market Failures		
(A) Risk Selection	a. Require open enrollment, prohibit medical underwriting b. Establish risk-adjusted premiums	Social insurance is usually regulated, but not private insurance

(continued)

TABLE 11.4. Regulation of Insurance   *(continued)*

CATEGORY OF REGULATIONS	HIGH-INCOME NATIONS	LOW- AND MIDDLE-INCOME NATIONS
	c. Reinsure high-risk individuals by transferring funds retrospectively from insurers with lower average risks to those with higher risks	
	d. Require insurance to set premiums on a community-wide basis	
(B) Adverse Selection	Disclosure by enrollee of medical history and condition	Very few regulations
(C) Monopolistic Pricing	Require minimum loss ratio; i.e., a minimum percentage of premiums must be paid out for health service benefits	Very few countries regulate
Correct Unacceptable Market Results		
(A) Free-Rider	Compel all eligible population to enroll in social insurance	Same, but less effective enforcement
(B) Cost-Effectiveness	Regulate benefit package of compulsory insurance	Similar

The United States is the only high-income country that relies primarily on voluntary private insurance to fund health care. It therefore has the most experience in its regulation. Most insolvency of private insurance firms is due to mistakes in setting prices compared to claims payments, poor investment of insurance reserve funds, or fraud. After witnessing a number of bankruptcies (in which insurers could not meet their contractual obligations), the national government pressured states, who are responsible for regulating private insurance, to tighten their fiscal requirements substantially. As a consequence, states now commonly require insurers to meet certain minimum capital and surplus standards, limit their investment options, and comply with established financial reporting standards. Various rules control pricing, reinsurance, reserves, asset-liability matching, and transactions with affiliates and management, and reporting on financial statements. Countries that have established private insurance without such controls (e.g., the Czech Republic) have seen a substantial number of bankruptcies due to poor business practices.

Governments also establish minimum standards for the qualifications of those who perform key technical tasks in the insurance industry. For example, actuaries who determine premium rates and reserves (Skipper 1992) are often subject to state or professional society regulation.

Regulation of sales and marketing practices

Much private insurance is sold through agents who receive a commission for each sale. Because of the complexity of insurance contracts, private insurance plans and their agents can use deceptive sales practices to sell their products. High-income countries regulate potential deception by regulating the form and contents of insurance contracts. Insurance plans must file their policy forms for approval by regulatory authorities (Fuenzalida-Puelma 1996). Often, sales literature and advertising are also regulated. Furthermore, to prevent private insurance plans from paying excess commissions to their sales agents and staff to promote sales, high-income countries establish loss ratio requirements that restrict the percentage of premiums that can be used for administration, sales expenses, and profits.

Enhance Equity

Regulation of risk pooling

In a fully competitive insurance market, the "equilibrium price" would reflect the expected payout (the risk) for each individual. This means that the healthy would pay smaller premiums, and the less healthy much higher premiums. To promote equity, however, many countries require high and low risks to be pooled for an entire community (community rating), instead of having different premium rates for different groups or individuals. This approach is used in Australia, for example. Reinsurance is also used as a mechanism to pool risks across a larger population.

In recent years, Germany has required the payroll tax rate of each sickness fund to be the same for all members, coupled with a reinsurance arrangement to even out the risks across sickness funds (Saltman and Figueras 1997). In the United States, many states require Blue Cross, a nonprofit health insurance plan, to base its premiums on community rating (Chollet and Lewis 1997).

Pay health premiums according to ability to pay

Even when a nation uses community rating to pool risks, a flat premium charge would require low-wage workers to pay a larger portion of their earnings for health insurance than high-wage workers. For equity reasons, many high-income nations have created social insurance schemes where premiums are based on a uniform percentage of wages instead of a flat amount. Where multiple parastatal, nonprofit, or for-profit funds operate, they are often required to set premiums in this way, as in Chile. Colombia has gone one step further. Besides a wage-based premium rate, it adds a surcharge to the rate for workers' social insurance contribution and uses this revenue to subsidize insurance for the poor (Londoño 1994).

Correct Market Failures

Regulation of risk selection

As we discussed in Chapter 8 on financing, insurance plans have an incentive to engage in risk selection, to insure healthy people and reject the less healthy. To counteract these practices, governments sometimes require that plans accept anyone who chooses to enroll during an open enrollment period. In addition, governments can reduce risk selection by prohibiting medical underwriting, restricting the exclusion of pre-existing conditions, and requiring insurers not to cancel policies for those who become sick. In the United States, risk selection remains a serious problem in many markets, because insurers have numerous subtle ways to encourage the less healthy to leave and enroll with another insurance plan. To address such problems, New York State had to create a reinsurance mechanism by transferring funds retrospectively from insurers with low risks to firms with higher risks.

Regulation of adverse selection

Sophisticated consumers who know they are relatively healthy may not be impressed when they calculate the costs and benefits of the insurance plans offered to them. If the rates they are offered reflect average risks, they may choose not to buy. Meanwhile, those who know they are sick will rush to be covered. Such *adverse selection* (as discussed in Chapter 8) does not allow insurers to pool the costs of covering healthy persons with the less healthy. Premiums—based on the costs of covering the less healthy—could then become unaffordable for most people. Compulsory insurance is often used to deter adverse selection and to pool the risks between the old and the young, the healthy and the less healthy.

Correct Unacceptable Market Results

Regulation of free riders

Many nations provide subsidized public-health services for those who are uninsured and cannot afford to pay for services. This arrangement may encourage people who are eligible for insurance coverage, but who have to pay a premium, not to sign up for insurance. To correct such *free-rider* problems, many nations require all eligible persons to enroll in an insurance program. Then the risks are pooled across a large population, which is one of the major advantages of social insurance.

Regulation of cost-effectiveness

In spite of public education efforts, purchasers of insurance may not have an adequate understanding of the benefits of certain preventive services. As a result, they may not buy insurance that covers such services. Governments, therefore, often use regulation to specify which minimum health services must be included in the benefit package.

Conditional Guidance

Just as other control knobs may require regulatory efforts to be effective, so, too, regulation often needs other control knobs to supplement it. One reason for this is the nature of regulation. Most regulations forbid or limit what organizations and individuals want to do. Yet regulation is limited, because it relies on the coercive power of the state to enforce compliance—and that power, too, is limited. Combining efforts to influence customer and provider behavior with incentives is one way to enhance voluntary compliance.

These considerations often seem to have been overlooked in the current push by international organizations for ministries of health to relinquish their financing role and rely instead on regulatory enforcement. Giving up the potential for incentives, as offered by the financing and payment systems, can be a grave strategic error for health-sector reformers. Combining regulation with incentives, on the other hand, can make rules more flexible and increase voluntary compliance.

There is a great tendency for low- and middle-income nations to attempt to transplant the regulations of certain high-income nations and make them their own. This approach seems like a quick and inexpensive way to develop a national program. Unfortunately, these nations are unlikely to enjoy regulatory success, unless they have taken into account their own particular circumstances.

We stressed at the beginning of this chapter that the success of regulation depends on cultural attitudes, government capacity, and political support. Regulatory success is more likely in countries where there is less corruption, more popular deference to formal authority, a well-functioning bureaucracy, and effective police and court systems. Successful regulatory enforcement will depend on the design of regulatory institutions and processes. Many practical features are relevant, including the resources regulators have, their technical competence, the available data, the processes for detecting violations and imposing sanctions, and the degree of voluntary compliance. The better-off a country is in these regards, the more likely it is that the regulatory system will function effectively and actually modify behavior. Simply put, the task of regulators is not the same in Swaziland as in Switzerland.

As part of developing a regulatory strategy, reformers should conduct a careful analysis to assess the political costs and benefits and the technical and administrative feasibility of the proposed regulations. Since the political and organizational resources required to legislate and implement regulations are limited, there is a need to decide where the largest gains are likely to be made and to develop an overall plan for how to proceed. The plan should include an assessment of the political feasibility of various interventions, and political strategies for passing the regulations, establishing appropriate regulatory bodies, and implementing the new rules.

In developing their strategic analysis, reformers should carefully consider issues of enforceability. Enforcement difficulties often differ for the four categories of regulations we have identified. Rules that define the basic conditions for market exchange, such as specifying property rights and rules for buying and selling, are easier to enforce than other kinds of regulation. The victims of violations of such rules will often be sophisticated economic actors, and they are likely to complain and initiate remedial action. On the other hand, regulation to promote equity is less likely to be effective. Requiring private clinics and hospitals to give free services to the poor, for example, will often be resisted, and the victims will frequently be socially or economically marginalized and unable to protest effectively. Similarly, it is difficult to use regulation to move doctors into underserved areas. The doctors in question ignore clinic hours, treat patients rudely, lack critical supplies, and sometimes just relocate elsewhere. The monitoring and enforcement problems in such cases are formidable. Hence, the state may have to rely on another control knob, such as financing or organization, to achieve its equity goals (see Chapters 7 and 10).

Regulation to correct market failure (e.g., to assure the quality and safety of water, food, and pharmaceuticals) typically enjoys great social acceptance and public support in high-income countries. In these areas, there are few alternatives to state action, and governments in such countries often have the needed technical and administrative capacity to act effectively. This is a good example of the principle that cultural attitudes have a major impact on regulatory enforceability. On the other hand, many low-income countries will find such regulatory activities difficult to establish. Popular attention may be focused on other issues, and the necessary political support and administrative capacity may be lacking.

Regulation designed to correct market failures can have a significant impact on the quality and efficiency of health services and on the functioning of insurance markets. The need to correct such market failures, however, depends on how much a nation relies on the market and for what. We have seen how many kinds of interventions are available here, from information, to certification, to licensing, to process controls on medical practice. Again, the more complex approaches will be beyond the capacity of many low-income countries. But some efforts to improve service delivery—for example, by publishing ratings and reports on hospitals—can have an impact in all but the poorest settings. And while the harm caused by some market failures (e.g., cream-skimming in private insurance markets) is primarily financial, and may be confined to upper-income groups, other kinds of quality failures do produce direct health-status impacts.

Regulation and Equity

Because we ourselves are egalitarians, we want to offer some concluding comments to reformers who share our values and specifically consider how regulatory efforts relate to equity concerns. The first point is that the poor, uneducated, and socially marginalized are often the populations that are most vulnerable to exploitation in the marketplace. Yet, they are also populations that are less likely to benefit from certain regulatory initiatives—especially those focused on informational strategies like product labeling, report cards, and disclosure rules. Limited sophistication and a diminished sense of personal efficacy can make it more difficult for the marginalized to use such information effectively. Such initiatives should not be avoided for this reason; but reformers need to be acutely sensitive to the differential effectiveness of regulatory approaches for disadvantaged populations.

By the same token, efforts to restrict the range of products or services available in the marketplace—by controlling unsafe drugs or incompetent providers, for example—are more likely to benefit less-sophisticated buyers. For such individuals are less able to defend themselves through their own purchasing decisions. At the same time, such restrictions also are likely to restrict the supply of lower-cost goods and services available to low-income households. Hence, regulators need to strike a careful balance between protecting buyers from the genuinely harmful and using their regulatory authority in ways that reinforce the monopoly position of organized professional groups and established corporate interests.

Moreover, poor households often rely, not just on the market, but also on the public sector for services. Hence, the most important initiatives for improving both clinical and service quality for them will often lie within the scope of the organization control knob—as discussed in the previous chapter. Indeed, better service in the public sector will serve to protect vulnerable populations from exploitation by private sellers because it will shift their consumption away from such suppliers.

Poor households may also need to be protected in other ways as well. A recent study of kidney sales in India revealed that such sales did not provide long-term economic benefits to sellers, and did lead to health-status declines among the disproportionately poor persons who engaged in such sales (Goyal et al. 2002). Similar issues may arise in the context of clinical trials of new pharmaceuticals.

Another realm of regulation that may be necessary in some contexts, but that does not do much from an equity point of view, involves the regulation of private insurance. As we discussed in the chapter on financing, as well as earlier in this chapter, such financing schemes are economically regressive. They also require substantial regulatory intervention to assure financial viability and to help promote the kind of risk-sharing that leads to real risk-protection. For these reasons, we are generally not advocates of such financing schemes—in part because they put a great burden on what is often a limited governmental regulatory capacity. Where they are used, however, we believe the needed regulation should be undertaken, albeit that such efforts will generally benefit the middle and upper-income groups, who will be the predominant purchasers of such insurance.

A final equity domain in the regulatory arena involves the regulation of the pharmaceutical industry, to assure the availability of affordable, safe, and effective medicines. It is now widely recognized that major global inequities exist in access to medicines between rich and poor countries, for many important diseases (Reich 2000). Regulation has an important role in determining these inequities in access and in shaping policy solutions.

First, many governments around the world regulate drug prices, in a variety of ways (Ess et al. 2003). Some countries set prices at the retail level, according to different classes of products, as occurs in India. Other countries, such as Japan, set reimbursement rates for individual products and for payment to dispensing physicians and health facilities. In Europe, a common system involves "reference prices," where government sets a purchase price for each class of drugs, based on prices in the marketplace, and the patient or supplemental insurer pays the difference if a more-expensive drug is prescribed (López-Casanovas and Jönsson 2001). Such systems are mostly used in the context of social insurance schemes that pay for a significant share of drug purchases. The regulation of drug prices is intended to ensure the availability of needed medicines for patients while containing the costs for government and other payers.

A third major regulatory approach to medicines involves the domestic manufacture or importation of lower-priced generic alternatives to patented drugs. This approach has depended, for many countries in the past, on national laws that did not recognize patents for pharmaceutical products. The recent round of international trade negotiations, however, agreed to introduce product patents for pharmaceuticals around the world, with some delays in implementation for the poorest countries, under the Trade-Related Aspects of Intellectual Property Rights Agreement, better known as TRIPS (Foster 1998). The interpretation of several key clauses in TRIPS—covering policies for pharmaceutical products—has become a major source of international controversy, with important ethical, political, economic, and public health implications (Velásquez and Boulet 1999). One key question is which diseases should be covered under rules that would loosen patent restrictions and allow the world's poorest countries facing a public health crisis to produce or import generic versions of medicines still under patent in developed countries (Fleck 2003). The United States stalemated the talks by seeking to restrict the scope to infectious diseases (such as HIV/AIDS, malaria, and tuberculosis), while other countries have sought to include noninfectious diseases (such as asthma, cardiovascular conditions, and obesity).

These regulatory issues of prices, formularies, and patents have been pushed into the international trade arena by the highly-publicized case of antiretroviral treatment for HIV. In that case, the equity implications were starkly presented for all to see: AIDS mortality dropped precipitously in rich countries when triple-drug therapy became widely available, while the vast majority of the world's AIDS patients, in poor countries, continued to die, because of continued lack of access to the same antiretroviral medicines. After substantial public and political pressures were applied, a number of pharmaceutical companies decided to lower their prices in the poorest countries—although access remains far below what is needed. For other diseases as well, efforts have been made, through public-private partnerships, to expand access to new medicines for such diseases as onchocerciasis, trachoma, and lymphatic filariasis (Reich 2002). While these efforts can be very helpful to recipient nations for specific populations, the programs are not a long-term solution to pharmaceutical access problems in poor countries.

Unfortunately, we cannot explore all the complex issues raised by these examples of pharmaceutical regulatory options. But we would be remiss not to note the potentially important links between regulation and equity.

Summary

In sum, the regulation control knob can be an effective measure to improve the performance of a health system, particularly when it is combined appropriately with incentives, behavior change, and suitable organizational arrangements. While it may seem relatively easy to establish regulations, the technical challenges of doing this well can be formidable, and the organizational and political obstacles to enforcement can be even more difficult. Regulation can significantly change behaviors in some situations, but its impact can be insignificant in others.

Health-sector reformers who want to make a real difference need to think carefully about the likely enforcement process, the available resources, legal capacity, political support, data and monitoring systems, and the incentives that regulation will generate, before pursuing the regulatory route.

While we have repeatedly cautioned the reader about the possibility of regulatory failures, we equally stress the large inefficiencies and inequities caused by market-driven systems without adequate regulation (Herrin 1997, Hsiao 1994, Nittayaramphong and Tangcharoensathein 1994). Therefore, reformers face a complex balancing act between what is desirable and what is feasible in devising the best strategic approach to regulation.

References

Ayres, Ian; and John Braithwaite. 1992. *Responsive Regulation: Transcending the Deregulation Debate.* Oxford Socio-Legal Studies No. 39. New York: Oxford University Press.

Bennett, Sara; and Ellias E. Ngalande-Banda. 1994. *Public and Private Roles in Health: A Review and Analysis of Experience in Sub-Saharan Africa.* SHS Paper Number 6, Geneva: World Health Organization.

Bennett, Sara; George Dakpallah; Paul Garner; Lucy Gilson; Sanguan Nittayaramphong; Beatriz Zurita; and Anthony Zwi. 1994. "Carrot and Stick: State Mechanisms to Influence Private Provider Behavior." *Health Policy and Planning* 9(1): 1–13.

Bhat, Rau. 1996. "Regulating the Private Health Care Sector: The Case of the Indian Consumer Protection Act." *Health Policy and Planning* 11(3): 265–79.

Brahams, Diana. 1989. "Monitoring Equipment and Anaesthetic Failures." *Lancet* 1(8629): 111–2.

Bunker, John P.; Frederick Mosteller; and Benjamin A. Barnes, eds. 1977. *Costs, Risks, and Benefits of Surgery.* New York: Oxford University Press.

Chassin, Mark R.; Edward L. Hannan; and Barbara A. DeBuono. 1996. "Benefits and Hazards of Reporting Medical Outcomes Publicly." *New England Journal of Medicine* 334: 394–8.

Chollet, Deborah J.; and Maureen Lewis. 1997. "Private Insurance: Principles and Practice." In: George J. Schieber, ed., *Innovations in Health Care Financing: Proceedings of a World Bank Conference.* World Bank Discussion Paper No. 365. Washington, DC: World Bank, March 10–11.

De Geyndt, Willy. 1995. *Managing the Quality of Health Care in Developing Countries.* World Bank Technical Paper No. 258. Washington, DC: World Bank.

Donabedian, Avedis. 1980. *Explorations in Quality: Assessment and Monitoring, Volume I: The Definition of Quality and Approaches to Its Assessment.* Ann Arbor, MI: Health Administration Press.

Ess, Silvia M.; Sebastian Schneeweiss; Thomas D. Szucs. 2003. "European Healthcare Policies for Controlling Drug Expenditure." *Pharmacoeconomics* 21(2): 89–103.

Feldman, Penny; and Marc Roberts. 1980. "Magic Bullets or Seven Card Stud: Understanding Health Care Regulation." In: Richard S. Gordon, ed., *Issues in Healthcare Regulation.* New York: McGraw-Hill.

Fleck, Fiona. 2003. "U.S. Blocks Deal on Cheap Drugs." *British Medical Journal* 326: 9.

Flanagan, Anne. 1997. "Ensuring Health Care Quality: JCAHO's Perspective." *Clinical Therapeutics* 19: 1540–54.

Foster, George K. 1998. "Opposing Forces in a Revolution in International Patent Protection: The U.S. and India in the Uruguay Round and Its Aftermath." *UCLA Journal of International and Foreign Affairs* 3: 283–323.

Fuenzalida-Puelma; L. Hernan. 1996. *Regulation of Health Insurance: Conceptual Framework, Case Studies on Hungary and Turkey, Notes on Croatia and Lithuania*. Washington, DC: World Bank, Human Development Department.

Fuller, Lon L. 1978. *The Morality of Law*. Revised ed. New Haven, CT: Yale University Press.

Goyal, Madhav; Ravindra L. Mehta; Lawrence J. Schneiderman; and Ashwini R. Sehgalet. 2002. "Economic and Health Consequences of Selling a Kidney in India." *JAMA* 288(13): 1584–93.

Graham, Cosmo. 1994. "Self-Regulation." In: Genevra Richardson and Hazel Genn, eds. *Administrative Law and Government Action: The Courts and Alternative Mechanisms of Review*. Oxford: Clarendon Press.

Hannan, E. L.; J. F. O'Donnell; H. Kilburn, Jr.; H. R. Bernard; and A. Yazici. 1989. "Investigation of the Relationship Between Volume and Mortality for Surgical Procedures Performed in New York State Hospitals." *JAMA* 262: 503–10.

Heriot, Gail L. 1997. "An Introduction: The Symposium on Law, Human Behavior and Evolution." *Journal of Contemporary Legal Issues* 1: 1–2.

Herrin, Alejandro. 1997. "Private Health Sector Performance and Regulation in the Philippines." In: William Newbrander, ed., *Private Health Sector Growth in Asia: Issues and Implications*. Chichester, England: Wiley.

Hsiao, William C. 1994. "Marketization—The Illusory Magic Pill." *Health Economics* 3(6): 351–7.

———. 1995. "Abnormal Economics in the Health Sector." *Health Policy* 32: 125–39.

———. 1999. *International Comparison of Health Systems—Special Report No. 2*. China: Government Printing Office, Hong Kong Special Administrative Region.

Irvine, Donald. 1997. "The Performance of Doctors 1: Professionalism and Self-Regulation in a Changing World." *British Medical Journal* 314: 1540–42.

Kelly, John T.; and James E. Swartwout. 1990. "Development of Practice Parameters by Physicians' Organizations." *Quality Review Bulletin* 2: 54–7.

Kessel, Reuben A. 1958. "Price Discrimination in Medicine." *Journal of Law and Economics*, 1: 20–53.

Kohn, Linda T.; Janet M. Corrigan; and Molla S. Donaldson, eds. 2000. *To Err Is Human: Building a Safer Health System*. Washington, DC: National Academy Press.

Laffont, Jean-Jacques; and Jean Tirole. 1993. *A Theory of Incentives in Procurement and Regulation*. Cambridge, MA: MIT Press.

Landy, Marc K.; Marc J. Roberts; and Stephen R. Thomas. 1990. *The Environmental Protection Agency: Asking the Wrong Questions*. New York: Oxford University Press.

Londoño de la Cuesta, Juan L. 1994. *Carga de la Enfermedad en Colombia*. Santafe de Bogota, Colombia: Ministerio de Salud.

López-Casanovas, Guillem; and Bengt Jönsson, eds. 2001. *Reference Pricing and Pharmaceutical Policy: Perspectives on Economics and Innovation*. Barcelona, Spain: Springer.

Ministry of Health, Government of Singapore. 1993. *Affordable Health Care*. Singapore: Ministry of Health.

Musgrave, Richard A.; and Peggy B. Musgrave. 1989. *Public Finance in Theory and Practice*. New York: McGraw-Hill.

Nittayaramphong, Sanguan; and Viroj Tangcharoensathien. 1994. "Thailand: Private Health Care Out of Control?" *Health Policy and Planning* 1: 31–40.

North, Douglass C. 1990. *Institutions, Institutional Change and Economic Performance*. New York: Cambridge University Press.

Oakeshott, Michael. 1975. *On Human Conduct*. Oxford, England: Clarendon Press.

OECD. 1996. *Regulatory Reform: Overview and Proposed OECD Work Plan*. Paris: Organization for Economic Cooperation and Development.

Palmer, R. H.; A. G. Lawthers; J. DeLozier; N. J. Banks; L. Peterson; and B. Duggar. 1995. *Understanding and Choosing Clinical Performance Measures for Quality Improvement: Development of a Typology*. Washington, DC: Agency for Health Care Policy Research.

Palmer, R. Heather; and Lee J. Hargraves. 1996. "Summary: Methods, Findings and Discussions." *Medical Care* Suppl(34) 9: 3–11.

Reich, Michael R. 2000. "The Global Drug Gap." *Science* 287: 1979–81.

———. 1994. "Bangladesh Pharmaceutical Policy and Politics." *Health Policy and Planning* 9(2): 130–43.

———. ed. 2002. *Public-Private Partnerships for Public Health*. Cambridge, MA: Harvard Center for Population and Development Studies, distributed by Harvard University Press.

Roberts, Marc J.; and Susan Farrell. 1978. "The Political Economy of Implementation: The Clean Air Act and Stationary Sources." In: Ann F. Friedlaender, ed., *Approaches to Controlling Air Pollution*. Cambridge, MA: MIT Press.

Rosen, Harvey S. 2002. *Public Finance*. Boston, MA: McGraw-Hill/Irwin.

Saltman, Richard B.; and Josep Figueras. 1997. *European Health Care Reform: Analysis of Current Strategies*. WHO Regional Publications, European Series No. 72. Copenhagen: World Health Organization, Regional Office for Europe.

Scrivens, Ellie. 1997. "Assessing the Value of Accreditation Systems." *European Journal of Public Health* 7: 4–8.

Shklar, Judith. 1987. "Political Theory and the Rule of Law." In: Alan C. Hutchinson and Patrick J. Monahan, eds., *The Rule of Law: Ideal or Ideology*. Toronto: Carswell.

Skipper, Harold D., Jr. 1992. *Insurer Solvency Regulation in the United States*. Research Report 92–4. Atlanta, GA: Georgia State University, Center for Risk Management and Insurance Research.

Stigler, George J. 1971. "The Theory of Economic Regulation." *The Bell Journal of Economics and Management Science* 2(1): 3–21.

Transparency International. 2000. *Corruption Perception Index* (CPI 2000). Berlin: Transparency International. Available from www.transparency.org. Accessed June 2002.

Velásquez, Germán, and Pascale Boulet. 1999. *Globalization and Access to Drugs: Perspectives on the WTO/TRIPS Agreement*. Revised. DAP Series No. 7. Geneva: World Health Organization, Action Programme on Essential Drugs.

Weiler, Paul C.; Howard H. Hiatt; Joseph P. Newhouse; William G. Johnson; Troyen A. Brennan; and Lucian L. Leape. 1993. *A Measure of Malpractice: Medical Injury Malpractice Litigation, and Patient Compensation*. Cambridge, MA: Harvard University Press.

Williamson, Oliver E. 1985. *The Economic Institutions of Capitalism: Firms, Markets, Relational Contracting*. New York: Free Press.

Yip, Winnie. 1998. "Physicians' Response to Medicare Fee Reductions: Changes in the Volume and Intensity of Supply of Coronary Artery Bypass Graft (CABG) Procedures for the Medicare and Provider Sectors." *Journal of Health Economics* 17(6): 675–99.

12

Behavior

Health-system performance and health status are affected by individual behavior in many ways. Sexual practices and needle-sharing have major impacts on HIV/AIDS. Whether people conscientiously take their medicines affects the success of tuberculosis control programs. Vaccination rates influence infant mortality. Physician prescribing habits for antibiotics influence the cost and the effectiveness of diarrheal disease control programs and the growth of microbial resistance. Driving habits and seatbelt use affect traffic deaths. In short, individual behavior can have a major impact on both personal health and health-system performance.

As providers and patients, eaters and drinkers, drivers and lovers, individuals respond to many forces. Some of these forces are determined by other control knobs: the financing and payment systems and organization and regulatory structures. But behaviors are also grounded in culture and social structure, in habits, values, perceptions, beliefs, attitudes, and ideas. This chapter describes the fifth control knob: methods for changing individual behavior through population-based interventions. Our primary concern is how the behavior control knob can be used to improve health-system performance and promote public-health goals.

In this chapter, we first introduce the basic concepts of behavior change in relationship to health-system performance and then explore four categories of individual behavior that are important to that performance. Next, we present advice about how to achieve behavior change, through a discussion of the basic elements of social marketing. We conclude with a discussion of the strengths and weaknesses of different behavior-change strategies in the context of health-sector reform.

The *behavior* control knob involves the design, implementation, and evaluation of programs intended to change individual behavior in order to improve health-system performance. Various approaches in the fields of information, education, and communication (IEC) and social marketing are all relevant. In particular, we use the term "*social marketing*" to mean a conceptual framework for designing interventions based on marketing principles. This framework will be a major focus in what follows.

In addition to messages aimed at individuals, changing individual behavior often can be helped by the coordinated application of one or more of the four other control knobs. For example, a behavior-change campaign might want to supplement an educational campaign with monetary incentives (payment) to providers, or rules governing their behavior. Similarly, the organization of the health-care system can be altered to influence patient utilization of specific health facilities. In discussing the behavior control knob, we will thus want to refer to the four other control knobs where these are relevant. But this chapter does not consider strategies to influence the political acceptability of health policy proposals, since these issues are addressed in Chapter 4.

Our understanding of options for the behavior control knob draws heavily from the field of social marketing, and we use many of its concepts in this chapter. The field of social marketing began in 1969, with a seminal work by Philip Kotler and Sidney J. Levy (1969), who observed that marketing methods were being used throughout American society to sell everything, from soap, to colleges, to politicians. They argued that all organizations confronting marketing challenges could benefit from using marketing approaches, whether the organization was selling a tangible commercial product or an intangible social idea. In this chapter, we have adapted the Kotler and Levy approach to social marketing to the issues of health reform.

Efforts to change individual behavior for public-health goals occur in the context of pervasive commercial marketing, which seeks to shape behavior for private profit. Commercial marketing invades all aspects of modern life, selling everything from cigarettes, to coffee, to computers, to condoms, to cough syrup. It explicitly advances commercial goals rather than public interests, although some commercial marketing (e.g., for condoms) can contribute to public-health goals. Such commercial marketing can have significant consequences for health-system performance, as exemplified by the marketing of fast food, infant formula, and tobacco products. Countries in transition from state-socialist to market-oriented systems have experienced a surge in commercial marketing, with dramatic changes in the patterns and amounts of private and public health expenditures. Sales of pharmaceutical products, for example, exploded in the largely unregulated market of Vietnam's transitional economy in the 1990s (McManus 1998). Marketing by private medical practitioners and private hospitals also shapes public expectations about medical services and can lead to expanded use of high-technology medical equipment and services (such as CAT scanners) and expanded demands on tertiary hospitals, as has occurred in Korea (Yang 1996).

The behavior control knob provides a way for health policymakers to counter-balance the negative health consequences of all this commercial marketing and to redirect individual behaviors in ways that promote public-health goals. The perva-siveness of commercial marketing leads to some of the behaviors that health-sector reformers would like to change, yet also creates political and practical challenges to its successful utilization.

Efforts to improve health-system performance by changing individual behavior can benefit from the lessons of commercial marketing. Like commercial market-ing, behavior-change efforts must recognize the central role of the customer and understand that the easiest way to change behavior is by helping to meet the cus-tomer's wants and needs. Health reformers need to work with the values, beliefs, and perceptions of customers, because these, after all, are the factors that shape health-related attitudes, knowledge, and behavior. Interventions that support or coincide with deeply rooted cultural values have a better chance of success, while those that challenge such values have a high risk of failure (as we noted similarly for regulation, in Chapter 11).

To be effective, health reformers need to combine different kinds of behavior-change approaches. In general, reformers should not seek to "push" certain practices or ideas on people; instead, they should find ways to "pull" new, desired concepts to existing values held by the individual.

Approaches to changing individual behavior vary from relatively low-coercion approaches like simply providing information, to relatively high-coercion efforts like regulation and prohibition (Table 12.1). The strategies covered by this control knob are somewhere in the middle. Social marketing can be more coercive than simply providing information, because it prepares, packages, and presents messages with the intention of producing specific behavioral changes. It often uses influence and persuasion based on emotion and symbolism, unlike the simple provision of infor-mation. Do note that there is some coercion involved in purposively supplying biased or incomplete information. The degree of coercion incorporated in behavior-change interventions can raise important ethical concerns, which we discuss later.

TABLE 12.1. Approaches to Change Individual Behavior

Information	Less Coercive
Marketing	↑
Incentives	
Restriction	
Indoctrination	↓
Prohibition	More Coercive

In designing behavior-change strategies, health reformers confront three common marketing challenges (Kotler and Levy 1969). First, they need a clear definition of the *product*, including both tangible products (including goods and services) and intangible products (such as ideas and beliefs). Second, they need to consider the product's relationship to specific *consumers* in the health system. Various kinds of consumers should be considered: clients (or direct consumers of the product), decision-makers (or policymakers for the health system), key stakeholders (who have a specific interest in the product), and the general public (all those whose attitudes might affect the product's use in some way). Third, health reformers need to identify *tools* that can promote the product's acceptance by the consumers. In this chapter, we examine tools for changing health behaviors in relation to the *four Ps of marketing*: To develop "the right *product* backed by the right *promotion* and put in the right *place* at the right *price*" (Kotler and Zaltman 1971).

The first widespread applications of social marketing involved family planning organizations in developing countries in the late 1960s and early 1970s. At that time, contraceptive distribution in developing countries became a high priority for the U.S. Agency for International Development and for private foundations, and they promoted the new methods of social marketing. The first national social-marketing effort was the Nirodh Condom Project, which was initiated by the government of India with assistance from the Ford Foundation (Altman and Piotrow 1980). These projects commonly used commercial distribution channels, with government support and social marketing strategies to expand consumer demand. The projects also gave rise to many consulting organizations that specialized in social marketing for family planning and health. In 1997, 60 large-scale contraceptive social-marketing projects operated in 55 countries around the world. These projects sold a total of 937 million condoms and 54.5 million cycles of pills in 1997, and reported a 13% increase in the number of couples served from the previous year—outcomes that have been attributed to the successful application of social marketing methods (DKT International 1998).

To date, behavior-change approaches have not been fully exploited to improve health-system performance. They have been directed mainly at fostering the adoption of particular health-related products or practices: contraception, breastfeeding, tobacco, bed nets, immunization, and oral rehydration salts. Behavior-change efforts focused on getting people to reduce their use of something have been less widespread and less successful. In part, this reflects our earlier point about how marketing works best when it meets people's deeply felt needs. Unfortunately, there is a limited availability of good substitute products to enable the "de-marketing" of risky behaviors (such as smoking and certain sexual practices). Where such products do exist (such as smoking cessation patches and condoms), they are often less effective in meeting those needs than the products they are trying to replace.

Another problem that has limited the effectiveness of behavior change is that individual problem-by-problem interventions have not been systematically connected to broader issues of health-system performance. Health-reform efforts have sometimes included the development of "communication plans," but these have usually been directed at the processes of *adopting* a reform proposal (processes we considered in Chapter 4 on politics), rather than as part of health reform itself. We argue that many opportunities exist to influence individual behaviors within health-reform plans, and that behavior change needs to be considered a basic control knob for health reform, to improve overall health-system performance and assist in achieving the core criteria.

Categories of Individual Behavior

Where can the behavior-change control knob be used in health-reform efforts? Here it is important to consider four categories of individual behavior:

- treatment-seeking behaviors
- health professional behaviors
- patient compliance behaviors, and
- lifestyle and prevention behaviors.

Each category can be related to important objectives for health-sector reform, including core criteria and intermediate criteria.

Treatment-Seeking Behaviors

Consumer decisions on when, where, and how to seek treatment are an important area for improving health-system performance. These treatment-seeking decisions include the kind of health professional (e.g., specialist versus generalist), the level of health facility (primary care versus teaching hospital), the timing and location of the treatment, and the use of traditional versus Western medicine. These consumer behaviors often involve interaction with a health professional, including physicians, midwives, traditional healers, and private drug sellers. Treatment-seeking behaviors are important for acute health problems (e.g., trauma and fevers) as well as chronic health problems (e.g., diabetes and health disease).

Because this is not an area of extensive experience, we will use a hypothetical example to illustrate its potential. Imagine, for example, a campaign to encourage patients to visit local clinics before seeking care at a regional hospital. The goal would be to enhance the efficiency of the referral system, diminish overcrowding at regional centers, and provide care in less costly settings where possible. All of this would enhance the technical efficiency of the system as a whole. To be successful, this campaign would require research into the reasons that patients avoid the local primary-care clinic, including perceptions of and real problems with the quality, cost, and availability of services at those sites. Suppose that research revealed that the advantages people saw with local centers were their accessibility (less travel and waiting time) and their less imposing size and less rigid bureaucratic system of operation. The negatives were lack of staff availability during clinic hours and concerns about quality. Then you might imagine a social marketing campaign that included slogans like "Go first to your local health center— Good doctors close to you" or "Go where they know you—Use your local health center first." But efforts would also be needed to improve the quality of services at primary-care clinics (through the organization control knob). For getting people to go to the centers—only to have them disillusioned by what they encounter there—would not convince them that your suggestion will meet their basic needs.

Of course, persuasion does not have to work alone. It could be combined with more-coercive initiatives. For example, the payment control knob could also be used, by raising patient co-payments at the tertiary-care facility and providing free treatment at the primary-care facility. By using a gatekeeper mechanism (an example of the regulation control knob), the effort could also require patients to receive approval from the primary-care physician before being seen at the tertiary-care facility.

Health Professional Behaviors

Provider decisions about treatment represent a second important category of individual behavior that can be addressed through this control knob. Important provider decisions include the nature of the treatment, including adherence to practice guidelines; the amount of attention given to preventative care; the location of treatment (a public hospital versus the provider's private office); and the referral of patients to other providers. Nor is government the only potential actor here, since issues of professional ethics can be addressed by behavior-change campaigns directed by professional societies and targeted at their members.

There is a huge literature on quality improvement for health services, frequently involving changes in provider behavior. One example in developing countries is the PROQUALI project, which seeks to improve the quality of reproductive health services in two states of Brazil. The project moves beyond conventional notions of clinical quality to a "new client-oriented model" of quality improvement. The PROQUALI approach involves organizational changes within the clinic, combined with external assessment for accreditation, followed by community recognition through an awards ceremony. The project also includes community mobilization to enhance local demand for quality performance (PROQUALI 2000).

This program is based on the realization that interpersonal dynamics of provider–patient relations can be significant determinants of perceptions of service quality and can affect health-seeking behavior, thereby influencing health status and consumer satisfaction. Changing the attitudes and behaviors of health providers, therefore, can make a major difference in how patients seek care and respond to treatment.

Many behavior-change strategies have been directed at the prescribing patterns of physicians and pharmacies. Drug prescribers are one of the main targets for commercial pharmaceutical marketing in the health sector. Partly in response, the practice of "academic detailing" has been developed to provide information to physicians, using a social marketing approach in order to change their prescribing behavior and improve the quality and cost-effectiveness of the medicines selected (Soumerai and Avorn 1990).

In developing countries, strategies to promote the rational use of drugs have included efforts to change the prescribing practices not only of physicians but also of commercial pharmacies, especially in environments where products are sold without a physician's prescription and often without the consultation of a trained pharmacist. For example, campaigns have targeted drug sellers to encourage the sale of oral rehydration salts and discourage the sale of antibiotics for cases of diarrhea (Ross-Degnan et al. 1996). Other campaigns have sought to discourage the use of injections, even though patients may want and expect this form of treatment as part of a medical visit.

These efforts illustrate a conflict that can arise between the goals of enhancing consumer satisfaction and improving health status. Injections may be the treatment that consumers prefer, but they may not be necessary or cost-effective, and can even cause health problems through the reuse of needles that transmit infectious diseases such as hepatitis and HIV. Successful social marketing efforts, aimed at patients and doctors, can help lessen this potentially unhelpful tension.

Patient Compliance Behaviors

The third category of individual behavior involves patient decisions on whether to follow the treatment instructions of health professionals. These behaviors include the use of pharmaceutical prescriptions, pursuing referrals to other health providers, and other kinds of treatment-following behaviors.

Many strategies aimed at changing patient compliance behaviors involve medications. Examples of behavior-change strategies in this area include efforts to encourage patients to take the full prescription of antibiotics (to decrease the development of antimicrobial resistance), and efforts to encourage patients with chronic diseases (such as schizophrenia, hypertension, and diabetes) to take their medications on a regular and timely basis. In some cases, behavior-change strategies may be combined with direct regulation of individual behavior to assure compliance, as occurs for tuberculosis, with directly observed treatment, short-course, known as DOTS (WHO 1999). In directly observed therapy, health-care workers watch patients take their medications, to ensure that the right combination of drugs is taken for the right period of time.

Behavior-change strategies have also been directed at persuading mothers to follow certain procedures in breastfeeding. For example, a social marketing program was introduced in traditional rural communities in Gambia to combine traditional beliefs and modern knowledge in ways that would yield optimal breastfeeding practices, such as early initiation of breastfeeding, feeding of colostrum, and exclusive breastfeeding for six months (Semega-Janneh et al. 2001). The study found the interesting result that behaviors like breastfeeding emerged from a complex social network. Therefore, attempts to change the breastfeeding habits of mothers need to take into account the attitudes and influence of husbands and elders, and especially the mothers of those childbearing mothers. This is an important lesson for program designers to remember—especially when working in relatively close-knit communities, as often occurs in rural areas of low- and middle-income countries.

Lifestyle and Prevention Behaviors

The fourth category of individual behaviors is consumer decisions on lifestyle habits that have major impacts on their health, especially in preventing disease. Examples of these behaviors include individual decisions about exercise patterns, food consumption, smoking, sexual relations, and contraceptive usage. These behaviors do not necessarily involve interaction with a health professional or a health facility. Indeed, they are often subject to a complex set of influences, from modern commercial marketing to the force of traditional cultural expectations.

One example of a successful program to change lifestyle behaviors is the Harvard Alcohol Project's Designated Driver campaign (Winsten 1994) designed to change the social behavior of driving after drinking. The project persuaded Hollywood television writers to incorporate references to *designated drivers* in top-rated television programs. These short messages within popular television stories influenced people's perceptions of appropriate behaviors and provided social models of how to behave in specific situations. The project also found that friends and peers have critical influence on teenagers' behavior, so it designed messages to connect to the existing values of teenagers, such as "Friends Don't Let Friends Drive Drunk."

The tobacco-control field has many examples of social marketing aimed at changing lifestyle behaviors. Evaluations have shown several factors that raise the effectiveness of such antismoking campaigns. "Advertisements that directly attack the tobacco industry as the source of the tobacco problem; expose the way in which the industry manipulates, deceives, seduces, and addicts children and adolescents; and highlight the way the industry maintains adult smokers as lifelong drug addicts to make profits are effective in challenging the legitimacy and credibility of the industry" (Siegel 1998, 130). Experiences from antismoking campaigns show how social marketing can be used in conjunction with regulation, payment, and financing to promote behavior change, and how evaluative research can help develop effective strategies that can be widely applied in different settings.

Basic Elements of Social Marketing

For health reformers, social marketing provides a useful conceptual framework for thinking about behavior change and developing practical strategies. Two other major approaches to behavior change are addressed by other control knobs: incentives (by the payment control knob), and restriction and prohibition (by the regulation control knob). In this section, we review the basic elements of social marketing—organized around the four Ps of marketing: *product, promotion, place*, and *price*—as critical dimensions that any individual behavior-change plan must include. We also emphasize that health reformers need to consider interventions apart from media-based tactics, including group interventions and other innovative approaches, in order to have the greatest impact on individual behavior.

We believe that health reformers would be well advised to design their efforts at behavior change based on a core conclusion of social marketing: that changing basic values is extremely difficult. Behavior-change strategies, therefore, work best when they build on existing values. This strategy serves as the foundation for commercial marketing as well. Getting a population to adopt your product requires that you design the product to meet the wants and needs of that population. This objective can be achieved by determining the wants of the population and then following the four Ps of marketing.

Product

The first step in social marketing is to define the product for a specific audience. This process is more complicated than it might seem, because it requires significant analysis of different potential audiences. Three principles guide the definition and design of the product.

First is the principle of *consumer orientation*. To design an effective product, the marketer must know the consumer. Both quantitative methods (such as population-based surveys) and qualitative methods (such as focus groups) can be employed. Information about the consumer is essential for product and message design, as well as for creating distribution and communication strategies. This kind of *formative* research helps define both the product and the audience for a social marketing effort.

This principle of consumer orientation provides the foundation for behavior-change strategies. To be effective, efforts to change individual behavior should be based on a multidimensional understanding of the wants and needs of recipients, and the product should be designed to meet (not change) those basic wants and needs.

A second principle of product definition involves *audience segmentation*. Marketers have learned that populations are often quite heterogeneous and that one message cannot respond to the various wants and needs of all the potential target groups. Instead, each product should be designed for a specific population group.

For our purposes, this means that the broad potential audience for behavior change should be divided into segments, with an assessment done of each segment's particular interests, wants, and needs. Separate products should then be shaped for each market segment. For example, a Brazilian breastfeeding-promotion program identified eight target audiences: *(1)* the doctor, *(2)* the health services, *(3)* the hospital, *(4)* the infant formula industry, *(5)* industry (in general), *(6)* the community, *(7)* government officials, and *(8)* the mother. Different products were designed for each audience. In this case, the doctors were informed about the medical benefits of breastfeeding, and the community was encouraged to offer psychological support for families and to provide support facilities for breastfeeding mothers (Manoff 1985, 48).

Audience segmentation is typically based on the psychosocial profile of a population (called "psychographics" by marketers). This involves identifying core values through an analysis of lifestyle, personality, communication habits, readiness for change, and perceived needs. These psychosocial characteristics can also be related to other factors that are useful for audience segmentation, including "geography (region, county, census tract), demography (age, gender, family size, occupation, race, social class), and social structure (worksites, churches, voluntary agencies, families, legislative bodies)" (Lefebvre and Flora 1988, 304).

Qualitative and quantitative research of potential audiences can be used to create profiles of personality types for specific population segments. These profiles (e.g., "Traditionalist male in a low-income Filipino community") can then be used in designing social marketing messages for family planning (Piotrow et al. 1997, 42). Health reformers can use various techniques of consumer analysis to define the target audience, identify specific population segments, and describe the audience's core values. Market research and focus groups are important tools to understand how people think and feel about their health needs and the health system, and to define relevant subgroups in the population. Identifying the right audience segments is critical for defining products and messages for each target audience, and for proposing specific methods to reach each group.

The third basic principle of product design is to *meet basic needs* rather than simply to provide a material object or a particular service. This principle also follows a commercial marketing tenet, a point made by Kotler and Levy (1969) in their classic article on social marketing. For a soap company, the product is not just soap, but cleaning; for a cosmetics company, the product is not just makeup and lipstick, but beauty or hope; for a publishing company, the product is not just books, but information.

Similarly, to be effective, health reformers should view their product in functional terms as meeting basic needs and values. For a family-planning organization, the product is not just condoms or contraceptives, but quality of life and reproductive control. For an AIDS-prevention program, the product is not just safe sex practices, but freedom from disease and control over one's own destiny.

TABLE 12.2. Product, Benefit, and Core Values for the Desired Action Among a Target Audience

DESIRED ACTION	PRODUCT/BENEFITS	CORE VALUES
Prevent smoking initiation	Freedom from nicotine addiction	Freedom
	Independence from tobacco industry manipulation	Independence Control
	Rebellion against an industry that is trying to trick you, seduce you, addict you, and kill you	Rebellion
Practice safe sex	Freedom from AIDS	Freedom
	Independence from the virus that is afflicting your friends and communities	Independence
	Control over your destiny	Control Rebellion
Exercise more often	Identity as a physically strong and attractive person in control of your appearance	Freedom Independence

Source: Siegel and Doner, 1998, p. 53.

Thus, the control knob for behavior change is concerned both with *tangible products* (such as condoms for contraception, or medications for chronic diseases) as well as *intangible products* (such as changing views about safe sex, or changing perceptions about quality of care). In short, health reformers need to learn how to define both kinds of products to appeal to the core values of a population segment in a specific society.

Table 12.2 provides some examples of how public-health products can be connected to core values for particular segments of the population. For example, in considering smoking initiation by teenagers in developed countries, the core value of rebellion may be connected to decisions to start smoking (as adolescents rebel against their parents and their social norms). The challenge for social marketing is to connect the same core value of rebellion to a rejection of smoking (as an effort to rebel against the tobacco industry and its desire to hook teenagers on cigarettes). These core values need to be identified for population segments in specific countries, since values can vary across subpopulations and across cultures. A major challenge is to connect the desired changes to existing values in specific audiences.

Place

Once the products and audiences are defined, the social marketer next works on how to bring the product to the audience. Where can audiences be reached with the product? Making a decision on place involves the selection of appropriate *channels* through which the product can be delivered or made available to the audience. As Lefebvre and Flora (1988, 305) noted,

Any person, organization or institution having access to a definable population is a potential channel for health communication. Thus, schools, worksites, social organizations, churches, physicians' offices, and various nonprofit agencies can all be viewed as potential channels of communication. Identification of "life path points"—such as laundromats, grocers, restaurants, bus stops—can also uncover potential channels to reach certain audiences.

Health reformers need to think creatively about channels to reach the target audience, especially if the group is socially disadvantaged, as commonly occurs with public-health campaigns for immunization, AIDS, or tuberculosis in developing countries.

Communication channels are commonly sorted into three broad categories: *interpersonal* channels, including family, friends, and health-care providers; *group* channels, including the mobilization of community and civil society organizations; and *mass media* channels, including print, radio, and television (Piotrow et al. 1997, 73). Research has demonstrated that greater impact can be achieved by combining different kinds of channels in order to repeat and reinforce key messages.

For example, a campaign in Kenya designed the slogan *Haki Yako* ("It's Your Right") to emphasize the basic human right of women and men to control their own fertility, and then used multiple channels to disseminate that message: "radio spots and a radio serial drama to publicize the slogan; community visits by field workers to reach rural areas; posters and billboards to create a visual image of men and women talking together; and T-shirts to stimulate more interpersonal communication and to encourage advocacy by satisfied users" (Piotrow et al. 1997, 73–74). A follow-up survey found that no single channel reached more than half the population, but the combined exposure from all five channels was 83% of a national sample survey. The goal for reformers is to reach target groups in different places through various channels, to raise the chances of changing knowledge, attitudes, and behavior.

The availability of diverse channels allows for imaginative approaches to connect the product and the audience. Health reformers need to consider methods beyond conventional media approaches (such as radio), including advertising, personal contacts, social groups, and environmental changes (see Table 12.3).

TABLE 12.3. Channels for Reaching Target Audiences

Advertising
Free media (e.g., endorsements)
Events
Organized groups
Personal contacts
Entertainment

Specific audience segments have different characteristics and habits that affect where they can be reached. For example, public-health promotion campaigns often use health centers to make available child-survival products. But if there are problems in access and utilization of health centers—as commonly occurs in many developing countries—then using health centers for product distribution will not be very effective. Audience research for oral rehydration salts has identified other places as more effective for product promotion, such as private pharmacies (in Egypt and Indonesia) and small general stores (in rural areas of Honduras)— because the target population actually uses these facilities on a regular basis (Rasmuson et al. 1988, 11).

In some cases, special events can be organized to attract a particular population group in order to deliver a message or a product. Social groups can also be used to promote and maintain behavior changes. For example, the Indonesian Family Planning Program (BKKBN) used village women's groups for promoting contraception and organized village "acceptor clubs" to provide support through social and economic programs.

In the United States, the first statewide condom-distribution program used social marketing methods to decide on locations where condoms would be available (Cohen et al. 1999). The program selected health facilities (public health clinics, community mental health centers, and substance-abuse treatment sites) to give authority and credibility to the role of condoms in disease prevention, through distribution by "a trusted health-care provider." In addition, the program provided free condoms in more than 1000 private businesses in neighborhoods with high rates of sexually transmitted diseases and HIV, focusing on convenience stores, bars, nightclubs, liquor stores, beauty salons, barbershops, tattoo parlors, dry cleaners, and low-cost motels. The evaluation found an increase in self-reported condom use, without being associated with increases in the number of sex partners or decreases in private condom sales.

Price

Setting the price for behavior-change interventions is a critical step that affects whether the product will be adopted and used. Deciding on the price involves managing both the monetary and nonmonetary costs of product adoption, including social costs, time costs, and physical costs. These different costs can combine to create substantial barriers to the use of a product or service or the adoption of a new idea or value. Applied research can be used to identify and measure these different costs for each product and audience and to find ways to overcome these costs to enhance the product's acceptance.

Price can also serve as a symbol of value to potential users. In some cases, a high price compared to similar products can attract purchasers who interpret that price as reflective of high value. A low price can similarly lead potential users to avoid the product, out of concerns about low value. Setting the monetary price at zero, as a free product, can reduce financial barriers to access, but may result in unnecessary usage and waste. As noted in our discussion of the financing control knob (in Chapter 8), economists are concerned that free products can encourage allocatively inefficient overuse. In other words, customers may use free health services even when the value to them is below the cost of production, indicating that more value could result if the resources were used to produce other goods or services in the economy.

Price has another function as well. It influences the nature of the relationship between patient and provider. In using a free service, patients may feel powerless— as recipients of a gift. As buyers, however, they are in control of the transaction and have a different relationship with the doctor. Anecdotal evidence suggests that such feelings of powerlessness, coupled with the reality of poor quality of service, can reduce the willingness of even poor people to use public clinics in some countries.

In deciding on a price for the product, social marketers need to think about their goals and the market in which they find themselves. Three main sources of information are relevant for price-setting: an assessment of the costs involved, the prices for similar products from competitors, and the price-sensitivity of the target audience (Kotler and Roberto 1989, 177). Each of these kinds of data requires research, and the results must then be combined in ways that reflect the overall pricing objectives and goals of the behavior-change endeavor.

In setting the price for a social marketing effort, reformers must take into account the broader objectives of price policy. Nagle (1987) has identified five pricing objectives, all of which are relevant to different kinds of behavior-change efforts, and each of which leads to different pricing strategies.

Maximizing the number of product adopters

If the aim is to maximize the number of people to adopt a social product, then products and services can be offered at *low prices or for free*. Examples include free immunization for children, as is commonly done in immunization campaigns, and free prenatal care for pregnant women, as South Africa introduced in 1994 with the new post-apartheid government.

As noted above, however, free products or services can sometimes create the perception of low quality, which can discourage use, thereby reducing the level of product adoption. Alternatively, a low price can encourage overuse and waste, thereby creating inefficiency. Health reformers also need to think about the final price to consumers. Subsidized price discounts may not reach consumers, since middlemen and retailers may sell the product at the normal price and pocket the discount as part of their profits (Manoff 1985, 137). Also, as we noted in previous chapters, nominally free services may not be free in practice, once we consider time and travel costs, the need for patient-provided supplies, and under-the-table payments. Thus, reformers may not be able to lower prices as much as they might desire, if use-maximization is a goal.

Social equity

If a behavior-change campaign seeks to achieve equitable distribution, then reformers can adopt a *graduated price structure* for the same product, with higher-income groups paying more and low-income groups less. Examples of this pricing strategy include surgical procedures and the use of insurance premiums based on income level. Some community-financing schemes also give payment exemptions to the poorest members of the community. As mentioned in Chapter 8, this kind of price discrimination is often used by medical practitioners who operate in a fee-for-service environment and charge high prices to rich patients and low prices to poor patients (thereby achieving increased access for poor patients and increased income to providers).

This pricing strategy can be used to reduce financial barriers to poor patients, while not offering subsidies to rich patients who can pay for care. A graduated price structure, however, requires a method for determining the economic status of buyers, which can be administratively costly and subject to favoritism or corruption. These problems can sometimes be addressed by innovative strategies for product targeting, such as offering low-priced products in particular geographic districts where rich customers are unlikely to go (as has been done for subsidized food products). An alternative is to have price vary with quality and allow upper-income people's preference for high quality lead them away from subsidized services—as is done with different levels of hospital rooms in Singapore.

Cost-recovery

If cost-recovery from customers has a high priority, then a *fixed price* can be selected to defray a suitable part of the costs. An example of this pricing strategy is a flat fee for a provider visit at hospitals, regardless of the patient's income level, as a user fee to recover some of the operating costs. User fees have been adopted in many health-sector reforms to allow public health facilities to recoup some of their costs directly from patients (in addition to government-provided resources). One tension that often occurs is between higher cost-recovery, which is intended to promote program sustainability, and lower (even zero) cost-recovery, which is designed to achieve greater product adoption by consumers.

The introduction of user fees, however, raises major questions about the consequences for poor patients, who can be discouraged from utilizing health services (reflecting the price elasticity of demand for different income groups). For example, the introduction of fees to treat bed nets with insecticides (for malaria prevention) in The Gambia reduced utilization and increased mortality rates to the levels before free treated nets were available (D'Alessandro et al. 1995). Where equity is a consideration, social marketing efforts must be careful not to set prices that can result in reduced access for poorer patients.

De-marketing

For certain types of products (such as tobacco and alcohol), social marketers deliberately set *high prices* in order to reduce use considered undesirable on objective utilitarian or communitarian grounds. For example, this pricing strategy is used when a government imposes high taxes on alcohol and cigarettes, with the goal of reducing consumption, especially for price-sensitive groups like adolescents. High prices can also be used to reduce demand for medical services that do not contribute to the goal of health maximization, such as cosmetic surgery. Again, there can be equity concerns if use of the high-priced good is heavier among lower income groups. A proposal for a cigarette tax in China sought to address this issue by varying the tax with the price of cigarettes (since they differ greatly in price), instead of setting a fixed tax per cigarette.

Profit maximization

While the pricing strategy of profit maximization is not commonly used for social products, one can imagine an organization that provides a social product, such as drug-abuse rehabilitation, and also seeks to maximize its profits (Kotler and Roberto 1989, 176–7). The classic monopoly strategy that can be adopted in such cases is *price discrimination*. Different prices are set for different market segments—based on each segment's price elasticity of demand. The less sensitive a market segment is to price increases, the higher the price they face. Where they can do so successfully, private companies often try to follow this approach. Multinational pharmaceutical companies, for example, set different prices for the same product in different countries, according to market conditions and income levels, in order to maximize their overall profits.

Promotion

Having selected the product, place, and price, health reformers next must deal with promotion—getting their message across to the target market segments. They need an explicit promotion plan. The objective of promotion is to enhance the probability that consumers will accept the product. The promotion plan identifies specific activities and materials that will help achieve the campaign's overall goals.

The most important tasks in designing the promotion plan are to decide on the content of the message, how to present the message, and which channels of communication to use. To create an effective communication strategy that will reach the target audience and produce the desired change in behavior, health reformers need to bring together prior decisions about the product and the audience, the place to reach the audience, and the price of the product. Here we will discuss some of the critical elements of these three key decisions.

Social marketers typically develop multiple messages about a particular social product in order to reach different market segments in the most effective way. The content of the message can draw on information about four different aspects of the product (Kotler and Roberto 1989, 225):

- physical/technical features (size, weight, shape, and other observable qualities)
- sensory features (qualities that people can feel, smell, see, hear, or taste)
- functional benefits (how the product will help the target audience)
- emotional/psychological benefits (how the target audience feels about the product's benefit for them).

The next task in developing a promotion plan is to decide how to present the message. Here customer-orientation is critical. Health reformers need to learn the basic rule of salesmanship: "Don't sell what you want, sell what they want" (Kotler and Roberto 1989, 227). In designing the messages, marketers recommend a strategy of *emotion followed by logic*, or beginning with the product's benefits to the customer, and then moving to the product's features. Structuring the order of information in the message will depend on the specific target group and their responses to different kinds of information. Health reformers, therefore, need to know their consumers and how they react to information, images, and emotions.

Experiences with antismoking campaigns show that messages need to be empathetic and believable to persuade people to accept the discomfort and risks of behavior change. By combining emotions and facts, an effective message can illustrate the consequences of behavior change. Some of the most effective antismoking messages evoked strong negative emotions (fear and sadness) by focusing on the consequences of smoking: "one [smoker] who had died, two who had lost their vocal cords to throat cancer, and one in which a baby who is exposed to secondhand smoke is coughing relentlessly" (Biener et al. 2000, 406). This example demonstrates again the importance of research on target consumer groups in designing the behavior-change efforts and evaluating the impacts of different interventions.

The third step in the promotion plan is to decide on the channel of communication. Two main strategies are mass communications (to reach large target audiences) and personal communications (to reach individuals and small group audiences). Most social marketing programs use a combination of these approaches. Since they are mutually reinforcing, they are generally more effective when used together (Kotler and Roberto 1989, 190). A third approach to communication, known as "selective communication," involves direct mail and telemarketing (Kotler and Roberto 1989, 212–20). This approach is less relevant for health-sector reform in most low-income countries. Low literacy rates, sporadic mail service, and limited telephone availability, particularly in poor and rural areas, all limit the usefulness of such strategies.

Mass communication

In using mass communications, health reformers face two basic choices: between *paid* or *free* coverage. Paid coverage (i.e., advertising) allows reformers to control the content and timing of messages. Budget constraints can reduce the effectiveness of this approach, although in some cases it may be possible to obtain free public-service announcements. The more usual form of free media involves media coverage of the social marketing message in the form of news stories. This is less reliable and controllable than advertising, and subject to the potential distortion or bias of the media involved (e.g., in a newspaper controlled by the political opposition). But it also may be more credible to readers than advertising, and it is typically much less expensive.

In working with mass communications, it is important to develop good *media relations*. By preparing materials and meeting with reporters, health reformers can frame the content of media reports. These efforts include preparing press releases (print, audio, and video), organizing press conferences, and conducting one-on-one briefings with key reporters. One way to obtain free media coverage is to organize a *social event* that can provide a "hook" for reporters to write an article and thereby give public attention to a particular message. *Television and radio programs* can also be used to deliver health messages directed at individual behavior, such as the Designated Driver campaign in the United States, mentioned above, which appeared in many Hollywood television programs.

Personal communication

The main point of personal communication is to deliver the message to target individuals in ways that enhance its credibility and acceptability. This means choosing a *place* and a *messenger* that will have an impact on the group you are seeking to reach.

Suppose, for example, we have identified lowering HIV transmission as a key health-reform priority, and we want to increase safe sex practices among young men. Suppose, too, our research shows that they fear such use will label them as somehow unmanly. *Social events* like sporting events (that can lead to media coverage) might provide a good occasion to reach this particular target audience. For example, we could distribute condoms and information on safe sex practices at a football (soccer) game. One can imagine going even further and have the *players* distribute the condoms (packaged in team colors)—say, by throwing packages into the crowd—before the game. A star player could also make a statement to the crowd endorsing the distribution. After all, if you are trying to convince young men that one can still be tough and macho while using condoms, what better person to deliver that message?

A peer or respected authority can be effective in reaching certain audiences— an approach known as *personal selling*. For example, it can be more effective to

have a teenager speak with schoolmates on the issue of violence and about negotiation strategies than to have a schoolteacher do the same. *Entertainment* can
also be used to deliver health messages to particular groups, including traditional
forms of entertainment, such as puppet shows that tour rural villages in India
on the dangers of chewing tobacco. *Social groups* can also be used to provide a
mechanism for both introducing and reinforcing new behaviors, and for assisting
individuals with the transition to new habits. Examples of this approach include
women's organizations that promote oral-rehydration therapy or contraception, as
well as Alcoholics Anonymous.

One example of an entertainment-based promotion plan was the 1993 multimedia
campaign to promote family planning in Mali (Kane et al. 1998). This project combined traditional theater and music forms, along with traditional proverbs in local
languages and familiar settings, with broadcasts on radio and television. The objective was to change knowledge, attitudes, and practices related to contraception—to
connect traditional social values with new contraceptive methods. The specific messages provided information about modern contraceptive methods, the need for male
sexual responsibility, the health and economic advantages of family planning, the
need for communication between spouses, and that Islam (the predominant religion
of Mali) does not oppose family planning. A comparison of the situation before and
after the intervention found increases in desired knowledge, attitudes, and self-
reported practices along the lines sought by the social marketers. The authors concluded that the impact "may reasonably be considered to be both positive and
significant" (Kane et al. 1998, 320).

Triggers

The final step in the promotion plan is to decide on actions that will *trigger* the
adoption of the product. These trigger actions involve different kinds of incentives to persuade the customer to adopt the product (Kotler and Roberto 1989,
240–241), and can involve the payment as well as the organization control knobs.
For example, incentives can be money (cash payment), social status (an award or
seal of approval), or something material (a radio or some other gift). One trigger
technique is to provide a *free sample* of the product or the service to induce the
customer to try the product. Another is to organize *contests and sweepstakes* for
persons who agree to adopt the product, with the offer of prizes, including money,
merchandise, or free services. A third trigger technique is to create *continuity programs*, in which adopters collect coupons each time they use a product or service,
with a reward after a certain number of uses.

Conditional Guidance

The behavior control knob has the potential to address difficult public-health
problems by producing changes in individual behavior. Individual behavior patterns

shape the utilization of health services, including, for example, decisions to go directly to regional hospitals rather than use local health centers, decisions to depend on traditional healers or medicine sellers rather than seek care from licensed physicians, and decisions to avoid seeking outpatient care until a medical condition has become quite serious. They also have a large impact on the utilization (or under-utilization) of important services like immunization, prenatal care for pregnant women, and disease-prevention for infectious as well as chronic diseases. This control knob also holds the promise of reducing high-risk individual behaviors, like smoking and drunk driving, and of promoting protective behaviors, ranging from helmet-wearing to physician hand-washing.

The examples of behavior change in this chapter illustrate that this control knob involves more than simply selling a product or redesigning a product for sale. The behavior control knob requires an iterative process of discovering the values of the target audience, creating goods and services consonant with those values, and evaluating the impact of strategies designed to enhance the products' acceptability. The example of encouraging villagers to use insecticide-treated bed nets to prevent malaria in rural Tanzania shows how this approach can be effectively applied in practice on a large scale (Schellenberg et al. 2001).

One example where behavior-change approaches have been used to improve health-system performance is the Delivery of Improved Services for Health (DISH) project in Uganda. DISH used many of the techniques discussed in this chapter to change behaviors that can contribute to improved health-system performance, especially for the health of women and children (DISH 2001). The project seeks to improve performance through a series of "Best Practices," including the introduction of integrated reproductive-health services, providing one-stop shopping in a client-oriented approach, and holding low-cost community events, which are recorded and broadcast as radio shows, to create wider audiences for DISH messages. While the project does not include the entire health system in its objectives, DISH does provide several examples of how behavior-change approaches can be successfully applied to achieve concrete improvements, especially in the core criteria of health status and customer satisfaction.

Behavior change, however, is not a magic wand. Social marketing methods present both problems and challenges, especially when compared to conventional commercial marketing. A list of some difficulties is presented in Table 12.4.

The Limits of Behavior-Change Efforts

Researchers concerned with behavior change are increasingly aware that social and cultural environments influence individual decisions, especially for complex health behaviors involving intimate matters such as sexual relations (Green 2003). Efforts to develop effective AIDS prevention programs have responded to this realization by emphasizing the importance of designing culturally appropriate

TABLE 12.4. Problems and Challenges in Social Marketing

Market-Analysis Problems: Social Marketers

Have limited primary data available about the consumers they are targeting.
Have difficulty obtaining valid, reliable measures of salient variables.
Have difficulty sorting out the relative influence of identified determinants of
   consumer behavior.
Have difficulty getting consumer research studies funded, approved, and completed
   in a timely fashion.

Market-Segmentation Problems: Social Marketers

Face pressure against audience segmentation, especially if segmentation leads to
   ignoring certain segments.
Frequently do not have accurate behavioral data to use in identifying segments.
Often target consumers who are negatively predisposed to the proposed changes.

Product-Strategy Problems: Social Marketers

Tend to have limited flexibility in shaping their products or offerings.
Have difficulty in formulating product concepts.
Have difficulty selecting and implementing long-term positioning strategies.

Pricing-Strategy Problems: Social Marketers

Find that the development of a pricing strategy primarily involves trying to reduce
   the monetary, psychic, energy, and time costs incurred by consumers when
   engaging in a desired social behavior.
Have difficulty measuring their prices.
Tend to have limited control over consumer costs.

Channel-Strategy Problems: Social Marketers

Have difficulty utilizing and controlling desired intermediaries.

Communications-Strategy Problems: Social Marketers

Usually find paid advertising impossible to use.
Often face pressure not to use certain types of appeals in their messages.
Usually must communicate relatively large amounts of information in their messages.
Have difficulty conducting meaningful pretests of messages.

Source: Bloom and Novelli, 1981.

interventions that will be accepted and supported by specific communities (Sweat
and Denison 1995). But this cultural embeddedness raises serious issues about
the limitations of behavior-change efforts that health-sector reformers need to
recognize.

   Public health policymakers need to recognize that it is very difficult to use the
behavior control knob to change the basic values of a target population, rather

than to change its behavior. Private advertisers have learned how difficult it is to change people's basic values, leading them to focus instead on identifying preferences and designing products to connect with existing values. Indeed, trying to change basic values can undermine a social marketing campaign's ultimate effectiveness. It may be that the adoption of new products can lead to broader social change, as has been argued for the birth control pill in American society. But broad social changes most often occur at times of multiple historical shifts, which makes it difficult to draw clear linkages from causes to differences in specific individual behaviors.

Even when they do focus on behavior, public-health professionals have a tendency to approach behavior change from an expert-driven or product-driven perspective ("We know what they need"), rather than seeking to understand and respond to consumer needs (Levebre and Flora 1988, 302). This pattern reflects the bias of traditional medical culture, with its low emphasis on psychology and a tendency toward professional arrogance. The expert-driven approach to behavior change, in connection with international assistance projects, can also lead to charges of "cultural imperialism," where "foreign" projects are perceived as seeking to alter "local" behaviors. This can both diminish the acceptability of the reforms and, because of a lack of awareness of local conditions, lead to programs that do not actually promote the well-being of the target group. Population-control programs in particular have been criticized for these problems. Post-partum sterilization, for example, was promoted for women when they were least able to make a real choice, and many women later regretted the decision.

Expert-driven efforts often ignore the basic consumer-oriented methods of social marketing, and they often neglect to conduct enough research among consumers to design an effective program for behavior change. This perspective also tends to underestimate the importance of "pretesting . . . ideas, messages, and methods with representatives of the target group[s] *before* implementation" (Levebre and Flora 1988, 304). The requirement to *know the consumer* (with both quantitative and qualitative methods) cannot be overestimated in efforts to use behavior change in health reform.

The Ethics of Behavior-Change Programs

Use of the behavior control knob raises a number of ethical issues. The first of these concerns the balance among alternative ethical imperatives. Suppose a traditional cultural practice leads to decreases in health status—e.g., lack of school attendance by girls. This might seem an obvious target for a social marketing campaign. But this issue also involves a potential clash between objective utilitarian concerns for effectiveness and relativist communitarian respect for tradition. The same issue arises with respect to feeding patterns that give preference to male children, or for female genital cutting. As egalitarian liberals, we see preservation of a minimum level of opportunity as more important than the preservation of past social practices—but that is only our view. We recognize that there are genuine issues here, and that health-sector reformers can confront serious disagreements about such questions when they use this control knob.

In a sense, as with all reform efforts, these ethical issues raise basic questions of process. Any consequentialist argument always runs the risk that it is based on poor science, or that unanticipated and undesirable side-effects will occur. For example, some health promotion campaigns may not have enough good scientific evidence to support the proposed changes in lifestyle, such as certain dietary changes. In other cases, social marketing campaigns may unintentionally perpetuate certain values that can undermine public-health goals in the long run. For example, the use of gender stereotypes to sell condoms—based on macho stereotypes—can reinforce asymmetrical power relations between men and women and thereby help undermine HIV-prevention programs. These efforts raise serious questions about who decides which behaviors are desirable or legitimate and which are not, and how those decisions fit with broader social values about democratic processes and community control (Fitzpatrick 2001).

A second ethical issue involves how far the state can go, how coercive it can be, once it has identified behaviors it believes should be changed. We believe that the degree of coercion that is justifiable depends in part on the nature of the problem and the values of the society. Coercion may be more acceptable for behaviors that involve harm to others (e.g., unprotected sexual behavior by a person who knows he is HIV-positive), that involve harm to self (for example, the decision by a motorcycle rider not to use a helmet), or that involve financial cost to society (for example, the health costs of illnesses due to tobacco smoking). As an empirical matter, behaviors that provoke cultural disapproval (for example, homosexuality or drinking in some societies) are also likely to be dealt with more coercively. Some societies are also reluctant to use coercive methods for intimate behavior (such as condom use) as distinct from public behavior (such as seatbelt use) (Steinbock 1999). Here again is a set of issues reformers need to confront honestly.

The use of incentives to promote certain behavior changes also raises a number of ethical questions about coercion. In particular, what level of incentive in the promotion plan is considered coercive? Some people have argued that any use of incentives is coercive. Others contend that if an incentive works to persuade someone to adopt a behavior they would otherwise not do (such as a vasectomy, in order to receive a radio), then that offer is coercive and ethically inappropriate. The counter-argument—from subjective utilitarians—is that no one is *forced* to accept the radio. If the exchange is not in the recipients' interest, they would not accept the bargain. The question of whether the choice really is free, of course, is central to this point of view.

In general, the degree of coercion that is considered justifiable will depend on a reformer's philosophical viewpoint. The most coercive perspective is the objective utilitarian. If individual behaviors are detrimental to health status, then a high level of coercion is seen as justified in seeking to change those behaviors. In short, the ends (better health) justify the means (coercion to change behavior). An objective utilitarian would favor the use of more-coercive interventions, such as regulation and prohibition of specific behaviors, as well as quarantine (or incarceration) for recalcitrant individuals, as long as the approach would improve aggregate health.

On the other hand, a liberal would oppose efforts to limit individual autonomy, even if respect for individuals resulted in unhealthy behaviors. But liberals would not object to the provision of information, as long as the autonomy of individual choice is respected. The problem is that the provision of information alone tends to be ineffective in changing ingrained personal behaviors important to public health (such as sexual practices, selection of health providers, water-use habits, and decisions about medication). In contrast to liberals, a communitarian would accept behavior change approaches to persuade providers and patients to comply with community values and would approve of using more-coercive techniques to change behaviors that violate cultural expectations.

These differences on the role of coercion, according to philosophical position, reflect one of the central ethical questions in public health: How much and what kinds of coercion are justified in seeking to change individual behavior for collective goals? This discussion of behavior change illustrates the importance of ethical reflection and analysis for health reformers who use the behavior control knob.

Behavior Change and Equity

Of particular concern for the ethics of behavior-change efforts are the equity aspects of such efforts. We see two major issues here. The first has to do with the ethics of incentives just discussed. In general, poor individuals are more likely to be influenced by incentives than those at higher income levels. A poor tribal woman in India is more likely to undergo sterilization in return for a sari than her middle-class counterpart, even when both have "free" choices. How can we think about this?

One appealing argument is that incentives that depend on granting or withholding a person's basic rights are illegitimately coercive (Nozick 1974). If I say, "You can choose sterilization or slavery," then I am clearly coercing you. We believe there is an analogy here to significant financial incentives to people whose baseline economic level does not allow them a decent range of opportunity. Such incentives are likewise coercive. They constitute an offer that the individual in a realistic sense cannot afford to refuse. Ironically, then, incentives to poor people need to be small enough to be refusable if they are to avoid the problem of coercion and be ethically acceptable. (Of course, the deeper equity issue is the poverty of the target group to begin with. But that cannot easily be addressed within the context of health-sector reform.)

The second ethical issue involves the vulnerability of the culturally marginalized to behavior-change efforts. Again, we noted above the relativist communitarian concern that expert-driven public-health efforts would ride roughshod over
traditional practices. Around the world, marginal groups seem especially vulnerable to such efforts because they lack the political power to protect themselves and
their cultures (e.g., the Roma in Eastern Europe or the Maya in Mexico). The difficulty is that such groups may also maintain cultural practices that have significant adverse health consequences (Fonseca 1996), thereby posing sharp ethical
questions about the limits of behavior-change interventions.

Summary

In closing this chapter we want to make three points. First, changing individual
behavior is critical to the successful implementation of health-reform plans. The
behavior control knob, however, has limits to its effectiveness and thus needs
to be used in conjunction with other health-system changes in financing, payment, organization and regulation in order to achieve the desired improvements in
health-system performance.

A second point is that this control knob seeks to change individual behavior but
does not seek to change the social structure or power dynamics of public-health
policy. Yet marketing methods are nevertheless critical in public policy debates, in
shaping public perceptions about the nature of social problems and appropriate
policy solutions, and in influencing the acceptability of proposed policies. (We
dealt with these issues in Chapter 4 on political strategies.) But many of the lessons we discussed in this chapter can also be helpful to reformers in managing the
political context.

A third point is that making behavior change work demands that health reformers mobilize a high level of commitment and substantial marketing expertise.
The conditions when social marketing produces health behavior change have not
been adequately specified (Walsh et al. 1993, 115–16). In particular, we need additional studies on the kinds of behavior-change approaches that work best for
health reform and the conditions under which these approaches are most likely to
succeed. But enough evidence is available to suggest that poorly thought-out or
badly implemented efforts, which ignore the lessons we have reviewed, are unlikely to contribute much to successful health-sector reform.

References

Altman, Diana L.; and Phyllis T. Piotrow. 1980. "Social Marketing: Does It Work?" *Population Reports* J-21(January).
Biener, Lois; Garth McCallum-Keeler; and Amy L. Nyman. 2000. "Adults' Response
to Massachusetts Anti-Tobacco Television Advertisements: Impact of Viewer and
Advertisement Characteristics." *Tobacco Control* 9: 401–7.

Bloom, Paul N.; and William D. Novelli. 1981. "Problems and Challenges in Social Marketing." *Journal of Marketing* 45: 79–88.

Cohen, Deborah A.; Thomas A. Farley; Jean Roger Bedimo-Etame; Richard Scribner,
William Ward; Carl Kendall; and Janet Rice. 1999. "Implementation of Condom Social Marketing in Louisiana, 1993 to 1996." *American Journal of Public Health* 89:
204–8.

D'Alessandro, U.; B. O. Olaleye; W. McGuire; P. Langerock; S. Bennett; M. K. Aikins;
M. C. Thomson; M. K. Cham; B. A. Cham; B. M. Greenwood. 1995. "Mortality and
Morbidity from Malaria in Gambian Children after Introduction of an Impregnated
Bednet Programme." *The Lancet* 345(8948): 479–83.

DKT International. 1998. *1997 Contraceptive Social Marketing Statistics.* Washington,
DC: DKT International.

Fitzpatrick, Michael. 2001. *The Tyranny of Health: Doctors and the Regulation of Lifestyle.*
London: Routledge.

Fonseca, Isabel. 1996. *Bury Me Standing: The Gypsies and Their Journey.* New York: Random House.

Green, Edward C. 2003. *Rethinking AIDS Prevention.* Westport, CT: Praeger Publishers.

Horsburgh, C. Robert Jr. 2000. "The Global Problem of Multidrug-Resistant Tuberculosis:
The Genie Is Out of the Bottle." *JAMA* 283(19): 2575–6.

Kane, Thomas T.; Mohamadou Gueye; Ilene Speizer; Sara Pacque-Margolis; and Danielle
Baron. 1998. "The Impact of a Family Planning Multimedia Campaign in Bamako,
Mali." *Studies in Family Planning* 29(3): 309–23.

Kotler, Philip; and Sidney J. Levy. 1969. "Broadening the Concept of Marketing." *Journal
of Marketing* 33: 10–5.

Kotler, Philip; and Gerald Zaltman. 1971. "Social Marketing: An Approach to Planned Social Change." *Journal of Marketing* 35: 3–12.

Lefebvre, R. Craig; and June A. Flora. 1988. "Social Marketing and Public Health Intervention." *Health Education Quarterly* 15(3): 299–315.

Manoff, Richard K. 1985. *Social Marketing: New Imperative for Public Health.* New York:
Praeger.

McManus, Joanne. 1998. *The Future of the Pharmaceutical Industry in Asia.* New York:
Economist Intelligence Unit.

Nagle, Thomas T. 1987. *The Strategy and Tactics of Pricing.* Englewood Cliffs,
NJ: Prentice-Hall.

Nozick, Robert. 1974. *Anarchy, State and Utopia.* New York: Basic Books.

Piotrow, Phyllis Tilson; D. Lawrence Kincaid; Jose G. Rimon II; and Ward Rinehart. 1997.
Health Communication: Lessons from Family Planning and Reproductive Health.
Westport, CT: Praeger Publishers.

"PROQUALI Improves Health Services in Brazil." *Communication Impact!* No. 10,
August 2000.

Rasmuson, Mark R.; Renata E. Seidel; William A. Smith; and Elizabeth Mills Booth.
1988. *Communication for Child Survival.* Washington, DC: Healthcom, June.

Ross-Degnan, D.; S. B. Soumerai; P. K. Goel; J. Bates; J. Makhulo; N. Dondi; Sututo;
D. Adi; L. Ferraz-Tabor; and R. Hogan. 1996. "The Impact of Face-to-Face Educational Outreach on Diarrhoea Treatment in Pharmacies." *Health Policy and Planning*
11(3): 308–18.

Schellenberg, Joanna R.M.A.; Salim Abdulla; Rose Nathan; Oscar Mukasa; Tanya
J. Marchant; Nassor Kikumbih; Adiel Mponda; Hapiness Minja; Hassan Mshinda;
Marcel Tanner; and Christian Lengeler. 2001. "Effect of Large-Scale Social Marketing

of Insecticide-Treated Nets on Child Survival in Rural Tanzania." *The Lancet* 357(9264): 1241–7.

Semega-Janneh, Isatou Jallow; Erik Bohler; Halvor Holm; Ingrid Matheson; and Gerd Holmboe-Ottesen. 2001. "Promoting Breastfeeding in Rural Gambia: Combining Traditional and Modern Knowledge." *Health Policy and Planning* 16(2): 199–205.

Siegel, Michael. 1998. "Mass Media Antismoking Campaigns: A Powerful Tool for Health Promotion." *Annals of Internal Medicine* 129: 128–32.

Siegel, Michael; and Lynne Doner. 1998. *Marketing Public Health: Strategies to Promote Social Change.* Gaithersburg, MD: Aspen Publishers.

Soumerai, Stephen B.; and Jerry Avorn. 1990. "Principles of Educational Outreach ('Academic Detailing') to Improve Clinical Decision Making." *JAMA* 263(4): 549–56.

Steinbock, Bonnie. 1999. "Drug Prohibition: A Public-Health Perspective." In: Dan E. Beauchamp and Bonnie Steinbock, eds., *New Ethics for the Public's Health.* New York: Oxford University Press, pp. 150–79.

Sweat, M. D.; and J. A. Denison. 1995. "Reducing HIV Incidence in Developing Countries with Structural and Environmental Interventions." *AIDS* 9(Suppl A): S251–7.

Wallack, Lawrence; and Lori Dorfman. 1996. "Media Advocacy: A Strategy for Advancing Policy and Promoting Health." *Health Education Quarterly* 23(3): 293–317.

Walsh, Diana Chapman; Rima E. Rudd; Barbara A. Moeykens; and Thomas W. Moloney. 1993. "Social Marketing for Public Health." *Health Affairs* 12(2): 104–19.

Winsten, Jay A. 1994. "Promoting Designated Drivers: The Harvard Alcohol Project." *American Journal of Preventive Medicine* 10(3 Suppl): 11–4.

World Health Organization. 1999. *What Is DOTS? A Guide to Understanding the WHO-Recommended TB Control Strategy Known as DOTS.* Geneva: WHO.

Yang, Bong-min. 1996. "The Role of Health Insurance in the Growth of the Private Health Sector in Korea." *International Journal of Health Planning and Management* 11: 231–52.

13

Conclusions

In the preceding chapters, we provided a set of tools and concepts that we believe can help health reformers be more effective in their own countries. We have avoided providing a specific recipe, but instead have presented more general guidance on the art and science of how to "cook up" a reform. Given these skills, we hope that readers can now go forward to develop their own recipes, ones that suit their local conditions and particular ethical commitments. We have also sought to be transparent about our own philosophical and scientific views, so that readers can calibrate our presentation and add "a grain of salt" where they find it necessary.

We have repeatedly addressed the fact that getting health reform right is not an easy task. Interest groups, political parties, and bureaucratic agencies will have different priorities and favor different policies. Entrenched forces will resist change. The complexity of health systems means that almost any policy is likely to produce unintended consequences. Economic instability, political turmoil, and social and cultural developments will also influence what seems possible or necessary. Indeed, there is no single way to get health reform *right*; our guidance, therefore, has always been *conditional* on many different factors.

We also believe, however, that it is possible to do things differently—and better— than they are often done now. Honest self-critical analysis can help reformers improve the results of health-sector reform. The concepts and methods we have offered—the policy cycle, the ethical framework, specific performance criteria, political analysis, diagnostic trees, and the control knobs—are designed to contribute to such an analysis. They provide a framework for organizing work, exploring causes, and generating and evaluating options. They are obviously not self-implementing—but we believe they can be helpful.

The analysis presented in this book depends on a series of critical propositions about the structure and functioning of health-care systems and about the health-sector reform processes. In this concluding chapter, we will present these propositions and discuss their implications for the reform process. Then we will review some of the substantive lessons from Part II on the control knobs.

- *Health systems are complex socioeconomic entities that have evolved to suit different, often conflicting objectives.* The historical embeddedness of health-sector arrangements often produces inconsistent policies and self-contradictory structures. Like the varying rock layers underlying a geological formation, different eras of policy action have often been the product of varying political forces, which have moved the health system in different directions. Interest groups have often captured institutions and parts of the health system and bent them to their own purposes. It is not surprising, therefore, that the system does not effectively maximize some simple, specific, objective function.

- *Despite this complexity, the results produced by a nation's health system can be altered for the better by well designed and implemented public policy.* In recent years, research has helped clarify how the structure of a health system can be changed through intentional actions and the impact that various changes are likely to have. We have summarized these variables under the headings of our five control knobs, and the emerging body of evidence constitutes the scientific basis for health-sector reform. Yet the details of any reform proposal and how it is put into practice are critical to the results it produces.

- *Designing an effective reform package requires a deep understanding of the particular system being reformed.* We have repeatedly stressed that any health system can be understood through a combination of different kinds of analyses. But achieving that understanding is not easy, and deciding how to act, based on such insight, can be even more difficult. The diagnostic process we have described is critical to successful reform initiatives. Such a process needs to break through taboos and ritualized ways of thinking if it is to reveal the true structure of a situation. And while international experience can be helpful in this process, knowledge of local conditions, customs, capacities, and attitudes is equally essential.

- *Failure to engage in reforms designed to improve outcomes, however understandable, will only perpetuate poor performance.* Many in the health-care system do *not* in fact want to change the system to improve its performance. Instead, they want to increase their incomes, or gain political power, or provide benefits to local constituents—in other words, they want to protect their own interests. While such motives may be understandable, they often perpetuate a system that does not achieve desired levels of performance. Given this opposition, change advocates must often be prepared to devote great effort and take significant personal and professional risks if they are to succeed in the reform process.

Critical Tasks

How, then, should reformers go about producing effective reform? Our advice is rooted in the health reform cycle we presented earlier in this volume. It provides a way of identifying the critical tasks reformers need to undertake, and some guidance on their relationship to each other.

Clarify Your Goals

Health-sector reform is not about solving a single well-defined set of problems. Instead, it is a messy, contentious process, often initiated in response to some external shock. Typically there will be much disagreement—not only about the answer, but even about the question. Therefore, if reformers are going to improve their health system's performance, they are advised to begin by *clarifying their goals*.

We have stressed throughout this book that the health system should be seen as a means to an end, and have offered performance goals and intermediate performance measures (Chapters 5 and 6) as a way of describing those ends. We have also stressed that different ethical theories (presented in Chapter 3) will lead to different priorities for different goals. Maintaining services to the poor is much more important to egalitarian liberal societies like Sweden or Denmark than it is in the more libertarian United States. By the same token, Singapore is much more willing to coerce its citizens, based on an expert-driven analysis of what will improve their health, than would be acceptable in the United States or the European Union.

Since the cycle of health-sector reform is often initiated in response to an external shock, reformers must be aware of how "the problem" is defined in the public arena, especially by the media and in political circles. Different definitions will often be promoted by specific economic or bureaucratic interests. Doctors will agitate for higher incomes; the social insurance fund will ask for increased subsidies; the ministry of finance will point to existing waste and inefficiency.

Rather than simply accepting any one of these, reformers need to craft their own definition of the problem, based on the priorities they set and the goals they identify. They need to articulate and promote their perspective in the muddled political world of policy debate. We have argued that they can best do this task—with clarity and coherence—by explicitly relating their performance goals to their own ethical position.

Clarifying goals is especially important because different goals are likely to imply different policies. Concentrating high-tech services in a national facility (like the National Heart Institute in Kuala Lumpur) can take advantage of economies of scale—but it will also reduce competition. Charging user fees for hospital use in Uganda will improve efficiency by discouraging low-valued usage—but it will also tend to exclude the poor. Trying to lower intravenous drug use via aggressive policing might (or might not) be effective in diminishing the spread of HIV—but it is also likely to constrain personal freedom.

Choosing reform priorities is best done strategically. Problems that emerge from an assessment based on an *ethical review* should be subject to a *political analysis* focused on the feasibility of getting an issue on the agenda and of getting an effective policy accepted, and a *technical analysis* of whether there are any feasible policy interventions that will have a positive impact on system performance. In doing this, various kinds of benchmarking can help set aspirations for improvement.

Carry Out an Honest Diagnosis

Once priorities have been identified and performance problems described, reformers next have to carry out an honest diagnosis. We strongly urge the drawing of one or more "diagnostic trees" to reveal patterns of causality and points of critical importance to the system. This is a practical method for giving life to the advice to "Ask 'why?' five times."

We have stressed the need for honest diagnosis because official reports and discussions often find it difficult to confront certain taboo features of the system. Widespread unofficial payments to doctors or the hiring of political supporters, physicians in rural areas who don't take up their posts, theft of hospital supplies, performance reports full of fictitious numbers—these are examples of the kinds of situations that diagnostic journeys need to honestly address.

We also recognize, however, that too much time and resources spent on analysis can delay, even paralyze, reform efforts. Instead, reformers should try to use existing studies and data where possible, and avoid the impulse to do everything again. Reformers need to know when to stop doing analyses. Data are always imperfect, and there is an art to balancing the gains from more study against the added costs. The window of opportunity for health-sector reform often remains open only for a limited time, and it can close suddenly.

A key aspect of our diagnostic advice is *not* to begin with your favorite solution. Instead, we urge that diagnosis follow an evidence-based approach, one that relies on data and science as opposed to slogans or preconceptions. For example, in many low- and middle-income countries, National Health Accounts studies reveal that the private sector provides the bulk of outpatient health care, even as reforms often focus almost exclusively on the public sector. An honest diagnosis of the causes of poor health status in such a country could not and should not make that mistake.

Develop a Plan that can Be Expected to Work in Your National Context

Solutions to national problems must fit the local context. Designing such solutions involves taking account of cultural, political, and institutional factors as well as a nation's level of economic development. If bureaucrats are likely to steal money from the social insurance fund (as they did in Kazakhstan), or if firms are likely to evade payroll taxes by shifting to noncash compensation for employees (as they did in Hungary), then such possibilities need to be addressed when programs are designed.

Our discussion of interventions has been arranged around five distinct control knobs, but we have repeatedly stressed that effective policy often requires coordinated action across these boundaries. Changing payment systems to hospitals to create incentives for efficiency will do little good if hospital administrators are not also provided with the skills, incentives, and authority they need to respond to those incentives. A social marketing campaign to encourage the use of local primary-health-care centers is more likely to succeed if we simultaneously improve their clinical and service quality through effective managerial reforms.

Even within a control knob, we may need to coordinate policy across a number of interventions. Few nations rely on only one financing mechanism, for example. Therefore, to achieve our overall financing goals, we may have to ensure that various sources are deployed in complementary ways. Similarly, if we want to use payment to create incentives to reduce inefficient care, we may need to redesign both how doctors are paid and how insurance is paid for.

In designing policy, reformers need to be realistic about what is possible. For example, realism reminds us that all the costs of health care must be paid for somehow. Hence, while a financing system can be designed to provide risk-protection for vulnerable groups, it cannot achieve the unattainable goal of allowing citizens to avoid the overall cost burden of their health-care system. Similarly, if local political leaders have a long record of using resources and authority for patronage purposes, we cannot assume that health-sector decentralization will improve customer service.

The art of effective reform requires a balance between being overly ambitious and overly pessimistic. Both kinds of mistakes are possible. Trying to design a perfect plan—that addresses all contingencies and problems—is likely to take too long, be too complicated, and then not succeed because of unanticipated consequences. Instead, it may be better to implement some reforms quickly, while the opportunity for change presents itself, and amend the details incrementally—as Singapore has done with its medical savings account system. On the other hand, focusing only on obstacles and difficulties can lead reformers to attempt too little.

Pushing the envelope and taking calculated risks is often necessary for producing change—again, with the chance to amend and adjust in later policy cycles.

Reformers can learn much from international experience. The control knob chapters are full of examples from various countries, both positive and negative. But we urge caution in using such experience. Be evidence-based, not ideology-driven. Consider your own national context: social values, political feasibility, and technical and administrative capacity.

Finally, reformers need to recognize that the process used to develop reform plans influences both their effectiveness and their acceptability. The participation of key actors and interest groups can produce valuable input, create legitimacy, and co-opt potential opponents. On the other hand, reform plans do not require unanimous support, which is a good thing, since genuine reform cannot please everyone. Negotiate? Yes. Turn the chicken coop over to the foxes? No.

Reformers do have to consider how the foxes are going to react if a reform plan is in fact implemented. They are liable to try to avoid taxes, evade regulation, "game" new reimbursement arrangements and resist meaningful reorganization. All this suggest that the policy needs to be designed so that it is seen as legitimate, that the relevant agencies need sufficient resources and competent management, and that the needed data (for payment, enforcement, monitoring, etc.) are reasonably easy to collect. In short, policies should be designed in ways that raise the chances of their being implemented effectively.

Embrace Politics

Reform is not just a technical process, but also a profoundly political matter. Politics pervades all stages of the reform cycle. This means reformers need to embrace, not shun politics. They need to do the kind of explicit political analysis and strategy development discussed in Chapter 4. Differences in ethics, interests, and beliefs will inevitably lead to different views about reform. Political processes of one sort or another will inevitably be deployed to resolve these disagreements, no matter what a nation's government structure.

Because of the cyclical nature of the reform process, the politics of reform always evolves. Reform will strengthen some interest groups and weaken others, and groups will seek to influence the implementation and redesign of reform policies. New external shocks will occur, changing both the reality and public perceptions of the problems each nation faces. Just as reformers need to re-evaluate their technical analyses, they need to redo their political analyses as the reform process moves forward.

Successful reform thus is not just a matter of the merits of an argument: It is also a matter of symbolism and language, of political skill and personal commitment. We have urged realism about the prospects for reform—but we also are aware that reformers can easily conclude that change is impossible, or at least unlikely.

The forces defending the status quo are often well organized, active, and committed. But reform does happen. Colombia does have a new insurance system, Korea is separating the roles of doctors and pharmacists, and Hungary is paying hospitals differently. These successes have been achieved by reformers who are willing to use political processes shrewdly to advance their policies.

Focus on Implementation

Successful implementation often requires leadership and attention to detail. If local authorities are to receive more responsibility for decisions, they may need additional training (as was done in Kerala, India). If fiscal decentralization is to improve interregional equity (as it did in Chile), as opposed to undermining it (as it did in Bosnia), interregional reallocation systems need to be carefully defined.

Successful implementation requires performance measurement. Here again, realism is critical. Some districts in India have reported 120% immunization coverage (defined as doses delivered divided by the eligible population). A closer look revealed that 40% of the children were receiving, on average, three doses each. Lean too hard on a measurement system and you risk dishonesty in reporting or unintended distortions in behavior. In the United States, clinics that do in-vitro fertilization report their success rates in a standardized way that is reliable—but few will do difficult cases, because it would lower their reported performance. These situations remind us of the need to focus on performance, not reports; on outcomes, not inputs; on results, not merely efforts made.

Institutions (and people) resist change out of both self-interest and anxiety. Staffs need to be helped through the reform process by leaders who are both credible and committed and who understand the dynamics of organizational change. Implementation does not just happen; it needs to be planned and guided. Critical tasks need to be identified and likely obstacles anticipated—although, of course, not everything can be. Managers need to adapt as experience accumulates.

Especially at senior (ministerial) levels, there is often rapid turnover. As a result, those who design reforms may not be in place long enough to oversee implementation. This gap can undermine reform efforts, if those who design a new program do not think far enough ahead to the practical challenges of making their bright idea a living reality.

Learn from Your Mistakes

Even successful reform often leads to new problems. Reformers, therefore, must be prepared to learn from their mistakes. Evaluation systems need to be built into the reform effort. Providers and insurers need incentives to report data accurately. There may well be reasons to consider an experimental approach, and there is always a need to collect baseline information before beginning implementation.

Reformers should expect that some of the details (and maybe even some of the major features) of the system will not be optimally designed the first time.

The inevitability of mistakes helps explain why the policy cycle is a *cycle*. Reform is not a one-time effort or a one-off activity. The larger context will continue to evolve. Technology will continue to advance. Expectations will increase. Costs will go up. Economic turmoil will occur. Political coalitions will unravel and regroup. All this makes it highly desirable for reformers to commit themselves to the process for the long run. For it is only in the long run that the success or failure of health-sector reform efforts will be determined. And it is only in the long run that the lessons from any one round of reform can be applied to modify and improve earlier reform initiatives.

Lessons from the Control Knobs

At the end of each of the control knob chapters in Part II, we offered a variety of comments we called "conditional guidance." The impulse behind these comments is our realization that saying "It depends" to would-be reformers is insufficient. Instead, it is our obligation to say something about how policy should depend on each nation's situation; to clarify what aspects of that situation matter and in what ways. While we do believe that a nation's factual situation and value commitments should influence its policy choices, we do not believe that all policy options are created equal. International experience over the years has taught us a good deal. And in this section of our concluding chapter we would like to highlight for the reader some of what we believe those conclusions to be, drawing special attention to the situations with serious equity implications.

Financing

The point of departure for our financing discussion is the fact that a nation's ability to finance its health sector is limited by its level of economic development. That is why in much of this chapter that distinction informed our analysis. Even with an optimally designed financing system, a healthy citizen with an average income will have to pay, directly or indirectly, the costs of their own routine care, plus something for risk-pooling and an amount for redistribution to the poor as well. How much such an individual can and will pay is obviously limited by their economic circumstances.

In general we observed that to truly provide risk protection, a universal system based on ability to pay is required. That allows the rich to cross-subsidize the poor and the healthy to pay for the sick. It is no surprise, then, that middle- and upper-income countries mostly rely on social insurance or general revenue to finance their health-care systems. As countries move up the development scale, social insurance is often especially attractive because the social contract implicit in such a system often improves tax compliance.

In poor countries, household surveys reveal that even poor people pay substantial amounts out-of-pocket for care—either for private providers or for fees, drugs, and "gratuities" in the public sector. To more effectively utilize these funds we believe community financing and other forms of decentralization have much to offer. We also believe, however, that only improved management in the public sector and improved quality of care will lead citizens to be willing to make financial commitments to a system that provides at least some measure of risk protection.

Finally, we view with some trepidation the growth of private insurance in upper–middle-income nations. Such systems have very high transaction costs, require sophisticated regulation, and offer only limited risk-sharing—especially where they allow individuals to withdrawn from social insurance pools. We realize that many countries are under pressure from their own elites to allow the creation of such schemes, which give the rich access to better care than the public system can offer. We also understand that the temptation of mobilizing the willingness to pay of upper-income individuals to raise additional funding for the health-care system is very great. For nations that follow a private insurance route, instead of an opting-out model, as in Chile, reformers might want to consider an Australian-style approach where such insurance is in addition to, not a substitute for, public coverage.

Payment

Our payment discussion emphasized the power of the incentives generated by payment systems. No payment system is perfect. All distort provider behavior in one way or another, and reformers have to consider which distortions they are most comfortable with. In that context, our general advice to reformers is to try to avoid fee-for-service reimbursement for physician services, in order to minimize the inflationary effects of supplier-induced demand. Similarly, per diem payments for hospital care encourage overly long lengths of stay, even as traditional budget systems create few incentives to improve quality. We do realize the political and technical difficulties of more-sophisticated alternatives—like capitation or per admission payments where the money follows the patients—but we believe they are preferable on incentive grounds in many situations.

The more sophisticated and market-oriented providers become, the more important payment methods become, for such providers respond more aggressively to price signals and to variations in their own price–cost margins. Thus the relative prices for providing various services or treating various patients will require close attention. Otherwise the sickest or the most difficult to deal with may face increased barriers to care—an outcome that raises serious equity concerns.

Then there is the question of payment levels. International experience suggests that providers are never satisfied with their level of payment—no matter what they are paid. The resulting conflicts over payment levels should be anticipated by reformers and considered in the institutional design of the payment-setting process.

There has been a good deal of attention paid in the economic literature to the issue of overuse if fees to patients are too low. While this may be a concern in some contexts (such as free drugs), in lower-income countries the opportunity costs of seeking care, and the ancillary costs of drugs, bribes, etc., are high enough to generally discourage overuse. Thus we favor paying great attention to the possible use-discouraging effects of high out-of-pocket fees, especially on the poor—for these work directly counter to risk-protection and health status goals.

Organization

Our analysis of health-sector organization turned on what we called the Six Keys to Organizational Performance. Successful reform has to both give managers reasons to function more effectively and the authority and skill they need to respond to those incentives. Thus any proposal for restructuring the public sector—like autonomization, corporatization, or decentralization—has to be analyzed to see what difference it would make for workers and managers. That is why the motto "The devil is in the details" is especially relevant to such proposals.

When reformers do consider changing who-does-what in the delivery system, they need to be aware of both the efficiency and access effects of their decisions. Large scale can both lower cost and improve clinical quality—even while it reduces the effective availability of services. This can be especially important for poor and marginalized groups who can find the travel time, out-of-pocket cost and bureaucratic remoteness of centralized services a serious barrier to their use.

Our discussion of using private providers and private markets centered on the need to ensure competition if the potential benefits of such an approach are to be realized. We argued that when buyers are sophisticated and the goal of government is customer satisfaction, competitive markets are more likely to be appropriate. But substantial government regulation is often required for such markets to function properly in the health sector. Hence, the capacity to undertake such regulation has to be present if the potential gains from markets are to be fully realized. Moreover, reformers must understand that the more competitive private sellers become, the less they will respond to social priorities (like caring for the poor) unless either paid or compelled to do so.

Many reorganization proposals such as autonomization, decentralization, or purchaser–provider separation pose distinct challenges for central administrative agencies. Their functions will not end, but they will be transformed. And the new skills and attitudes that will be required are often not easy for ministries to develop.

The same can be said at the institutional level of the changes that are required to improve the functioning of the usual type of public-sector institution. These are both obvious and fly in the face of profound political objections because they undermine the patronage structure characteristic of many public delivery systems. This fact may explain why such changes are not more widely implemented. Yet, without more effective management at the level of delivery organizations, approaches like TQM or contracting-out are unlikely to have much impact.

Regulation

Regulation is often difficult to implement exactly because it involves using the coercive power of the state to get people to do what they do not want to do. Instead, they resist—and seek to capture, corrupt, or otherwise undermine the process. Thus regulation works best when most of the society, including both regulators and regulatees, sees the goal of the process as generally legitimate. This greatly facilitates voluntary compliance, which in turn significantly increases the deterrence effect of enforcement efforts. For the same reason, ongoing political support is likely to be required to preserve a regulatory agency's effectiveness.

We analyzed health-care regulation in terms of establishing markets, perfecting markets, and doing what markets cannot do. The pervasiveness and variety of the last two forms of regulation testify to the limits of the market approach in health care, for in this sector, buyers are often ignorant and the agency problem is extremely strong. We have pointed out that informational and certification strategies are more likely to benefit those with the education, decision-making skills, social status, and sense of personal efficacy needed to make use of such data. Hence they are less likely to be useful to marginalized groups than to the middle and upper classes. We also noted, however, the paradox that quality-oriented regulation designed to limit the practice of less-educated providers is also likely to adversely impact the accessibility of services to these same vulnerable populations.

Many forms of regulation require substantial scientific, legal, and economic expertise. Reformers therefore have to be strategic and consider their available administrative capacity, data requirements, enforcement processes, and inspection resources in deciding what regulatory initiatives to undertake. They should also consider using professional societies, NGOs, or certification processes, instead of regulation, to conserve those resources and minimize opposition from those being regulated.

Behavior

Health-sector reformers, in our view, often both under- and overestimate the potential role that efforts to change individual behavior can play in health-sector reform. The overestimates come in the form of unrealistically ambitious plans to influence citizens' basic values and attitudes—which, in fact, are extremely difficult to change. The underestimate comes from failing to pay any attention to these possibilities.

We stressed throughout the need for a customer-focused approach to behavior change. Reformers need to market their ideas in ways that meet or resonate with customers' existing needs and values. This means they have to begin with empirical research on those customers and learn how they vary so that appropriate market segments can be identified. Then a plan that unites the four Ps (place, product, price, and promotion) can be developed. Such plans require skill and sophistication to develop—whether aimed at individual patients or at providers within the health-care system.

Final Thoughts

If health-sector reform is so difficult and demands so much from reformers, readers who have journeyed so far with us may now be asking themselves, Why take on the challenge? We have discussed just this point with many participants in courses and workshops around the world in the last five years. The answer, of course, depends on the individual values of each person who participates in the process. But we do want to pass on some thoughts that have arisen repeatedly in the conversations we have had on the subject.

First, health really is an important component of both opportunity and well-being for all individuals in a society. So those who work to improve health status are doing genuinely important work from almost any ethical perspective. The same goes for efforts to protect individuals against the financial risks of illness—risks that can cause great anxiety and deprivation for those who lack such protection.

Second, providing such gains to those who are most vulnerable in a society is, in terms of our own ethics, an especially urgent and praiseworthy task. Improving access to the extraordinary advances of modern medical science could make an enormous difference to the lives of millions, if not billions of our fellow human beings. We hope that the fact that we come from an industrial country in the world that does a particularly poor job in this regard does not undermine our credibility on this point—for we are hardly defenders of the American system, in part because of its poor equity performance.

Third, for all of its difficulty and frustration, health-sector reform, we believe, is an arena in which intelligence, energy, passion, and critical thinking can make a difference. It is an arena that calls upon many aspects of a person—analytical and intra-personal, creative and purposive. It requires an appreciation of many aspects of human life—from politics and economics to cultural forces, biological processes, and philosophical commitments. It offers opportunities for leadership and craftsmanship, for doing work that is truly worth doing. For those who choose to participate, we hope this book can serve as handbook and guide, as tool kit and design manual, and that the methods and observations we have offered will improve your chances of getting health reform right in the years ahead.

Index